Natural Products for Treatment of Skin and Soft Tissue Disorders

Edited by

Heba Abd El-Sattar El-Nashar
Department of Pharmacognosy
Faculty of Pharmacy
Ain Shams University
Cairo, Egypt

Mohamed El-Shazly
Department of Pharmacognosy
Faculty of Pharmacy
Ain Shams University
Cairo, Egypt

&

Nouran Mohammed Fahmy
Department of Pharmacognosy
Faculty of Pharmacy
Ain Shams University
Cairo, Egypt

Natural Products for Treatment of Skin and Soft Tissue Disorders

Editors: Heba Abd El-Sattar El-Nashar, Mohamed El-Shazly & Nouran Mohammed Fahmy

ISBN (Online): 978-981-5124-36-1

ISBN (Print): 978-981-5124-37-8

ISBN (Paperback): 978-981-5124-38-5

need for a court order if at any point you breach any terms of this License Agreement. In no event will any delay or failure by Bentham Science Publishers in enforcing your compliance with this License Agreement constitute a waiver of any of its rights.

3. You acknowledge that you have read this License Agreement, and agree to be bound by its terms and conditions. To the extent that any other terms and conditions presented on any website of Bentham Science Publishers conflict with, or are inconsistent with, the terms and conditions set out in this License Agreement, you acknowledge that the terms and conditions set out in this License Agreement shall prevail.

Bentham Science Publishers Pte. Ltd.
80 Robinson Road #02-00
Singapore 068898
Singapore
Email: subscriptions@benthamscience.net

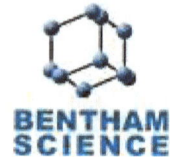

BENTHAM SCIENCE

CONTENTS

FOREWORD

I am very happy and honored to write a foreword for the book titled "Natural Products for Treatment of Skin and Soft Tissue Disorders" which will be edited by three prestigious scientists, Dr. Heba Abd El-Sattar El-Nashar, Dr. Mohammed El-Shazly, and Dr. Nouran Mohammed Fahmy and published by Bentham Science Publishers.

The book will be very useful as an important textbook and guideline in the field of natural products for skin care and disorders. It is a comprehensive book with content from tiny acne to serious cancer, from natural products to nanoparticle formulation, as well as from protection to clinical treatment. In addition to professional editing, many distinguished professors will be involved and contribute their knowledge and promising ideas to this cherished book.

I am very honored to introduce and recommend this book edited by my good friends. They are not only excellent scientists but also professional and talented in scientific writing that will fulfill readers' expectations.

Fang-Rong Chang
Graduate Institute of Natural Products
Kaohsiung Medical University (KMU)
Taiwan

PREFACE

Mother Nature has always been the treasure trove for biologically active compounds that helped humanity to survive and thrive. Medicinal plants have played a major role in the development of human civilizations. Since antiquity, humans searched for natural sources to cure diseases, and they found their target in medicinal plants. The Egyptian, Greek, Indian, Chinese, and Aztec civilizations relied heavily on the use of medicinal plants to cure human and animal ailments. Medicinal plants have been used to treat all types of disorders, including cardiovascular, digestive, skin and kidney disorders. Skin disorders differ from other disorders by being external, can be detected by the naked eye, medicinal plant extracts can be easily applied to the disorders and the healing effect can be easily tracked. Skin is the largest organ in the human body and the first line of defense against traumas, infections and radiation. Skin is a dynamic organ with millions of cells dying and regenerating regularly. It is affected by a plethora of disorders and should be treated to avoid the spread of invasion to internal organs.

Medicinal plants have been used to treat skin disorders and to improve skin condition. They have also been used in cosmetic preparations to remove wrinkles, black spots and provide a radiant appearance. In the current book, we take the reader on an enjoyable journey of medicinal plants treating skin-related disorders. The first chapter deals with "Eczema, etiology and treatment". Eczema is not a condition but a group of skin diseases that cause skin inflammation and irritation. It exists in seven different forms with different signs and symptoms. Eczema, also called Atopic dermatitis (AD), is its most prevalent and popular form, with a high global burden in morbidity and health-care costs. It is a chronic recurrent skin inflammatory disorder characterized by itching, redness, and burning sensation of dark or light patches or crusting eruptions of the skin. The second chapter discusses "Superficial mycoses as a challenging skin disorder". Superficial mycoses of skin, nails and hair caused by dermatophytes, non-dermatophyte molds, yeasts and yeast-like fungi are among the common morbidities that invade particularly in tropical countries. Various antifungal agents, including polyenes, fluoropyrimidines, echinocandins, and azoles, have been commonly used, topically and/or orally, for the treatment of superficial mycoses. The third chapter focuses on "Acne and current possible treatments". Acne vulgaris is one of the skin diseases related to the sebaceous gland, characterized by multiple pathogenic factors. The treatment strategies involve the blockage of these pathological factors. Conventional therapies for the treatment of Acne vulgaris in controlling its pathological factors are still inadequate in providing therapeutic effectiveness and exhibit remarkable side effects. The fourth chapter concentrates on "Vitiligo and treatment protocols". Vitiligo is an abiding acquired skin disorder caused by the epidermal disappearance of pigment cells of localized and general skin mucosa, characterized by the appearance of symmetrical patches on the skin. The exact cause of this disorder is unknown, but genetic susceptibility, melanocyte growth factor deficiency, autoimmunity, and some neurological and environmental factors are believed to play a triggering role. The fifth chapter summarizes "Atopic Dermatitis Prevalence and How to manage it". Atopic dermatitis is a common inflammatory skin disorder characterized by recurrent eczematous lesions and intense itch. The disorder affects people of all ages and ethnicities, has a substantial psychosocial impact on patients and relatives, and is the leading cause of the global burden of skin disease. Moreover, the persistence of atopic dermatitis has been reported in 60% of adults who had the disease as children. The sixth chapter deals with "Epidemiology, diagnosis, and policy framework for prevention and treatment schemes of skin infections in developing countries". Skin disease (SD) infections are a common public health problem in developing countries. The prevalence is universal and can cause a significant economic burden. Besides, it is considered an essential source of morbidity among special groups like children and affects all ages and ethnicities globally. However, the impact of SD on the national public healthcare system is complex and poorly studied up-to-date, especially in developing countries. Moreover, the trends of SD have changed due to population aging, genetic and environmental factors. The seventh chapter discusses "Skin cancer as an emerging global threat and potential natural therapeutic". Global advancement is facing a huge threat due to rising cases of skin cancer and potential health-system costs. Perception of skin cancer prevalence is important for the treatment, prevention strategies, and administration of medical allowances. In addition to fair and tanned skin being a risk factor for the development of disease, sedentary lifestyle habits and reduction in physical activities have increased the mortalities worldwide. This effort signifies information on the incidence, risk factors and mortality rates across six continents. The eighth chapter summarizes "Skin ulcers as a painful disorder with limited therapeutic protocols". A skin ulcer is a type of open wound on the skin caused by injury, poor circulation, pressure, or infection. Specific forms of wounds are described using distinct terms, such as surgical incision, burn, and laceration. Skin ulcers can be extremely painful and take a long time to heal. They can become infected and cause other medical complications if left untreated. Treatment for skin ulcers is diagnosed on the basis of the ulcer as well as the underlying cause. However, there is still a shortage of efficient medicine in the skin ulcer treatment guidelines since wound management consists only of wound dressing, antibiotics, and pain control.

We covered in this book a wide array of skin disorders and how to treat them using medicinal plants. We included researchers from different countries to discuss their experience in using medicinal plants for the treatment of skin disorders. This book will guide researchers all over the world to understand the value of medicinal plants in treating skin disorders and how to move forward in their research.

ACKNOWLEDGEMENTS

The authors would like to express their deep appreciation for the professional assistance of the assistant editors and the publishing house. The authors are also grateful to their families for their continuous support and help, and to their colleagues for their insightful comments on how to improve the content of the book.

Heba Abd El-Sattar El-Nashar
Department of Pharmacognosy
Faculty of Pharmacy
Ain Shams University
Cairo
Egypt

Mohamed El-Shazly
Department of Pharmacognosy
Faculty of Pharmacy
Ain Shams University
Cairo
Egypt

&

Nouran Mohammed Fahmy
Department of Pharmacognosy

Faculty of Pharmacy
Ain Shams University
Cairo
Egypt

Dedication

To

THE SOUL OF MY FATHER,

Who taught me to trust in ALLAH,

encouraged me to believe in myself.

MY MOTHER,

A strong woman whose loving spirit always sustains me.

&

MY HUSBAND AND MY LITTLE ANGLE LAYLA

A constant source of love, concern, support, strength, never-ending motivation, and patience.

List of Contributors

Abdul Jabbar   Department of Veterinary Medicine, Faculty of Veterinary Science, University of Veterinary and Animal Sciences, 54000, Lahore, Punjab, Pakistan

Aqsa Arooj   College of Earth and Environmental Sciences, Faculty of Environmental Sciences, University of the Punjab, 54590, Lahore, Punjab, Pakistan

Areeba Akhtar   Department of Biotechnology, Kinnaird College, Lahore, Punjab, Pakistan

Bilquees Bhat   Department of Pharmaceutical Science (Pharmacology Division), University of Kashmir, Hazratbal, Srinagar, Jammu and Kashmir, 190006, India

Edith Filaire   University Clermont Auvergne, UMR 1019 INRA-UcA, UNH (Human Nutrition Unity), ECREIN Team, 63000 Clermont-Ferrand, France

Haroon Elrasheid Tahir   School of Food and Biological Engineering, Jiangsu University, 301 Xuefu Rd., 212013 Zhenjiang, Jiangsu, China

Haroon Khan   Department of Pharmacy, Abdul Wali Khan University, Mardan, Pakistan
School of Food and Biological Engineering, Jiangsu University, 301 Xuefu Rd., 212013 Zhenjiang, Jiangsu, China

Hassan Hussein Musa   Faculty of Medical Laboratory Sciences, University of Khartoum, Khartoum, Sudan

Humaira Bilal   Department of Pharmaceutical Science (Pharmacology Division), University of Kashmir, Hazratbal, Srinagar, Jammu and Kashmir, 190006, India

Idriss Hussein Musa   School of Medicine and Surgery, Darfur University, Nyala, Sudan

Jacques Peyrot   Cabinet de Dermatologie, 43 Rue Blatin, 63000 Clermont-Ferrand, France

Jean-Yves Berthon   GREENTECH, Biopôle Clermont-Limagne, 63360 Saint Beauzire, France

Mehnaz Showkat   Department of Pharmaceutical Science (Pharmacology Division), University of Kashmir, Hazratbal, Srinagar, Jammu and Kashmir, 190006, India

Nadia Mushtaq   Department of Life Sciences, Syed Babar Ali School of Science and Engineering, Lahore University of Management Sciences, 54792, Lahore, Pakistan

Nahida Tabassum   Department of Pharmaceutical Science, Dean School of Applied Sciences and Technology, University of Kashmir, Hazratbal, Srinagar, Jammu and Kashmir, 190006, India

Pharkphoom Panichayupakaranant   Department of Pharmacognosy and Pharmaceutical Botany, Faculty of Pharmaceutical Sciences, Prince of Songkla University, Hat-Yai 90112, Thailand

Taha Hussein Musa	Biomedical Research Institute, Darfur University College, Nyala, Sudan
Thongtham Suksawat	Department of Pharmacognosy and Pharmaceutical Botany, Faculty of Pharmaceutical Sciences, Prince of Songkla University, Hat-Yai 90112, Thailand
Tosin Yinka Akintunde	Department of Sociology, School of Public Administration, Hohai University, Nanjing, China
Wiwit Suttithumsatid	Department of Pharmacognosy and Pharmaceutical Botany, Faculty of Pharmaceutical Sciences, Prince of Songkla University, Hat-Yai 90112, Thailand
Yaseen Hussain	College of Pharmaceutical Sciences, Soochow University, Suzhou, Jiangsu, China

CHAPTER 1

Eczema, Etiology and Treatment

Humaira Bilal[1], Mehnaz Showkat[1] and Nahida Tabassum[2,*]

[1] *Department of Pharmaceutical Sciences (Pharmacology Division), University of Kashmir, Hazratbal, Srinagar, Jammu and Kashmir, 190006, India*

[2] *Department of Pharmaceutical Sciences, Dean School of Applied Sciences and Technology, University of Kashmir, Hazratbal, Srinagar, Jammu and Kashmir, 190006, India*

Abstract: Eczema is not a condition but a group of skin diseases that causes skin inflammation and irritation. It exists in several different forms, and each form has its signs and symptoms. Eczema is also referred to as Atopic dermatitis (AD), which is its most prevalent and popular form, with a high global burden in morbidity and health-care costs. It is a chronic recurrent skin inflammatory disorder that is characterized by itching, redness, burning sensation of dark or light patches, papular bumps and weeping or crusting eruptions of the skin. Pathophysiology of AD is complex and multifactorial, involving genetic predisposition, skin barrier defects, immunological dysfunction and regulation, microbial colonisation, neuroinflammation, altered lipid composition, food allergies and other environmental risk factors. Currently, available treatment regimens, which include corticosteroids, calcineurin inhibitors, antibiotics, immunomodulatory agents, UV therapy, may offer some relief to patients, but there is no permanent cure for the disease. Specific cases may additionally need psychosomatic counselling (in stress induces exacerbations), Monoclonal antibodies targeting T-helper 2 pathways and aeroallergens, which may improve the condition of associated asthma or rhinitis. To minimize the side-effects caused by conventional treatments such as skin atrophy, telangiectasia, lymphomas and malignancies, Novel jakus kinase (JAK) receptor inhibitors are under development which are believed to show promising effects in treating AD. Traditional Chinese herbs, used widely, have revealed some supplementary activity in reducing the severity of AD. Tapinarof, a naturally derived stilbene that activates aryl hydro carbon receptor (AHR) and triggers inflammation, has shown significant results in AD and psoriasis patients. Homeopathy, aroma therapy, essential oils, essential fatty acids, vitamins and minerals, have also been exemplified to aid clinical AD treatment.

Keywords: Atopic dermatitis, Calcineurin inhibitors, Corticosteroids, Cutaneous microbiome, Dupilumab, EASI, Eczema, Filaggrin, Immune dysregulation, JAK receptor inhibitors, Monoclonal antibodies, Phototherapy, SCORAD, Traditional herbs.

---

* **Corresponding author Nahida Tabassum:** Department of Pharmaceutical Sciences, Dean School of Applied Sciences and Technology, University of Kashmir, Hazratbal, Srinagar, Jammu and Kashmir, 190006, India; E-mail: n.tabassum.uk@gmail.com

Heba Abd El-Sattar El-Nashar, Mohamed El-Shazly & Nouran Mohammed Fahmy (Eds.)

INTRODUCTION

Eczema is not a condition but a reaction pattern associated with a group of skin diseases that causes skin inflammation and irritation [1]. Eczema is also referred to as Atopic dermatitis (AD), which is its most prevalent and popular form, with a high global burden in morbidity and health-care costs [2]. AD may or may not occur as Triad, *i.e.*, in association with asthma and hay-fever (Atopic march). It starts at an early age and thus predominantly affects children and infants more than adults. About $1/3^{rd}$ of children with AD develop asthma in later life [3]. It is a non-contagious, chronic recurrent skin inflammatory disorder, which is characterized by intense itching, redness, and burning sensation of dark or light patches, or popular bumps [4], and is associated with a dramatic decrease in the quality of life and high sleep disturbances [5]. It can exacerbate exposure to different things, including allergens, such as pet dander or dust mites and other common triggers, like harsh soaps, detergents, chemicals, perfumes, *etc*.

The pathophysiology of AD is complex and multifactorial. Immunologic findings in AD include raised immunoglobulin E (IgE), eosinophils, spontaneous histamine release from mast cells, and T-helper 2 (Th2) cells secreting interleukin-4 (IL-4) and IL-5, and decreased numbers ofTh1 cells secreting interferon-γ [6]. The "inside-out" hypothesis suggests that the disease is primarily cytokine-driven, with resultant reactive epidermal hyperplasia caused by immune activation. Corticosteroids and Calcineurin inhibitors are still the mainstays of treatment. However, novel treatment modalities along with herbal treatment, can provide alternate options for reducing disease progression.

Diagnosis

Diagnosis is mainly based on examining the patient skin and reviewing medical history. Following tests that detect specific IgE levels to allergins are conducted on patients to rule out other skin diseases or identify conditions that accompany eczema [6].

Atopy Patch Test (APT)

The APT is based on T cell–a specific response to the application of allergens on the healthy skin of the patient's back or forearm, where an eczematous reaction is read after 48 and 72 hours when it is positive. That method is used to assess sensitization for aeroallergens in AD patients and is not aimed for healthy individuals, asthmatic patients, or patients with rhinitis.

Skin Prick Tests (SPT)

The SPT value is variable in diagnosing food allergies. The history of the disease and the SPT values of specific IgE are important in the diagnosis of early sensitization, but the diagnosis is more problematic for the late type of allergic manifestation, especially to food allergens.

The late type requires a patch test, an APT skin application food test (SAFT), and an exposition test such as the open test, single-challenge test, or double-blind placebo-controlled food challenge test (DBPCFC). The latter is the gold standard procedure for diagnosing food allergies. A combination of SPT and APT significantly enhance the accuracy in the diagnosis of specific food allergies in infants with AD or digestive symptoms [7]. These methods are costly, time-consuming and often inconvenient to patients.

Severity Scoring of Atopic Dermatitis (SCORAD)

This method is used to detect the severity of AD, and it's useful for clinical trials. In this method, three elements of eruptions, *i.e.*, erythema/acute papules, exudation/ crusts, chronic papules/lichenification/nodules, are measured in the five areas of eruption head/neck, anterior trunk, posterior trunk, upper limbs and lower limbs. The severity score for each body region is given as 0 (for absent), 1 (for mild), 2 (for moderate), 3 (for severe) and 4 (very severe). The highest possible score is 20 (5 areas and 4 degrees). When the evaluation of the area of eruption is done considering all three elements for all five body regions, the highest score is 60 points [8].

Modern image processing and computer algorithm have also been used for automatic eczema detection and severity measurement models. This system can successfully detect regions of eczema and classify the identified region accordingly based on image color and texture features. Then the model automatically measures "Eczema Area and Severity Index (EASI)," by computing skin parameters - eczema affected area score, eczema intensity score, and body region score of eczema, allowing both patients and physicians to accurately assess the affected skin [9]. This method is non-invasive, fully automatic, precise, accurate, and efficient in diagnosing AD.

TYPES OF ECZEMA

The earliest classification of eczema was based on the presence/detection of IgE antibodies and was of 2 types intrinsic or non-allergic form and extrinsic or allergic form [10]. Later, Kursel *et al.* conducted a study in support of two variants of eczema, by providing generalised risk factors [11]:

- **Atopic Eczema:** Eczema occurring in early childhood (earlier known as extrinsic eczema) with additional IgE sensitivity. More likely found in males, the onset of rash developing in the first year, prolonged breast fed, and having a history of asthma, rhinitis, or food allergies.
- **Nonatopic Eczema:** Earlier known as intrinsic eczema, which shows normal IgE levels or no specific IgE, it is more prone in girls and children who attended day-care attendance in their early lives.

In 1992, another study proposed that there were 4 subtypes of eczema based on the results from skin prick tests and aeroallergen tests on patients with eczema [12]. Since then, types of eczema have grown in a multiplicative fashion depending on the number of tests available, infections spreading over erythematous eczema and many other tests that may not relate to underlying disease genesis. However, it is important to identify different types of eczema to establish a proper line of treatment. Depending on the underlying cause of disease, affected area/body part, and variation in appearance, diagnosis of eczema is broad and is differentiated as [1, 3]:

Contact Dermatitis: It may be Irritant dermatitis caused by repeated exposure to toxic substances or Allergic dermatitis caused by repeated exposure to some allergen which activates body's immune reaction and produces dermatitis. Initially affects the area that comes in contact with the trigger; other areas might get involved later.

Dyshidrotic Eczema: This is the formation of small blisters on the hand and feet. It is more common in women than men. It is caused by allergies, exposure to nickel, Cobalt, and Chromium salt, stress, and damp hands. In dyshidrotic eczema, fluid-filled blisters are formed on fingers, toes, palms and soles of feet. Skin becomes flaky and scaly.

Eczema Herpeticum: Also known as a form of Kaposi varicelliform eruption caused by the herpes simplex virus (HSV), it is an extensive cutaneous vesicular eruption that arises from pre-existing inflammatory skin disease. Usually AD characterised by an eruption of dome-shaped blisters and pustules, fever, malaise, and lymphadenopathy [13].

Hand Eczema: This type of eczema only affects hands. Hands become red, itchy and dry, and form cracks and blisters. Caused due to exposure to chemicals that irritate the skin. People working in hairdressing, healthcare, and laundry are more prone to this type of eczema.

Ichthyosis Vulgaris: It is the slowing down of skin's natural shedding process, which results in a chronic, excessive build-up of the protein in the upper layer of the skin (keratin). The skin becomes dry and scaly, in a color range from white to dirty grey or brown. It is sometimes called fish scale disease or fish skin disease, which can be present at birth, but usually, first appear during early childhood.

Impetigo: Mainly affects infants and children. Red sores are seen on the nose and mouth. The sores rupture, ooze for a few days then form a brownish crust.

Lichen Simplex Chronicus: It produces thickened plaques of skin commonly found on the shins and neck.

Netherton Syndrome: It is a rare inherited disorder characterized by red, inflamed, scaly skin, hair anomalies, increased susceptibility to atopic eczema, elevated IgE levels, and predisposition to allergies, asthma, and eczema. Newborns with this syndrome have reddened skin (erythroderma) and sometimes a thick parchment-like covering of skin (collodion membrane) [14].

Neurodermatitis: Similar to atopic dermatitis. Thick and scaly patches appear on the skin of arms, legs, back of neck, scalp, genitals, soles of feet, and back of hands. The exact cause is not known; stress can be a trigger.

Nummular Eczema: It differs from other types of eczema; as in this, coin-shaped itching spots are formed on the skin. It is triggered by a reaction caused by insect bites or reaction to chemicals.

Pityriasis Rosea: May be triggered by a viral infection and is characterised by the appearance of skin rash as a large spot on chest, back or abdomen followed by a pattern of smaller lesions.

Psoriasis: Formation of itchy, dry scaly patches on the knees, elbows, trunk and scalp.

Scabies: Caused by the infestation of the human itch mite and produce a rash similar to other forms of eczema.

Seborrheic Dermatitis: Rash is formed on the scalp, face, ears and occasionally the mid-chest in adults. In infants, the weepy, oozy rash is formed behind the ear, which can be quite extensive, involving the entire body.

Stasis Dermatitis: It is seen in people who have blood flow problems in their lower legs resulting from the inability of the heart to push blood through the legs causing fluid to leak out of the weakened vein into the skin, resulting in swelling, redness, itching and pain.

Xerotic Eczema: Skin becomes excessively dry and causes the skin to crack.

In many cases, where eczema is caused by exposure to reactive substances, it may be prevented by simply avoiding contact with that specific substance. Additionally, applying moisturizers or emollients to the affected area also prevents certain types of eczema.

Severity Classification of Atopic Dermatitis

Clinically adult AD may exist in three forms depending on the disease timespan and its severity. However, little is known about the transition mechanisms taking place in disease progression.

Acute Form: Vesicular, weeping, crusting eruptions of the skin.

Subacute Form: Dry, scaly, erythematous papules and plaques.

Chronic Form: Lichenified skin from repeated scratching, scales, crusts, and infiltered erythema.

In children, AD is mostly detected by pityriasis alba, which is characterized by hypopigmented, poorly demarcated plaques with fine scales initially on the scalp and face, which later spread to the trunk and extremities. Overtime, AD tends to involve the flexural surfaces of the body, anterior and lateral neck, eyelids, forehead, face, wrists, dorsal of the feet, and hands [4].

Severity is determined using SCORAD or EASI.

ETIOLOGY

The etiology of AD is complex, and it involves several factors, including genetics, dysfunctional epidermal barrier, skin microbiome abnormalities, type 2 immune dysregulation, altered lipid composition and neuroinflammation, but the interplay between genetic and environmental factors contribute to its development and maintenance. The exact basis of AD is perplexing and controversial, but advances in molecular biology have transformed the understanding of AD pathogenesis. These factors have availed to the development of novel therapeutic and preventative strategies that do not focus on a single pathological pathway of the disease, but on more complex molecular interactions that drive AD. New possible and effective trends for treating AD have also been observed mostly by focusing on the patient's Immunotype/genotype/phenotype.

Genetics

There are evidences for strong genetic susceptibility to AD. The strongest identifiable risk factor for developing the disorder, is having a familial history

[15]. AD also has strong heritability in twin studies of approximately 75%, suggesting strong genetic factors as an important contributor [16]. Worldwide discoveries in molecular biology have identified the involvement of 46 genes in AD, of which mutations of at least one positive filaggrin gene (FLG) have been demonstrated with an association of AD [17].

FLG is a highly unusual gene that is found within a cluster of more than 60 genes on chromosome 1q21, involved in epithelial differentiation (Epithelial Differentiation Complex-EDC). FLG encodes for seven S100 proteins – filaggrin, filaggrin 2, hornerin, trichohyalin, trichohyalin-like 1, cornulin, and repetin. All these proteins share a common protein domain organization having an S100 calcium-binding motif at the *N*-terminal with an extended, highly repetitive tail which is characteristic of 'fused' gene family [18]. EDC also contains several other gene families which encode for S100 proteins, loricrin (LOR), involucrin, small proline-rich proteins and late cornified envelop (LCE) proteins. LCE gene variations (deletion of LCE3B and LCE3C) have been implicated as a susceptibility factor for psoriasis [19] whereas, loricrin keratoderma is caused by an unusual gain-of-function mutation of loricrin [20]. There are 3 exons and 2 introns on FLG gene. Exon-1 is 15bp and non-coding. Exon-2 (159bp) encodes parts of the S100 domain and Exon-3 (12,753bp) is the largest axon in the genome at more than 12.7 kb, and it encodes for entire profilaggrin pre-protein which is processed by serine proteases to filaggrin monomers after translation (Fig. **1**) [21].

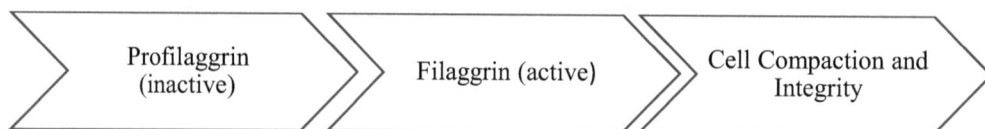

Fig. (1). Processing of profilaggrin to filaggrin.

Profilaggrin is the main constituent of electron-dense keratohyalin granules that are found within a granular layer of the epidermis, but itself has no keratin binding property, but filaggrin monomers bind to and condenses the keratin 1, keratin 10, and other intermediate filaments within the cytoskeleton of keratinocytes, and thereby contributes to the cell compaction and integrity process. Within the squames, filaggrin is citrullinated, which promotes its unfolding and further degradation into hygroscopic amino acids, pyrrolidone carboxylic acid and *trans*-urocanic acid, which constitute elements of natural moisturising factor (NMF) which may also contribute to epidermal barrier function retaining water and hence increasing flexibility of cornified layer [18]. This process involves caspase14 and other proteases. Filaggrin is, therefore, in the frontline of defence, and protects the skin from UV radiation, maintains the skin pH, and prevents the entry of foreign environmental substances that can otherwise activate aberrant immune responses [3].

Loss of functional mutation of FLG confers a higher risk of AD in individuals who have them than in individuals who do not. Loss-of-function mutations of profilaggrin or filaggrin lead to a poorly formed stratum corneum, which is also prone to xerosis due to water loss, leading to the most prevalent disorder of keratinization, called mendelian ichthyosis [22].

Besides skin, FLG is also expressed in: a) gastrointestinal system: in oral and upper esophageal mucosa b) respiratory tract: in the cornified epithelium of nasal vestibulum but not within the transitional epithelium covering the inferior turbinate bone [23]. Reduction or complete loss of filaggrin expression or functional mutation of FLG leads to enhanced percutaneous transfer of allergens and predisposes those individuals to allergic rhinitis and asthma [24]. FLG mutations are also associated with contact dermatitis [25], nickel allergy [10] and peanut allergy [26].

Skin Barrier Defects

Epidermis comprises epithelial cells, immune cells, and microbes which provide a physical and functional barrier to protect the human skin [27]. Epidermal barrier proteins, including FLG, transglutaminases (TGs), keratins, loricrin, involucrin, corneodesmosin (protein from corneodesmosomes which are important organelles for end-to-end adhesion), claudins (tight junctions that form insoluble barrier), and intercellular proteins are cross-linked to form an impermeable skin barrier [28]. Skin barrier defects facilitate allergen sensitization and lead to systemic immune responses such as increased IgE levels and airway hyperactivity [29]. FLG mutations play a key role in the development of skin barrier defects [30]. The free aminoacids obtained from the degradation of FLG maintain/lower skin pH and thereby prevents the activation of serine proteases and subsequent growth of bacteria [31]. In AD skin, there is overexpression of IL-4, IL-5, IL-13, IL-25, IL-17A, and IL-22, as keratinocytes send proinflammatory and pruritogenic signals, during the stress-induced conditions through IL-33 and thymic stromal lymphopoietin (TSLP) which activate Th2 cells and eosinophils. Lack of FLG causes impaired corneocyte integrity and cohesion by overexpression of Th2 cytokines through STAT6 signalling, as shown in Fig. (**2**) [32].

Hence, in both affected and unaffected skin of AD patients, there is elevated transepidermal water loss (TEWL) [33], increased pH [31], increased permeability to allergens [34], and reduced water retention. Increased pH activates pH-sensitive serine proteases, which results in premature degradation of corneodesmosome, and other lipid processing enzymes and activation of IL-α and

IL-β [35]. Besides FLG, microbial dysbiosis, type 2 immune activation causes secondary downregulation of skin barrier genes, exacerbating underlying barrier defects.

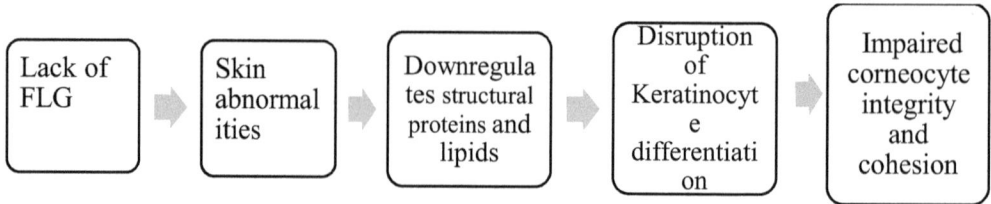

Lack of FLG		Skin abnormal ities		Downregula tes structural proteins and lipids		Disruption of Keratinocyt e differentiati on		Impaired corneocyte integrity and cohesion

Fig. (2). Mechanism of lack of filaggrin causing cellular abnormalities.

Microbial Colonization and Superinfection

In normal skin, commensal bacteria augment skin defensive mechanisms against infectious agents, by producing antimicrobial peptides (AMPs), defensins and cathelicidins (LL-37) which stimulate immunity. In AD skin, epidermal barrier defects lead to abnormal colonization *S. aureus,* which correlates with the severity of eczema [36]. Skin dysbiosis by pathogens affects skin immune responses and causes skin inflammation driven by type-2 helper T (Th2) cells [34]. Activation of Th2 cytokines in AD skin down-regulate AMPs, tight junctions (claudins) [37] and Corneodesmosin (CLDN1) by IL-4, IL-13, IL-22, IL-25, IL-31predisposing to recurrent microbial (fungal, viral, bacterial) infections and altering skin pH [35] and contributing to skin barrier defects. AD flare investigation of patients with severe AD has revealed greater colonization with *S. aureus* than in patients with less severe disease. *S. aureus* induced epidermal thickening and expansion in cutaneous Th2 and Th17 cells in these patients [38]. Additionally, *S. aureus* has reportedly shown inhibited expression of differentiation markers like FLG, loricrin, keratins, desmocollin-1, Th1, NK cells, Interferon-γ and overexpression of serine proteases, cytokines, lytic enzymes, IgE [39]. Futhermore, staphylococcal peptides and their superantigens have also been implicated in driving eczematous inflammation: staphylococcal delta toxin causes mast cell degranulation whilst alpha-toxin induces keratinocyte apoptosis; T cells are stimulated by staphylococcal enterotoxins; and certain staphylococcal surface proteins modulate inflammation [40]. FLG-degraded products play an important role in optimizing skin pH. An elevated pH of stratum corneum may lead to enhanced *S. aureus* adhesion and multiplication. In addition, urocanic acid and pyrrolidone carboxylic acid may contribute to a specific anti-staphylococcal effect by directly inhibiting bacterial expression of iron-regulated surface determinant protein A, which promotes bacterial adhesion to squames [31].

Environmental factors, detergents and scratching also contribute to bacterial colonization. Other pathogens which exacerbate or trigger cutaneous inflammation in AD include cutaneous yeasts like *Malasezzia* species, *Staphylococcus epidermidis, Molluscum contaginosum, H. simplex* virus (HSV), *H. zoster* virus, *Human Papilloma* virus (HPV), *Aspergillus fumigatus* [34, 38, 41].

Immunological Dysfunction or Regulation

Immune dysfunction is the key factor underlying the pathophysiology and etiology of AD. Cutaneous Inflammation of AD is triggered by mechanical injury, allergens, and microbes which activates the signal transducer and activator of the transcription (STAT-6) pathway, which ultimately leads to the release of proinflammatory cytokines (Tumor necrosis factor- TNF-α and IL-1) and chemokines (promote expression of adhesins on vascular endothelium and facilitate extravasation of inflammatory cells into the tissues) from keratinocytes as shown in Fig. (3). During this process, IgE production by B cells depends on the release of IL-4 and IL-13 by activated Th-2 cells, which are involved in humoral cell responses, promotes cutaneous inflammatory response and keratinocyte apoptosis [42]. The increased IgE levels are also associated with the increased cAMP levels, which correlates with the higher Phosphodiesterase enzyme, predominantly PDE4, which is widely distributed in the mast cells, eosinophils, neutrophils, macrophages and monocytes [43].

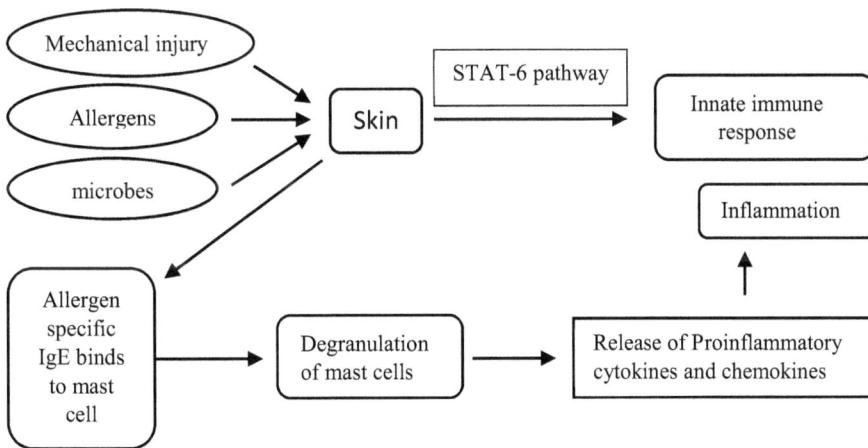

Fig. (3). Pathway of immune-activation in AD promoting inflammation.

Comparison between the lesional and non-lesional skin of AD patients has shown that in lesional skin, T cell infiltration is predominantly characterised by CD4 expression defined by the production of the cytokines IL-4, IL-13 (modulate IgE level class switching in B cells, induce expression of vascular adhesion molecules involved in eosinophil infiltration and downregulation of Th1 type cytokine activity) and IL-5 (promotes development, activation and survival of eosinophils) m-RNA expressing cells, but few Interferon-γ (inhibit the synthesis of IgE, the proliferation of Th2, and expression of IL-4 receptors on T cells) producing cells while non-lesional skin shows more subtle but similar T cell infiltrations as that of lesional skin, but there is fluid accumulation between cell (spongiosis) and immunohistological changes [44].

AD is characterised by the overexpression of cytokines: Th2 (IL-4, IL-10, IL-13) and Th22 (IL-22 has a role in epidermal hyperplasia). As the disease progresses, the skin becomes infiltrated with additional Th1, Th17 (IL-17 - a mediator of psoriasis) and IL-23 (activates and differentiates Th17 and Th22), further contributing to disease pathology [45]. Activated lymphocytes adopt a tissue-resident memory T cell phenotype facilitating rapid recall responses when exposed to the same antigens. Thus, patients with severe AD have increased IgE-reactivity to aeroallergens, food proteins, microbial antigens, or keratinocyte-derived auto-antigens. Besides, CD4+ T cells, other lymphocyte subsets are found in increased numbers, including type 2 cytokines (IL-4, IL-13, IL-31, TSLP) - producing CD8+ T cells and type 2 innate lymphoid cells (ILC-2) [46]. ILCs play a role in the early sensing of tissue damage, and initiation of inflammatory cascades prior to the development of antigen-driven adaptive immune responses. Inflammatory epidermal dendritic cells (IDEC), dendritic cells (DC) and Langerhans' cells (LC) directly process antigens and subsequently present them to Th2 cells. These cells also produce chemokines such as CCL5 (RANTES-regulation on activation, normal T cell expressed and secreted), CCL17 (TARC-thymus and activation regulated chemokine), CCL13 (MCP-4 – monocyte chemotactic protein-4), CCL22 (MDC- macrophage-derived chemokine), CCL27, eotaxin (eosinophil specific chemoattractant), IL-16 (chemoattractant cytokine)which further attracts Th2 cells and results in the amplification of type 2 responses, which inturn downregulate terminal differentiation markers- such as FLG, loricrin, periplakin, and claudins [47].

Activity exhibited by Treg cells is another important immunological factor contributing to the pathology of AD. Treg cells have a suppressive action on Th1 and Th2 cytokine profile, as shown in Fig. (**4**).

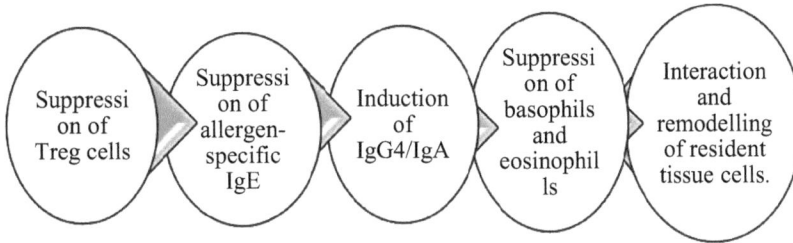

Fig. (4). Mechanism of Treg cell suppression.

A number of natural Treg cells have been identified and characterised by their phenotype CD4+CD25+, which develop under the control of transcription factor PFox in the thymus and periphery [48]. Reduced natural killer (NK)-cell-mediated immunomodulation has been proposed to be involved in the immune dysregulation in atopic dermatitis [49]. Other contributing factors to inflammatory response include reduced expression of antimicrobial peptides, such as cathelicidins and β-defensins, and expression of superantigens by colonizing pathogens.

Altered Lipid Composition

Lipids, such as ceramides, long-chain FFAs, and cholesterol, constitute the lipid matrix in which corneocytes (bricks) are organized in lamellar bodies (mortar) and play a crucial role in the epidermal permeability barrier. Precursor lipids are stored in lamellar bodies within the upper cell layers of the epidermis and extruded into the extracellular domain, during epidermal differentiation. Enzymatic processing of precursor lipids produces major lipids, which are necessary to maintain the integrity of the epidermal barrier [50]. A reduction in the lipid level in the stratum corneum gives rise to AD. Both lesional and non-lesional skin has shown a reduction in the ceramide content and lipid chain length. This is due to the altered expression of enzymes in the stratum corneum, essential for lipid biogenesis, such as acid sphingomyelinase (aSmase) or β-glucocerebrosidase (GBA). The activity of these enzymes depends on pH, and it has been suggested that a low pH in the stratum corneum is essential for lipid secretion and assembly [51]. Long-chains of omegahydroxy-ceramides are essential because their covalent binding with cornified envelope proteins contributes to the integrity of stratum corneum and accelerate recovery of damaged skin barrier function by stimulating differentiation processes. Th2 cytokines reduce levels of long-chain FFAs and omega hydroxy-ceramides in a STAT6-dependent manner. Altered levels of long-chain ceramides in patients with AD correlate with *S. aureus* colonization. TEWL negatively correlates with levels of these ceramides [52].

Neuroinflammation

Itch is the dominant symptom of AD induced by a number of pruritogens, including inflammatory lipids, cytokines, neuropeptides, neurotransmitters such as histamine and serotonin (5-hydroxytryptamine, 5-HT), proteases, proteinase-activating receptors, and opioid peptides which participate in 'itch-scratch' cycle [53]. Both the nervous and immune system in the skin is managed by the neuromediators. Skin immune cells such as mast cells and dendritic cells release neuropeptides: VIP and CGRP modulate the functions of macrophages, T cells and Langerhans cells, while substance P affects lymphocyte proliferation and mast cell degranulation. Histamine, a well-known pruritogenic found in high concentrations in AD lesions, activates H1 and H4 receptors, which causes itch and allergic inflammation. Histamine-induced pruritis is mediated by various endogenous and exogenous stimuli which activate itch-specific pathways through chemosensitive C-fibers. H1 antihistaminics have been widely used in urticaria, but their effects are limited in the treatment of chronic itch in AD. Itch in chronic pruritis maybe attributed to Type 2 cytokines, including IL-4, IL-13, IL-31, and TSLP, which stimulate afferent neurons *via* its receptors and Janus kinase (JAK) family and neurons expressing transient receptor potential cation channel subfamily member 1 respectively. The presence of IL4R-α (mediates the action of IL-4 and IL-13) in afferent neurons reinforces the role of type 2 cytokines in neural itch. IL-31 has been noted to cause sensory elongation and branching, promoting its sensitivity to minimal stimuli and sustained itch *via* IL31R-α [46, 54]. An increase in the number of stress-induced 5-HT receptive mast cells is seen in AD; patients have shown improvements in pruritis with antipsychotropic drugs that act on 5HT or have serotonin-modulating effects, implying the role of neuromediators in pruritis [53]. In addition, the activation of STAT3 in the astrogliosis of the spinal dorsal horn has been reported to be involved in chronic pruritus *via* the generation of lipocalin-2 [55].

Food Allergies and Other Environmental Factors

Skin barrier dysfunction predisposes to epicutaneous sensitization and food allergy. Adverse reactions from food proteins are particularly seen in children, which produce cutaneous reactions which might later extend to the gastrointestinal tract and respiratory system, producing ulcerative colitis and allergic rhinitis and asthma, respectively. Heat treatment, food processing, and digestion of these food proteins may result in the formation of new allergenic epitomes. The mechanism underlying unique protein allergy remains unclear. Resistance to proteolysis in gastric or intestinal fluids, post-translational glycosylation, and non-specific enzymatic activation of immune cells may correlate with allergenicity. However, similarities between the environmental allergens (pollen) and food proteins can cause IgE-crossreactivities, establishing a cytokine environment that could contribute to Th2-cell activation and cascading events, which has been suggested to represent a molecular basis for the allergic symptoms in patients with oral allergy syndrome (OAS) [56, 57].

Environmental factors are uniquely contributing to the growing rates of AD over the past five decades through epigenetic alterations. Factors that predispose to or aggravate AD are shown in Fig. (5).

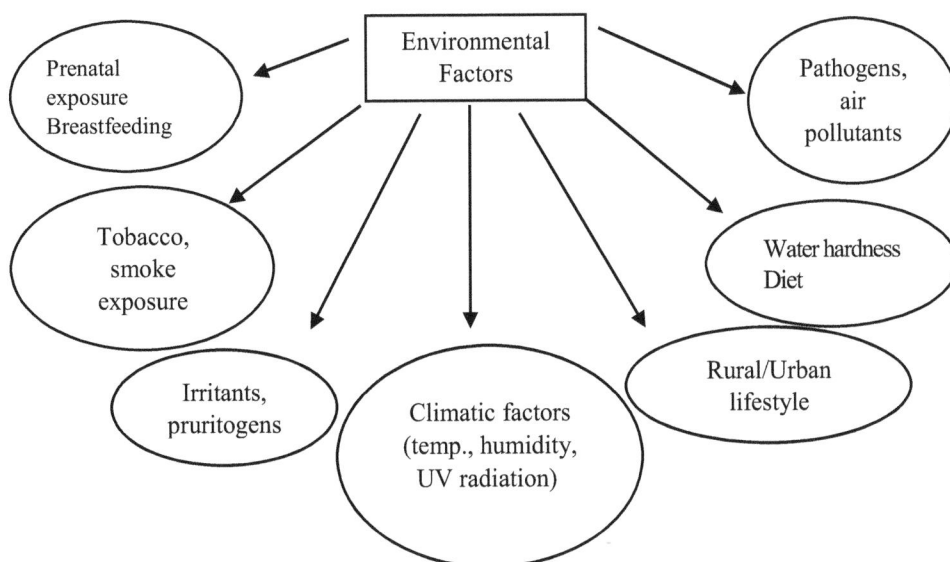

Fig. (5). Environmental factors involved in AD.

Early life exposures to dirt and pathogens, prenatal intake of omega-3 long-chain polyunsaturated fatty acids, Vitamin D, prebiotic and probiotics may reduce the risk of AD [58].

TREATMENT

Treatment has been given in three parts (Table **1**).

The objective of the treatment is [8]:

- To reach a no-symptom or minor-symptom stage, where the disease does not affect patient's quality of life.
- That no acute or intense exacerbations/eruptions are seen, if the disease persists.

So far, no drug with complete healing capabilities has been discovered. However, treatment radially focuses on symptomatic relief and long-term control.

Table 1. Treatment classification.

Conventional Treatment	Novel Treatment	Herbal Treatment
• **A. Topical Therapy** • Emollients • Corticosteroids • Calcineurin Inhibitors • Phosphodiesterase (PDE) Inhibitors • Antibiotics • **B. Phototherapy** • Broad-band UVB (BBUVB) • Narrow-Band UVB (NBUVB) • UVA1 • Combined UVA/UVB • Psoralens UVA (PUVA) • Excimer laserd for targeted areas • Blue Light (Novel) • **C. Systemic Therapy** • Immunosuppressive • Immunomodulatory • Antimicrobials	• Monoclonal Antibodies(MAbs) • Jakus Kinase (JAK) receptor inhibitors • Histamine-4 receptor (H4R) antagonists • PDE4 inhibitors • Aryl Hydrocarbon receptor (AhR) modulating agents • Transient receptor potential vanilloid-1 receptor (TRPV1R) antagonists • Oral Sphingosine-1 Phosphate (S1P) Modulators	• Traditional Herbs • Chinese Herbs • Essential Oils

CONVENTIONAL TREATMENT

Topical Therapy

Emollients

Emollients/Moisturizers are topical preparations that soothe skin and help in retaining and replenishing epidermal moisture and softness. Emollients serve as the first-line of therapy for both acute and remitting flares and in initial cases of dryness with no or little skin inflammation. Emollients fill in the cracks, thus, preventing skin drying and inflammation recurrence, adding to the barrier function and reducing the penetration of irritants. General recommendations are to use emollients with high oil and low water content. Additional application of moisturizers, two or three times daily after showering/bathing, is recommended, and its use should not be limited to post-bathing. Another recommendation is to use 250-300g emollient weekly. A suitable range of emollients are now found in markets which include physiological lipids (ceramides and free fatty acids) in their ingredients, adding anti-inflammatory, anti-pruritic, and anti-microbial effects to the moisturizers, but no superiority of these compounds over the others have been demonstrated. A case-control study suggests that emollients may penetrate the thin layer of neonates, cause irritation and damage the skin barrier, which may predispose to allergen sensitisation. Another randomised controlled trial study conducted on infants with familial history of AD suggested no significant occurrence of adverse effects. It is also suggested that early application of emollients in such patients may prevent the worsening of AD in the future, though the exact positive mechanism of emollients remains unidentified [59]. Emollients are safe and effective to use and, unlike corticosteroids, do not necessarily have steroid-sparing effects when used as adjuvants.

Natural Emollients

Plant-Derived Products: Aloe vera, Coconut oil.

Animal-Derived Products: Lanolin, Horse oil.

Other Excipients: Ceramides, Natural moisturizing factors (carboxylic acids, aminoacids, glutamic acid), Antimicrobial peptides, Ectoin.

Topical Corticosteroids (TCs)

For mild, moderate and severe flare-ups of AD, corticosteroids are used as the first line of treatment when emollients alone cannot control AD symptoms. Due to their anti-proliferative, anti-inflammatory and immunosuppressive action, corticosteroids find wide application in skin-related disorders, including allergic ones. Topical safety therapy of corticosteroids is determined by the action potency, dose and site of application. The potency of the corticosteroid is also affected by its formulation. An ointment is more potent than a cream, which is more potent than lotions and gels.

Owing to their lipophilicity, corticosteroids penetrate the cell membrane easily and bind with their specific receptor in the cytoplasm. The transcription of mRNA becomes inhibited or stimulated, leading to a multidirectional activity causing a lower expression of adhesion molecules, limitation of T-cell migration, the decline in the synthesis of proinflammatory cytokines and stimulation of lipocortin's synthesis [60]. TCs induce Langerhans' cell apoptosis as well as indirectly reduce Langerhans' cell survival factors, such as granulocyte-macrophage colony-stimulating factor, in basal keratinocytes [61].

Side-effects such as skin atrophy, recurring bacterial/viral/fungal infections, purpura, striae, telangiectasias, dyspigmentation and facial acne forms mainly arise from the prolonged application of strong corticosteroids. Though uncommon, systemic absorption of high-potency TCs from topical sites may result in hypothalamic–pituitary–adrenal suppression, diabetes mellitus, moon face and growth retardation. Allergic contact dermatitis rarely occurs in response to corticosteroids [8].

Traditionally, Corticosteroids are applied 1-2 times daily, though there is no evidence of additional improvement with twice daily over once daily application. Low-potency steroids are the safest agents for long-term use, on large surface areas, on the face or areas of the body with thinner skin, and on children. More potent agents are beneficial for severe diseases and for areas of the body where the skin is thicker, such as the palms and bottoms of the feet. High- and ultra-high-potency steroids should not be used on the face, groin, axilla, or under occlusion, except in rare situations and for short durations. Chronic application induces tolerance and tachyphylaxis. Rebound phenomena characterized by the intensification of lesions occur with the sudden withdrawal of the corticosteroid therapy [62].

Topical Calcineurin Inhibitors (TCIs)

The steroid-free topical calcineurin inhibitors are used both as alternatives and adjuvants to corticosteroids, to avoid and limit the steroidal side-effects of the TCs. TCIs are effective, safe and cheap as compared to TCs and emollients. Tacrolimus and Pimecrolimus, are two macrolactam immunomodulators that are considered second-line therapy of TCIs. Tacrolimus is slightly more effective than pimecrolimus. TCIs exert their immunosuppressive action by inhibiting calcineurin-dependent T cell activation, suppressing mast cell activation and thereby decreasing the production of proinflammatory cytokines.

Pimecrolimus is a lipophilic molecule that binds to cytosolic receptor macrophilin-12 and inhibits the phosphatase calcineurin, which causes inhibition of dephosphorylation of the cytosolic form of the nuclear factor of activated T cells. As a consequence, it prevents the transcription and release of inflammatory cytokines such as IL-2, interferon-γ, IL-4, IL-10, and TNF-α, as well as cell proliferation, in T cells. In contrast to TCs, these do not have any depleting effect on Langerhans' cells, keratinocytes, endothelial cells, or fibroblast cell lines in human skin [61].

TCIs do not cause skin atrophy and hence can be used for thinner skin areas that show good cutaneous absorption. TCIs are generally reserved for short-term or intermittent long therapy in persons with moderate to severe AD when corticosteroids cannot be used. Additionally, tachyphylaxis is not seen with the continued use of TCIs. Other local side-effects related to TCIs include- burning sensations and hot flushes, which subside on repeated use. The incidence of bacterial, fungal and viral infections is not altered with TCIs. TCIs are largely safer drugs, though there is a risk of malignancies with long-term use of TCIs, in patients receiving TCIs post organ-transplant. Few reports of skin lymphomas are higher in eczema patients taking tacrolimus as compared to pimecrolimus [63].

Contraindicated in breast-feeding and pregnant women and children below 2 years of age; in patients with Netherton's syndrome, tacrolimus ointment is contraindicated as its increased cutaneous absorption may lead to increased blood concentration and result in renal disturbances [8]. 0.1% Tacrolimus ointment for adults demonstrates the same effectiveness as corticosteroids when used on the trunk and extremities.

Uses

Contact eczema, hand dermatitis, intertriginous psoriasis, seborrheic dermatitis, vitiligo and Netherton syndrome.

Phosphodiesterase-4 (PDE4) Inhibitors

Crisaborole, a phosphordiesterase-4 inhibitor approved by USFDA in 2016 as 2% crisaborole ointment for the treatment of mild to moderate AD of patients with age ≤ 2 years and psoriasis.

Crisaborole competitively and reversibly inhibits PDE4 active sites, which causes cAMP accumulation with subsequent activation of protein kinase A, resulting in inhibition of proinflammatory and T cell cytokines which contribute to immune dysregulation and skin barrier dysfunction [43]. Crisaborole is rapidly metabolized into inactive metabolites. Crisaborole ointment is generally well tolerated. A temporary burning or stinging sensation occurs on application. Few cases of hypersensitivity reactions probably because of butylated hydroxytoluene and gastrointestinal effects (nausea, vomiting), worsening of AD flare, and infections have been reported [64].

Topical Antibiotics

Reducing *S. aureus* colonization by controlling inflammation and improving barrier function are supposed to improve AD. Restoring the epithelial barrier using skin protective measures and anti-inflammatory therapy also results in reduced colonization with *S. aureus*. Topical antibiotics most commonly prescribed for mild/moderate secondary infections are gentamicin, fusidic acid and mupirocine. Topical antibiotics application reduces bacterial colonization, but no remarkable differences in the restoration of cutaneous microbiota are seen. Prolonged use of topical antibiotics should be avoided to reduce the risk of development of bacterial resistance, including FRSA and (fusidic acid-resistant *S. aureus*) MRSA (methicillin-resistant *S. aureus*).

Phototherapy

Phototherapy with UV light can be considered/ used as a second-line of treatment for moderate to severe AD when the disease cannot be controlled with topical agents. Ultraviolet phototherapy is effective for treating severe or refractory atopic dermatitis. Approaches of phototherapy in AD include:

Broad Band UV-B/ BBUVB (290-320nm)

Its use began in 1948, and contained carbon arcs in lamps. UV-B dosing depends on patient's pigmentation and tolerance to UV radiation. Dosing with 0.5-1.0 MED (Minimal erythema dose defined as the minimal UV-B radiation able to induce minimal erythema in the patient) leads to complete healing of lesions as compared to visible light. UVB radiation is confined to the epidermis and causes a significant reduction of *S. aureus* colonisation at the dose of 900 mJ/cm^2 than UVA [65]. BBUVB has erythemogenic potential and lower efficacy; it was soon replaced by UVA and NBUVB therapy [66].

Narrow-Band UVB/ NBUVB (311-313nm)

Most effective phototherapy in managing chronic flares of AD. NBUVB can damage DNA and induce apoptosis of epidermal T lymphocytes by activating death receptors. It also inhibits the release of cytokines and the Th1 response leading to a Th2 switch [67]. It is nowadays considered the first line of phototherapy treatment owing to its higher efficacy, safety, ease of administration, tolerability, and less carcinogenic potential. The usual treatment schedule with NB UV-B for AD is 3 sessions per week for 6 weeks. Based on the six skin phototypes (measured on the basis of skin pigmentation), the initial dose can vary from 130mJ/m^2 to 400 mJ/m^2 and the maximal achievable dose can vary between 2000 mJ/m^2 to 5000 mJ/m^2. A dose increment of 15 mJ/m^2 to 65 mJ/m^2 is used with progressive phototherapy [68]. NBUVB has been found to be more effective than visible light, UVA, medium dose UVA1 and PUVA. It is also more effective in managing managing pediatric AD [69]. The combined therapy of NBUVB with the Cys A has demonstrated a sustained improvement with a SCORAD reduction of 50% or more, compared to the baseline [70].

UVA-1 (340-400nm)

UV-A1 uses the lower frequencies of the UV-A light spectrum (between 340 and 400 nm). Higher dose UVA-1 radiation penetrates deeper into the dermis and into the superficial vascular plexus, increasing collagen synthesis, inhibiting calcineurin and suppressing TNF-α, IL-12 and interferon-γ. It also induces apoptosis of T-cells and mast cells [71]. UV-A1 can be administered either employing a high dose (80–130 J/cm^2), medium dose (40– 80 J/cm^2) or low dose (<40 J/cm^2). Medium-dose UV-A1 is highly effective and better tolerated than low-dose and high-dose UV-A1. Also, medium-dose UV-A1 has shown prompt improvement in clinical symptoms of AD as compared to UVA/UVB therapy. Usual treatment schedules with UV-A1 medium dose for AD are 3–5 sessions per week for 3–8 weeks with a maximum dose of 80 J/cm^2. Treatment times can range from 10 min to 1h per session. UVA-1 is essentially used in acute AD flares [72]. UVA1 therapy is not performed on patients with photodermatoses as there is a risk of the development of carcinoma [73].

Combined UVA/UVB (280+400nm)

UVA/B is a combination of UVA and UVB and is considered superior in all aspects to UVA and UVB therapy when used alone for the management of chronic-severe AD. UVA/B radiation is the emission device that emits two radiations of different wavelengths simultaneously from a single device. This allows better control of radiational doses [74]. Treatment duration was reportedly reduced when UVA/B was given in combination with cyclosporine-A therapy [75].

Psoralens+ UVA therapy (PUVA)

It is the use of UVA in combination with the highly reactive psoralen compound (8-methoxypsoralen) which causes interstrand DNA crosslinking, thereby leading to irreversible DNA damage. It causes alteration of lymphocyte function in the dermal infiltrate. Psoralens comes in various formulations oral pills, bath lotions, and creams. In Bath-PUVA, the UVA session is conducted post 20-30 minutes of bath exposure with 8-MOP, and in cream-PUVA, the same is conducted after 20-30 min after 0.0006% 8-MOP cream application [76, 77]. PUVA therapy is associated with rebound phenomena. Additionally, long-term use of PUVA is associated with an increased risk of developing cancer, possibly malignant melanoma, and risk of cataract formation requiring constant protection by sunglasses [78]. PUVA therapy should mostly be limited to patients, not TCs and UVA1 therapy. Der *et al.* reported no significant differences in PUVA as compared to NBUVB [79]. Another study suggests that 5-MOP (5-methoxypsoralen) is more effective in delaying remission times than PUVA therapy [80].

Excimer Lasers for Targeted Areas (el) (308nm)

It is targeted phototherapy, which uses a single wave-length light source. It requires sessions after very 1-2 weeks, and has a maximum irradiating area of 504 cm^2. This method has better patient compliance, and carries a lower risk of side effects. It has been found to be more effective than NBUVB in psoriasis [69]. Currently, data is insufficient to suggest the use of MEL in AD.

Blue Light (400-495nm)

A novel method could be used as an option for the management of AD. A randomised trial conducted by Becker reported blue light full body irradiation offers long-term control of disease, improvement in pruritus and quality of life [81]. A multicentre trial on 150 AD patients is being performed using blue light results, which are yet to be published [82].

Common Side- Effects of Phototherapy

Actinic damage, Increased skin aging, Local erythema and tenderness, Pruritus, Burning, Stinging, Dyspigmentation, Heat-induced flares, and Claustrophobia.

Uncommon Effects on Prolonged Therapy

Non-melanoma skin cancer, Melanoma, Lentigines, Photosensitive eruptions, Polymorphous light eruption, Lupus flare, B6 deficiency, Folliculitis, Folic acid depletion, Photo-onycholysis, HSV reactivation, Facial hypertrichosis, Cataract formation, Headaches, nausea, vomiting, Hepatotoxicity, Ocular toxicity.

Systemic Therapy

Topical therapy is the main stay, but patients with widespread moderate to severe atopic dermatitis who do not respond to topical and UV therapy may require systemic therapy. Rectification of underlying factors contributing to the pathogenesis of AD, such as the resolution of skin inflammation, restoration of the impaired skin barrier, and avoidance of trigger factors, can provide better control over the disease. This may be achieved by:

Immunosuppressive Therapy: Corticosteroids, Cyclosporine, Azathioprine, Mycophenolate mofetil, Methotrexate.

Immunomodulatory Therapy: Alitretinoin, Biologics (mAbs and Small Molecules), Interferons, Immunoglobulins.

Antimicrobials: Cephalosporine, Acyclovir, Ketoconazole.

Immunosuppressive Therapy

Oral Corticosteroids (OCs)

OCs may affect the transcription of several pathogenesis mediators of AD, including cytokines, chemokines and adhesion molecules, but these are unable to produce stable remission and long-term control of AD. Conventionally, an Initial dosage of 0.75–1 mg/kg/day is given, which should be tapered in 7–10 days [83]. Long-term therapy is not recommended, owing to its ability to cause potential side-effects *viz*; diabetes, hypertension, gastric ulcers, osteoporosis, skin atrophy, glaucoma, Cushing's syndrome, and growth retardation and serious relapses and rebound of the disease. Consequently, the use of systemic corticosteroids should be limited to exceptional cases such as short-term flare treatment or when starting another systemic therapy or during break-severe exacerbation of AD.

Cyclosporine (Cys A)

It is a macrocyclic compound that blocks T-cell activation and cytokine production by blocking the nuclear factor of activated T cells (NFAT)-dependent cytokine production. Cyclosporine is the only approved and the first choice of systemic immunosuppressant treatment, for moderate to severe AD patients not responding to topical therapy and oral anti-histaminics [84]. A typical starting dose is 5 mg/kg/day, and therapeutic response is seen within several days to 1 week. After 2 weeks, tapering may begin at 100 mg every other week, depending on the achievement of clinical benefits [85].

Common side-effects are nephrotoxicity, hypertension, tremors, headaches, paresthesia, nausea, diarrhoea, myalgias, electrolyte imbalance, hyperlipidemia, hypertrichosis and gingival hyperplasia [86]. Rarely, cutaneous T cell lymphoma, non-Hodgkin's lymphoma and lymphomatoid papulosis in adult AD patients on cyclosporine therapy may occur [87]. Detailed patient monitoring, especially of the renal status and blood pressure, is required before and after cyclosporine administration.

Interactions: CYP450 enzymes inhibitors like phenytoin, phenobarbital, carbamazepine, erythromycin, doxycycline, rifampin, trimethoprim ± sulfamethoxazole, azole antifungals, furosemide, thiazides and steroid hormones increase cyclosporin levels. Other drugs that can act synergistically to increase cyclosporin-induced nephrotoxicity: Diuretics, aminoglycoside antibiotics, trimethoprim±sulfamethoxazole, amphotericin B, and nonsteroidal anti-inflammatory drugs.

Recently, a topical formulation of CysA nanocapsules, able to potentially bypass the drawback, was developed, which has shown a marked reduction in inflammatory cytokines and preservation of skin barrier integrity. Thus, it can provide a novel tool for the management of AD [88].

Azathioprine

It is a purine synthesis inhibitor that inhibits the formation of RNA and DNA, and reduces leukocyte proliferation and inflammation. It has been used to treat severe AD in UK and USA. Adverse events of azathioprine include gastrointestinal disturbances, liver dysfunction and leukopenia. Myelosuppression is due to partial or total deficiency in thiopurine methyltransferase (TPMT) activity. Several studies have supplied evidence for its improvement in skin symptoms, pruritis, insomnia and reduction in *S. aureus* colonization. Several studies comparing azathioprine with methotrexate have shown azathioprine to be superior in comparison to the placebo, as it significantly improves disease severity and causes reduction by at-least 50% in the SCORAD [89, 90]. Azathioprine is used as an off-label drug, when cyclosporine cannot be used or is ineffective.

Methotrexate (MTX)

It is an antimetabolite, which interferes with folic acid metabolism, resulting in reduced production of purine and pyrimidine nucleotides required for DNA and RNA synthesis that regulates the immune system and inflammatory processes. Studies have shown MTX to be a well-tolerated and effective drug in the treatment of moderate to severe AD. A median dose of 15mg/week has resulted in the reduction of disease activity by 52% from baseline after 24 weeks and persistent improvement in some patients over 12 weeks after discontinuation [91]. Frequent side effects such as nausea, headache, fatigue, gastrointestinal effects, hepatotoxicity, hematological abnormalities, pulmonary toxicity and drug interactions often result in discontinuation of treatment. Liver and bone marrow toxicity need to be considered before starting MTX therapy. A study comparing MTX with CysA had reported MTX 15mg/week inferior to CysA 2.5 mg/kg/day at the 8th-week analysis when SCORAD50 was not achieved at the former concentrations, however, dose increment to 25mg/week has shown significant improvement comparable to that of Cys A, in treatment of moderate to severe AD at 20th week [92]. Since MTX is about equally effective to azathioprine, its use (off-label) may be recommended when cyclosporine is either not effective or contraindicated.

Mycophenolate Mofetil (MMF)

It is the prodrug of Mycophenolic acid (MPA). MMF is an antimetabolite that inhibits purine synthesis, which results in B and T cell proliferation. It is used as an off-label drug and several patients with severe AD not responsive to CysA have shown improvement with MMF. Monotherapy with MMF has led to a significant reduction in disease severity after 4-week therapy with the dose of 1g twice daily followed by 4-week therapy of 0.5g twice daily [93] MMF has a slower onset of action and can be used effectively in maintenance therapy (2g/day) or long-term therapy (1-2 g daily over 12-29 months) for patients with chronic eczema [94]. The main side effects reported during MFA therapy were nausea, fatigue, flu-like syndrome, liver enzyme alteration, and infections such as herpes zoster, herpes simplex, and staphylococcal infection [95]. A study has demonstrated that patients unresponsive to MMF have shown a direct correlation between UGT1A9 polymorphisms which is its main metabolizing enzyme [96].

Immunomodulatory Therapy

Alitretinoin

9-cis retinoic acid is an antagonist vitamin A derivate that binds to both retinoic acid receptors RAR and RXR, resulting in antiinflammatory and antiproliferative effects. Alitretinoin is licensed in some European countries for the treatment of severe hand eczema, so it is effectively used in atopic hand eczema [97]. Studies have reported improvement of palmar and extrapalmar lesions in six patients with AD with prominent hand involvement [98], lichen simplex chronicus and severe AD of the hands [99] with the administration of a standard dose of 30 mg daily of alitretinoin for 12 weeks. Treatment with alitretinoin should be considered in AD patients with prominent involvement of the hands, which are resistant to topical corticosteroids and calcineurin inhibitors. Headache, serum lipid and thyroid-stimulating hormone elevation were the most frequent adverse events occurring during alitretinoin therapy [100]. Moreover, since alitretinoin is teratogenic, all women of childbearing age must adhere to a strict birth control program. Overall, studies supporting alitretinoin efficacy in adult AD patients are limited.

Biologics

Biologic drugs are a class of pharmacological agents engineered to target specific mediators of inflammation (IL-4 and IL-13) involved in the pathogenesis of AD, driven by innate type 2 lymphoid cells and Th2 cells. Although none of these biologic drugs have been approved for the treatment of adult AD so far, dupilumab has received breakthrough therapy designation and has been accepted by the USFDA for the treatment of adult and pediatric patients with inadequately controlled moderate-to-severe AD, and different clinical trials are now being conducted to determine the efficacy, dosing and long-term safety of these promising therapies.

Dupilumab

It is a fully human monoclonal antibody against IL-4Rα, which is a component of both IL-4 and IL-13. It is the first biologic approved by USFDA, for the treatment of moderate-to-severe AD for both pediatric and adult populations. It is cost-effective and shows a favourable safety profile with no dose-limiting toxicity and few adverse effects, including nasopharyngitis, upper respiratory tract infections, headache, injection-site reaction and back pain. The incidence of conjunctivitis was higher in patients with AD, when treated with dupilumab. However, Conjunctivitis was not seen in patients with asthma receiving Dupilumab. Clinical improvements in pruritis, skin lesions, itching, sleep, mental health and overall health status have been reported [101].

Ustekinumab

It is a fully human immunoglobulin G1 (IgG1) monoclonal antibody which binds to the p40 subunit of IL-12 and IL-23, and suppresses Th1, Th17, and Th22 activation.It is FDA approved for use in psoriasis. Therefore, it may be useful in AD, which is increasingly recognized as a Th2- and Th22-centered disease with some contributions of the Th17 and Th1 axes. Significant reductions with Ustekinumab in EASI, SCORAD scores [102, 103], skin lesions and related symptoms [104] in various studies have been reported. Reports of increased exacerbations, and inadequate response of the patients to the drug have led to controversies on the use of the drug in AD. Increased risk of infection, headache, fatigue, injection site reactions, and myalgia are seen with Ustekinumab. Clinical trial data regarding the use of Ustekinumab in AD is insufficient and based on small case series.

Apremilast

Apremilast is an oral small-molecule PDE-4 inhibitor that modulates and inhibits multiple inflammatory pathways and has been approved by the USFDA in 2014 for the treatment of active Psoriatic arthritis in adults and of moderate-to-severe plaque psoriasis in patients who are candidates for phototherapy or systemic therapy. It is also used for the treatment of asthma, COPD. In an open-label pilot study in moderate-to-severe AD patients, apremilast has reported a significant reduction in the EASI scores. Most common side effect is nausea followed by diarrhoea and headache; an episode of herpes zoster during the treatment period was reported [105]. A recent study has demonstrated a significant improvement in

EASI score from the baseline, a reduction in mRNA expression of Th 17 and Th 22 markers with minimal changes in other immune axes. Besides common adverse effects, cellulitis was more frequent with patients receiving 40 mg dose [106]. Even though apremilast has been shown to be an interesting and promising drug, especially due to its safety profile, further studies are needed to clearly assess its efficacy in the treatment of moderate-to-severe recalcitrant adult AD.

Immunoglobulins

Intravenous immunoglobulins (IVIg) have been used for the treatment of severe autoimmune and inflammatory skin diseases, including severe AD, because of their immunomodulatory effects. The mechanism of action in AD is unknown but may relate to the blockade of Fc-receptors on splenic macrophages, alteration of cytokine production, or effects on Fas (CD95)-mediated apoptosis. IVIg therapy can also entail safety concerns as it is produced from pooled, purified human blood or plasma donations, and can induce adverse effects like immediate-type hypersensitivity reactions, hyperviscosity, aseptic meningitis, and potential transmission of infectious agents [107]. Adjunctive therapy with six cycles of high-dose IVIg 2 g/kg/month significantly improved skin symptoms in four of six patients with AD. Moreover, IVIg therapy allowed the reduction in concomitant systemic drugs in patients on long-term corticosteroid therapy. The benefit of IVIg therapy for patients with severe AD has controversially been discussed, as some reports revealed no or just slight improvement [95]. Administration of three cycles of IVIg 2 g/kg/month in children with severe AD has resulted in a significant reduction in disease activity and inflammatory markers like serum eosinophil cationic protein levels. IVIg can be considered in children with AD refractory to systemic immunosuppressive therapy.

Interferons

Recombinantinterferon-γ (rIFN-γ) leads to the normalization of the cytokine imbalance in AD by decreasing IL-4 and IL-6, while clinical improvement despite unchanged IgE levels highlights the unclear role of humoral immunity in AD pathogenesis. It is administered *via* a subcutaneous route daily or alternatively at doses of 50 μg/M^2 [108]. Long-term studies have demonstrated safety and efficacy for upto two years [109]. Generally, well tolerated. Flu-like symptoms are commonly reported.

Although mentioned in certain guidelines and reviews, rIFN-γ therapy became less important, most likely because of significant expense, inconvenience of subcutaneous administration, and 20% non-responder rate and availability of alternative drugs with better benefit–risk profiles. Due to this reason, rIFN-γ is not an appropriate first-line agent for AD but is an available effective therapy for moderate to severely affected patients who are refractory or intolerant to other systemic therapies [95].

Oral Antimicrobials

Systemic antibiotic therapy is a mainstay in the management of patients with AD who are likely to develop complications such as skin bacterial infections caused by *Staphylococcus* or hemolytic *Streptococcus* with oozing and yellow-crusted lesions of eczematous skin and Kaposi's varicelliform eruption caused by *H. simplex* virus, which is more typical for AD in childhood [95]. *Staphylococcal* isolates are invariably resistant to penicillin and usually to erythromycin, leaving oral cephalosporin and dicloxacillin as agents of choice, in doses of 250 mg four times daily for adults, or 125 mg twice a day (25±50 mg/kg/ day divided into two doses) for children. Systemic antiviral therapy, such as acyclovir and antifungal therapy, such as ketoconazole, can be used effectively used in AD patients who develop eczema herpeticum or infections related to Malassezia species, respectively [13, 110]. However, in most cases of yeast-triggered AD, mainly in the head-and-neck area, a topical antimycotic therapy seems sufficient, as it has been demonstrated for ciclopirox olamine cream [111].

Complementary and Alternative Therapies

Prebiotics and Probiotics

Prebiotics are non-digestible ingredients and Probiotics are live microorganisms that, when administered in sufficient amounts, that benefit the host by selectively stimulating growth or limiting some species of intestinal bacteria, such as *Bifidobacterium* and *Lactobacilli* that have the potential to improve the health of the host. Normally used probiotics are normal microbiota flora of *Lactobacillus* family: *acidophilus, sporogenes, lactis, reuteri* RC-14, GG, *L. plantarum* 299v or *Bifidobacterium* family: *bifidum, longum, infantis* or *Streptococcus* group: *thermophillus, lactis, fecalis*, and some non-bacterial organisms such as, non-pathogenic yeast *Saccharomyces boulardii*. Decreased incidence of AD in children under 5 years is reported with probiotic consumption during late pregnancy or lactation period (Pelucchi *et al.*, 2012). A limited number of studies suggest the efficacy of probiotic strains and prebiotic on the basis of reduction of SCORAD scores in preventing the onset of AD. Most meta-analyses suggest the administration of probiotics for atleast 8 weeks to improve SCORAD [112].

Vitamin D

Vitamin D was shown to affect both the innate and the adaptive immune system, and thus, low vitamin D levels might contribute to the main features of AD, such as defective skin barrier and chronic skin inflammation. Vitamin D stimulates AMP expression by endothelial cells; inhibits dendritic cell activation, antigen presentation, and cytokine production; and supports macrophages in defending against opportunistic infections. As most cells of the adaptive immune system express the vitamin D receptor, vitamin D exhibits broad effects, for example, it may inhibit T-cell proliferation, suppress Th17 cell, but increase regulatory T-cell functions, and blocks B-cell proliferation and immunoglobulin production.AD patients with very low 25 (OH) D3 levels (4 and 15 ng/ml) profited from vitamin D supplementation for 3 months, as assessed by a significant decrease in objective and subjective SCORAD [113]. The results on vitamin D status and therapeutic effects of supplementation are controversial, but a recent meta-analysis-based study suggested that vitamin D supplementation may help ameliorate the severity of AD, and can be considered a safe and tolerable therapy [114, 115].

Allergen-Specific Immune Therapy (ASIT)

It has widely been applied for other atopic diseases such as allergic rhinitis and asthma. In AD, ASIT has mainly been studied in patients sensitized to house dust mites and birch pollen. Sublingual immunotherapy has revealed significant improvement in AD severity in patients sensitized to house dust mites as assessed by SCORAD. Some patients with AD allergic to pollen experience acute exacerbations during pollen seasons. ASIT with birch pollen extract for 12 weeks was shown to significantly reduce skin symptoms and improve quality of life despite strong birch pollen exposure. Although a recent systematic review on ASIT for AD stated a significant positive effect, current data do not allow a broad recommendation so far [95].

Psychosomatic Counselling

Certain severe AD-affected patients suffer from psychosocial stresses such as social relations, workload, worries about the future and anxieties for independence, which may induce a habitual scratching behaviour, called "addictive scratching" or "scratch dependence"; this behaviour worsens their eruption. In such cases, mental and physical treatments become necessary, and psychiatric counselling may be required. Patients are mostly advised to make changes with respect to their daily routine and hygiene which include: regular bathing or showering to keep the skin clean, keeping their room clean and aerated and creating an environment with appropriate temperature and humidity, wearing clothes with little stimulation or no stimulation, regularly cutting fingernails to avoid skin damage by scratching.

NOVEL THERAPEUTIC TREATMENT

A detailed understanding of etiological factors has availed to develop novel therapeutic and preventative strategies that do not focus on a single pathological pathway of the disease, but on more complex molecular interactions that drive AD. New possible and effective trends of treating atopic dermatitis, mostly by focusing on patient's Immunotype, genotype, and phenotype have also been discovered, which would provide us with an increasingly broad range of therapeutic options.

Monoclonal Antibodies

Besides Dupilumab, which is the only currently FDA-approved biologic therapy for AD; Novel targeted biologics and small molecule agents are emerging as safer and more effective alternatives through ongoing clinical trials for patients with uncontrolled AD when conventional therapies topical therapies, phototherapy or immunosuppressant therapies fail or cannot be given, subjected to their wide-array of toxicities, malignancies, drug interactions, contraindications and requiring continuous monitoring. Targeted biologics are attractive treatment options for topical therapy refractory cases of AD and many MAbs have proven effective in patients, but the need for continuous study of additional biologic therapies is necessary to address the needs of diverse patients with severe uncontrolled AD [116]. Investigational MAbs are given in Table **2**.

Table 2. Investigational monoclonal antibodies.

Target (S-Systemic and T-Topical)	Agent	Trial Phase	Manufacturer	References
Anti-IL13 (S) prevents heterodimerization of the IL-4Rα/IL-13Rα1/IL3Rα2receptor subunits	Lebrikizumab Tralokinumab	Phase-3 Phase-3 recently completed	Hoffmann-La Roche, Basel, Switzerland MedImmune, Gaithersburg, MD	[117, 118]
Anti-IL31RA (S) blocks IL-31 mediated signaling Inhibits binding of IL-31 and Oncostatin-M (OSM) to OSMR-β	Nemolizumab KPL716	Phase-3 Phase-2 (adolescents) Phase 1a/1b	Chugai, Tokyo, Japan Kiniksa Pharmaceuticals Corp., Lexington, MA	[119, 120]
Anti-IL17C (S) blocks the interaction IL-17C with its high affinity receptor IL-17RE	MOR106	Phase-2	Galapagos NV;MorphoSys	[121]

(Table 2) cont.....

Target (S-Systemic and T-Topical)	Agent	Trial Phase	Manufacturer	References
Anti-IL22 (S) neutralizes / prevents cytokine binding with its receptor IL-22	Fezakinumab LEO 138559	Phase 2a Phase 1	Pfizer, New York, NY LEO Pharma, Denmark	[122]
Anti-OX40/ CD134 (S) inhibits T-cell expansion, survival, and functioning	GBR-830 KY1005 KHK4083	Phase 2b Phase 2b Phase 2	Glenmark, Mumbai, India Kymab Ltd., Cambridge, UK. Kyowa Kirin Co. Ltd., Japan	[123]
Anti-TSLP (S) inhibits production of type 2 cytokines (IL-4, IL-5, IL-13) and TNF-α	Tezepelumab	Phase 2b	Amgen, Thousand Oaks, CA	[124]

JAK Receptor Inhibitors

The Jakus Kinase JAK protein—JAK1, JAK2, JAK3, or tyrosine kinase 2 (TYK2) are intracellular, which, when activated by binding ofIL-4 and IL-13 to IL-4 receptor complex, phosphorylates and activates the transcription factors signal transducer STAT proteins—STAT1, STAT2, STAT3, STAT5A/B and STAT6 to dimerize and translocate to the cell nucleus to increase gene expression of Th2 which plays a key role in AD pathogenesis and other inflammatory mediators including periostin which stimulates keratinocytes to produce TSLP. Moreover, there is a downregulation of proteins essential for skin-barrier function, including filaggrin, loricrin, involucrin, and ceramides. TH2 cells also express IL-31, which acts on keratinocytes to potentiate the release of IL-24. This, in turn, leads to decreased FLG production, increased TEWL by interactions of a number of cytokines causing AD by stimulating the expression of IFN-γ, IL-31, IL-23, and IL-22, Increased IgE level that binds to the mast cell, angiogenic factors and chemokines for eosinophils; All these events in concert result promoting AD inflammatory process and skin barrier breakdown.

Several oral and topical JAK/SYK inhibitors have been shown to decrease AD severity and symptoms and are being actively investigated in the treatment of moderate to severe AD [125], which might have the potential to be comparable with dupilumab in terms of EASI score improvement. Some of the following agents (Table **3**) inhibit the whole family, *e.g.*, tofacitinib, ruxolitinib, and baricitinib, also called first-generation/ pan-jakinibs, while some are selective for particular JAK proteins *e.g.*, upadacitinib and abrocitinib also called as second generation jakinibs selectively inhibit JAK1. Cerdulatinib and Gusacitinib inhibit not only JAKs but also spleen tyrosine kinase (SYK) are also first generation jakinibs.

Table 3. Investigational JAK STAT inhibitors.

Target (S-Systemic and T-Topical)	Agent	Trial Phase	Manufacturer	Side-Effects	References
Non- selective JAK1/3, TYK2, JAK2 inhibitor (S/T)	Tofacitinib	Phase 2	Innovaderm, Montreal, Quebec, Canada	No potential side-effect detected in this phase.	[126]
Selective JAK1 and JAK2 (T)	Ruxolitinib	Phase 2b	Incyte Coorporation, US	Pain at the site of application.	[127]
Selective JAK1/2 inhibitor (S)	Baricitinib	Phase 2	Eli Lilly, Indianapolis, IN	Nasopharyngitis, headache.	[128]
Non-selective JAK1, JAK2, JAK3 (T)	Delgocitinib	Phase 3	Japan Tobacco Inc, Tokyo, Japan	Mild drop in WBC count, headache.	[129, 130]
Selective JAK1 inhibitor (S)	Upadacitinib	Phase 3	AbbVie, Inc,Lake Bluff, Illinois, United States	Upper respiratory tract infections.	[131]
Selective JAK1 inhibitor (S)	Abrocitinib	Phase 3	Pfizer, New York, NY	Upper respiratory tract infections, headache, nausea, diarrhoea.	[132]
Selective JAK1, JAK2, JAK3, SYK (T)	Cerdulatinib	Phase 2	Portola Pharmaceuticals	Diarrhoea, neutropenia.	[133]
Selective JAK1, JAK2, JAK3, TYK2, SYK (S)	Gusacitinib	Phase 1b	Asana BioSciences, Bridgewater, NJ	Headache, nausea, diarrhea, ehino-pharyngitis, backpain, mild hypertension, decrease in lymphocyte.	[134]

JAK inhibitors are effective and offer a desired oral form of delivery but there is always associated risk of side-effects. This may be attributed to the involvement of the JAK proteins in complex signaling cascades that regulate both acute inflammatory reaction and hematopoiesis, inhibition of which by JAK inhibitors may lead to serious adverse effects. Using selective JAK1 inhibitors (upadacitinib) in AD—may help minimize undesired side effects. However, the higher dosages required for the treatment of an autoimmune disease may overcome the selectivity of these agents at lower dosages. Non-selective agents with a wide scope of action may carry a greater risk of serious adverse events compared with agents with a narrow scope of action, such as single interleukin inhibitors.

H4R Antagonists

Histamine-4 mediates proinflammatory functions in a number of cell types involved in allergic inflammation, including T cells, mast cells, eosinophils and DCs. Selective H4 receptor antagonists have shown anti-inflammatory and antipruritic efficacy in various preclinical animal models, supporting the concept that they might represent a novel treatment for inflammatory skin diseases, including AD. Recently, a study conducted to evaluate ZPL-3893787 activity in moderate-to-severe AD patients has shown reduced EASI score and SCORAD. It is generally well tolerated, without any reductions in circulating granulocytes. These results have shown that a selective H4R antagonist was able to improve inflammatory skin lesions inpatients with AD, suggesting that the H4 receptor antagonist could be one choice of oral anti-histamine blockers in AD [135].

Topical PDE4 Inhibitors

OPA15406, like crisaborole is a PDE4 inhibitor with high selectivity for PDE4B. A phase II study performed on adult and adolescent patients with mild-to-moderate AD has shown topical OPA15406 to improve EASI score from baseline, which persisted for eight weeks. Its levels in blood were reported to be negligible and the incidence of adverse events was lower, with most events mild in intensity [136]. A recent study on pediatric patients with AD revealed the same results suggesting topical OPA application twice daily for 4 weeks as a safer and more effective option. Some benign transient hyperphosphatemia was occasionally observed in children under the age of 5 years [137]. E6005 is another novel topically active PDE4 inhibitor with low transdermal bioavailability to minimize systemic exposure caused by PDE inhibitors [138]. Taken together, topical PDE4 inhibitors demonstrate a favorable safety profile and remarkable improvement in efficacy, including overall disease severity and skin score. Both PDE4 inhibitors are currently in Phase 3 trials.

AhR Modulating Agents

Tapinarof cream is a novel topical nonsteroidal agent natural derived stilbene that targets and activates the aryl hydrocarbon receptor, leading to the downregulation of pro-inflammatory cytokines, including interleukin-17, and regulation of skin barrier functions and accelerating epidermal terminal differentiation by upregulating filaggrin expression. Phase 2b study on adolescent and adult patients with AD treated with tapinarof cream reported significant Investigation Global Assessment (IGA) responses on week 12 and 75%-90% improvement in EASI from baseline. Reported adverse events were mild or moderate [139].

Topical TRPV1R Antagonists

Transient receptor potential vanilloid 1 is a non-selective cation channel with high permeability to calcium and belongs to a superfamily of ion channels known as the transient receptor potential channels (TRPs). TRP1 receptors have a key role in AD and pruritis, which on binding specific agonists causes a release of the proinflammatory cytokines and pruritic mediators. PAC-14028 cream is a topically administrated TRPV1 antagonist, which improves skin barrier function and reduces allergic inflammation by suppressing signalling pathways, including IL-4, IL-13 mediated JAK-STAT, TRPV1 and neuropeptides. The recent vehicle-controlled study, in patients with mild-to-moderate AD receiving PAC-14028 cream, has demonstrated improved IGA, EASI and SCORAD scores as compared to the vehicle [140].

Oral S1P Modulators

S1P1 (selective sphingosine 1-phosphate) is a cell surface G protein-coupled receptor (GPCR) that regulates lymphocyte exit from lymph nodes and dendritic cell trafficking. Etrasimod is an oral S1P1 receptor 1, 4, 5 (S1P1, 4, 5) modulator which, upon binding to S1P1, inhibits receptor internalization, thereby preventing cell migration along S1P gradients, resulting in lymphocyte retention within lymphoid tissue, and a reduction in peripheral blood lymphocytes available to be recruited to sites of inflammation. It has effectively reduced ear skin inflammation and dermatitis in the FITC-induced hypersensitivity dermatitis mouse model. It has shown a reduction in the trafficking of dendritic cells and T cells out of lymph nodes into circulation, which produced a downstream reduction in immune cells, cytokine production, and dermatitis in the skin. These data encourage further study of etrasimod as a novel therapy for atopic dermatitis [141]. A similar mechanism is expected in humans.

HERBAL TREATMENT

As conventional medicines for moderate and severe AD patients have been reported to be associated with unwanted side effects, many patients with AD have sought herbal therapies.

Traditional Herbs

Althea Officinalis (Common Name: Marshmallow; Family: Malvaceae)

Marshmallow is a very valuable herb, as their soothing emollient properties make them very effective in treating irritations and inflammations of the mucous membranes and epidermis in the treatment of atopic eczema. The root, due to its demulcent properties, can also be used in an ointment for treating boils and abscesses [142]. In children with AD, *Althaea officinalis* 1% ointment decreases disease severity more in comparison to 1% hydrocortisone [143].

Arnica Montana (Common Name: Wolf's Bane; Family: Asteraceae)

It essentially contains numerous compounds which are beneficial in treating skin conditions such as, eczema, itching, irritation and other associated infections and forms an important ingredient of many seborrheic dermatitis and psoriasis preparations. It has been accepted by Commission E for topical treatment of skin inflammation [144]. Sesquiterpene lactones such as helanalin, 11α,13-dihydrohelenalin and chamissonolid are the main active constituents of this plant and suppress inflammation by impeding the transcription factor nuclear factor κB (NF-κB), which controls the transcription of many genes, including cytokines (IL, TNF-α), intercellular adhesion molecule 1, vascular cellular adhesion molecule1, and endothelial leukocyte adhesion molecule 1 and also inhibits many genes accountable for antigen presentation and activation of cyclooxygenase-2 (COX-2) [145].

Avena Sativa (Common Name: Oat; Family: Poaceae)

It has been used as a relaxing herb for a long time in order to alleviate itching and irritation associated with various xerotic dermatoses. Oats have compounds called avenanthramides, which are powerful anti-inflammatory agents and also display anti-oxidant activity [146]. Different clinical studies have been undertaken to investigate the effect of oats on eczema, all of which have shown a significant decrease in skin redness, dryness, scaliness, itching and erythema after the application of oat extracts in adults and children. *In vitro* , a colloidal oat extract has demonstrated anti-inflammatory activity–inhibited expression of phospholipase A2 (PLA2) and COX-2, the release of the arachidonic acid from phospholipids, and subsequent metabolism into prostaglandin and leukotrienes [147].

Glycyrrhiza Glabra (Common Name: Liquorice; Family: Fabaceae)

Liquorice is a traditional medicinal plant used in various ancient medicine systems to cure varieties of ailments. The most important active constituents of liquorice include oleanane-type triterpenes such as glycyrrhizin (glycyrrhizic or glycyrrhizinic acid), and its aglycone glycyrrhetinic acid. There are also various phenolics and flavonoids of the chalcone and isoflavone type, and many natural coumarins such as liqcoumarin, umbelliferone, glabrocoumarones A and B, herniarin, and glycyrin. It also contains polysaccharides such as glycyrrhizan GA, and a slight amount of volatile oil. The dried root and stolons of Liquorice possess anti-inflammatory properties, and are, thus, used topically in the treatment of atopic eczema and other inflammatory skin conditions. The anti-inflammatory properties of Liquorice are mostly due to glycyrrhetinic acid, which exerts mineralocorticoid and oestrogenic activity [148].

Linum Usitatissimum (Common Name: Linseed; Family: Linaceae)

Linumusitatissimum is cultivated as a food and fibre crop in regions with temperate climates. It contains fixed oil which is rich in essential fatty acids (EFA) such as triglycerides of α-linolenic and linoleic acids and mucilage polysaccharides. These EFA possess anti-inflammatory, emollient and demulcent properties, which aid a patient to recover from AD or atleast provide relief from itchiness and other related symptoms [149, 150].

Matricaria Recutita (Common Name: German Chamomile, Family: Asteraceae)

Matricariarecutita has long been used to treat gastrointestinal tract symptoms, dermatitis, and skin inflammation. It is either taken internally in the form of tea by mixing 2–3 teaspoons of dried flowers per cup of water or is used as a compress. However, topical preparations with cream or ointment bases have also been researched and are being used [151]. It has been observed that the efficacy of topical chamomile is comparable to 0.25% hydrocortisone and showed enhancement in sodium lauryl sulfate–induced contact dermatitis [152]. It has also been observed that ointment containing matricaria flower extract was more efficacious than 0.1% hydrocortisone in reducing chemically-induced toxic dermatitis [153]. The anti-inflammatory, antimicrobial, antispasmodic and wound-healing properties of Chamomile are mainly attributed to an essential blue oil that chiefly contains sesquiterpene alcohol, α-bisabolol, chamazulene, and flavonoids. These substances act by inhibiting COX and lipoxygenase *in vitro*. The flavonoids also act by inhibiting histamine release from antigen-stimulated human basophilic polymorphonuclear leukocytes [152].

Oenotherae Oleum (Common Name: Evening Primrose Oil; Family: Onagraceae)

It has been used by indigenous tribes in North America for hundreds of years as a food and medicinal plant. Active ingredients of this plant include triglycerides of fatty acids, mainly γ-linolenic and linoleic [154]. Oil of this plant is administered internally for the treatment of atopic dermatitis. It has revealed promising results in alleviating the symptoms of AD, such as inflammation, dryness, exfoliation and itching, which has been primarily attributed to an increase in the levels of dihomo-gamma-linolenic acid (DGLA). DGLA and its metabolite 15-HETrE are among the epidermis lipids, which are vital for keeping the correct structure and ultimately regulating epidermal barrier function [155, 156]. Administration of 2-4g oil daily for 12 weeks in a study has shown a 30-45% enhancement in the severity of eczema, including a substantial decrease of itching and scaling, in comparison to patients who received the placebo [154].

Stellaria Media (Common Name: Chickweed; Family: Caryophyllaceae)

The application of chickweed in the form of ointment or cream is mainly used to treat skin irritation. It is mainly used in pruritus, and is frequently added to topical eczema preparations for treating eczema and other inflammatory skin conditions. It works particularly well in combination with *Matricaria recutita,* due to its strong anti-inflammatory properties and has revealed very successful results in the treatment of mild to chronic eczema [157, 158].

Viola Tricolor (Common Name: Wild Pansy; Family: Violaceae)

It has been used for a very long as herbal and folk medicine, for epilepsy, skin diseases and eczema. Infusion of the wild pansy is recommended, especially in infants as a nontoxic treatment for seborrheic dermatitis. The infusion is made by mixing 1–2 tsp of flowers per cup of water and is used as a wet dressing. Salicylic acid, in concentrations of about 0.3%, appears to be the active ingredient. It also contains saponins and mucilage, which exerts softening and soothing effects [159, 160].

Chinese Medicine (CM)

CM is a traditional and widely used treatment for AD, psoriasis and acne in the western world. There are a number of studies that demonstrate the improvement of AD with traditional therapy. Conversely, studies on Chinese adults and children with AD treated with the same standardized CM formulation used in the earlier positive studies have found no benefit. A randomised study on moderate to severe AD patients has been conducted to estimate the potency of the Chinese herbal formula-Pei Tu Qing Xin Tang (PTQXT), composed of nine Chinese Herbal Medicines (CHMs), which has reported decrease in the SCORAD in all patients. PTQXT was found effective in reducing disease severity and improving quality of life [161]. Another Chinese medicine formulated into an ointment, TYO (Tzu-Yun) ointment composed of *sesame oil* (Ma you), *Angelica sinensis* (Oliv.) *Diels* (Dong qi), *Lithospermum erythrorhizon* (Tzu tsao), and yellow wax (Huang la) is clinically used for skin ulcers and pus discharge. TYO has successfully lowered EASI and TIS scores in patients with AD [162]. Assessment of CM therapy is difficult due to its heterogeneity. Standard regimens include a variety of herbs. Thus, rigorous scientific analysis of these medications becomes complicated. Long-term controlled studies are required to better define the safety and effectiveness of TCM in AD.

Essential Oils

Essential oils have widely been used in traditional medicines for their anti-inflammatory, moisture-retaining, soothing and reducing itching and other signs of eczema. Limited small-population studies have demonstrated the activity of essential oils, and more research is needed to determine their efficacy in eczema. One study has revealed essential oils of *Syzygium aromaticum, Cedrus deodara, Eucalyptus radiata, Cannabis sativa, Mentha citrate, Melaleuca alternifolia, Copaifera officinalis*, formulated into the gel base applied over a period of nine months have demonstrated instant relief in the itching, reduction in inflammation characterised by the reduced pain, edema, heat and may be used as an effective alternative to topical steroid therapy in individuals with acute dry or acute weeping dermatitis [163]. Steam Distillation extracted essential oil of *Chamaecyparis obtuse* applied over 4 weeks in clinical trials has shown improvement in AD. The antioxidant activities increased upto80μL/mL [164].

Salt Baths, Homeopathy and Acupuncture may help in reducing itching sensations and providing relief, but trialbase evidencesfor use in AD are lacking.

CONCLUSION

Atopic dermatitis is one of the most frequently occurring chronic diseases caused by complex interactions between a variety of genetic and environmental factors. Although many areas of uncertainty persist, discoveries from genetics, molecular biology, epidemiology, and clinical medicine have spurred new disease concepts, including the notion of endotypes and a broader understanding of health and psychosocial outcomes in AD. Novel treatments based on these pathological mechanisms or on subgroup classifications are under development that could considerably improve patients' quality of life. How much these innovative drug developments will allow us to alleviate symptoms by blocking distinct pathogenic aspects of AD is not yet fully known. However, the great success of biologics and novel small molecules in controlling a diverse spectrum of chronic inflammatory diseases is on hand. As the pathogenesis of AD is heterogeneous, a pathomechanism-specific and customized approach should be developed. Continued research to dissect the individual mechanisms will likely lead to the development of therapies that more directly influence the disease.

REFERENCES

[1] Gary W, Faad CMD. Eczema treatment, causes, types, definition, symptoms, 2020. Available from: https://www.medicinenet.com/eczema_facts/article.htm (accessed March 27, 2022)

[2]   Ring J. Atopic dermatitis: eczema - Johannes ring - Google Books. Springer Cham Heidelberg New York Dordrecht London: Springer International Publishing Switzerland, 2016.

[3]   Langan SM, Irvine AD, Weidinger S. Atopic dermatitis. Lancet 2020; 396(10247): 345-60.
[http://dx.doi.org/10.1016/S0140-6736(20)31286-1] [PMID: 32738956]

[4]   Berke R, Singh A, Guralnick M. Atopic dermatitis: an overview. Am Fam Physician 2012; 86(1): 35-42.
[PMID: 22962911]

[5]   Silverberg JI, Garg NK, Paller AS, Fishbein AB, Zee PC. Sleep disturbances in adults with eczema are associated with impaired overall health: a US population-based study. J Invest Dermatol 2015; 135(1): 56-66.
[http://dx.doi.org/10.1038/jid.2014.325] [PMID: 25078665]

[6]   Lipozenčić J, Wolf R. The diagnostic value of atopy patch testing and prick testing in atopic dermatitis: facts and controversies. Clin Dermatol 2010; 28(1): 38-44.
[http://dx.doi.org/10.1016/j.clindermatol.2009.03.008] [PMID: 20082949]

[7]   de Boissieu D, Dupont C. Patch tests in the diagnosis of food allergies in the nursing infant. Eur Ann Allergy Clin Immunol 2003; 35(5): 150-2.
[PMID: 12838776]

[8]   Saeki H, Furue M, Furukawa F, *et al.* Guidelines for management of atopic dermatitis. J Dermatol 2009; 36(10): 563-77.
[http://dx.doi.org/10.1111/j.1346-8138.2009.00706.x] [PMID: 19785716]

[9]   Alam MN, Munia TTK, Tavakolian K, *et al.* Automatic detection and severity measurement of eczema using image processing. 38th Annual International Conference of the IEEE Engineering in Medicine and Biology Society (EMBC), IEEE. 2016; pp. 1365-8.
[http://dx.doi.org/10.1109/EMBC.2016.7590961]

[10]   Novak N, Bieber T. Allergic and nonallergic forms of atopic diseases. J Allergy Clin Immunol 2003; 112(2): 252-62.
[http://dx.doi.org/10.1067/mai.2003.1595] [PMID: 12897728]

[11]   Kusel MMH, Holt PG, de Klerk N, Sly PD. Support for 2 variants of eczema. J Allergy Clin Immunol 2005; 116(5): 1067-72.
[http://dx.doi.org/10.1016/j.jaci.2005.06.038] [PMID: 16275378]

[12]   Imayama S, Hashizume T, Miyahara H, *et al.* Combination of patch test and IgE for dust mite antigens differentiates 130 patients with atopic dermatitis into four groups. J Am Acad Dermatol 1992; 27(4): 531-8.
[http://dx.doi.org/10.1016/0190-9622(92)70218-5] [PMID: 1401304]

[13]   Ring J, Alomar A, Bieber T, *et al.* Guidelines for treatment of atopic eczema (atopic dermatitis) Part II. J Eur Acad Dermatol Venereol 2012; 26(9): 1176-93.
[http://dx.doi.org/10.1111/j.1468-3083.2012.04636.x] [PMID: 22813359]

[14]   Netherton syndrome - NORD (National Organization for Rare Disorders) n.d https://rarediseases.org/gard-rare-disease/netherton-syndrome/ (accessed March 28, 2022).

[15]   Apfelbacher CJ, Diepgen TL, Schmitt J. Determinants of eczema: population-based cross-sectional study in Germany. Allergy 2011; 66(2): 206-13.
[http://dx.doi.org/10.1111/j.1398-9995.2010.02464.x] [PMID: 20804468]

[16]   Thomsen SF, Ulrik CS, Kyvik KO, *et al.* Importance of genetic factors in the etiology of atopic dermatitis: a twin study. Allergy Asthma Proc 2007; 28(5): 535-9.
[http://dx.doi.org/10.2500/aap2007.28.3041] [PMID: 18034971]

[17]   Barnes KC. An update on the genetics of atopic dermatitis: Scratching the surface in 2009. J Allergy Clin Immunol 2010; 125(1): 16-29.e11.

[http://dx.doi.org/10.1016/j.jaci.2009.11.008] [PMID: 20109730]

[18] Sandilands A, Sutherland C, Irvine AD, McLean WHI. Filaggrin in the frontline: role in skin barrier function and disease. J Cell Sci 2009; 122(9): 1285-94.
[http://dx.doi.org/10.1242/jcs.033969] [PMID: 19386895]

[19] de Cid R, Riveira-Munoz E, Zeeuwen PLJM, *et al.* Deletion of the late cornified envelope LCE3B and LCE3C genes as a susceptibility factor for psoriasis. Nat Genet 2009; 41(2): 211-5.
[http://dx.doi.org/10.1038/ng.313] [PMID: 19169253]

[20] Maestrini E, Monaco AP, McGrath JA, *et al.* A molecular defect in loricrin, the major component of the cornified cell envelope, underlies Vohwinkel's syndrome. Nat Genet 1996; 13(1): 70-7.
[http://dx.doi.org/10.1038/ng0596-70] [PMID: 8673107]

[21] Irvine AD, McLean WHI, Leung DYM. Filaggrin mutations associated with skin and allergic diseases. N Engl J Med 2011; 365(14): 1315-27.
[http://dx.doi.org/10.1056/NEJMra1011040] [PMID: 21991953]

[22] Wells RS, Kerr CB. Clinical features of autosomal dominant and sex-linked ichthyosis in an English population. BMJ 1966; 1(5493): 947-50.
[http://dx.doi.org/10.1136/bmj.1.5493.947] [PMID: 20790920]

[23] Brown SJ, Irvine AD. Atopic eczema and the filaggrin story. Semin Cutan Med Surg 2008; 27(2): 128-37.
[http://dx.doi.org/10.1016/j.sder.2008.04.001] [PMID: 18620134]

[24] Henderson J, Northstone K, Lee SP, *et al.* The burden of disease associated with filaggrin mutations: A population-based, longitudinal birth cohort study. J Allergy Clin Immunol 2008; 121(4): 872-877.e9.
[http://dx.doi.org/10.1016/j.jaci.2008.01.026] [PMID: 18325573]

[25] de Jongh CM, John SM, Bruynzeel DP, *et al.* Cytokine gene polymorphisms and susceptibility to chronic irritant contact dermatitis. Contact Dermat 2008; 58(5): 269-77.
[http://dx.doi.org/10.1111/j.1600-0536.2008.01317.x] [PMID: 18416756]

[26] Brown SJ, Asai Y, Cordell HJ, *et al.* Loss-of-function variants in the filaggrin gene are a significant risk factor for peanut allergy. J Allergy Clin Immunol 2011; 127(3): 661-7.
[http://dx.doi.org/10.1016/j.jaci.2011.01.031] [PMID: 21377035]

[27] Harding CR. The stratum corneum: structure and function in health and disease. Dermatol Ther 2004; 17 (Suppl. 1): 6-15.
[http://dx.doi.org/10.1111/j.1396-0296.2004.04S1001.x] [PMID: 14728694]

[28] Candi E, Schmidt R, Melino G. The cornified envelope: a model of cell death in the skin. Nat Rev Mol Cell Biol 2005; 6(4): 328-40.
[http://dx.doi.org/10.1038/nrm1619] [PMID: 15803139]

[29] Tang KT, Ku KC, Chen DY, Lin CH, Tsuang BJ, Chen YH. Adult atopic dermatitis and exposure to air pollutants—a nationwide population-based study. Ann Allergy Asthma Immunol 2017; 118(3): 351-5.
[http://dx.doi.org/10.1016/j.anai.2016.12.005] [PMID: 28126434]

[30] Howell MD, Kim BE, Gao P, *et al.* Cytokine modulation of atopic dermatitis filaggrin skin expression. J Allergy Clin Immunol 2009; 124(3) (Suppl. 2): R7-R12.
[http://dx.doi.org/10.1016/j.jaci.2009.07.012] [PMID: 19720210]

[31] Miajlovic H, Fallon PG, Irvine AD, Foster TJ. Effect of filaggrin breakdown products on growth of and protein expression by Staphylococcus aureus. J Allergy Clin Immunol 2010; 126(6): 1184-1190.e3.
[http://dx.doi.org/10.1016/j.jaci.2010.09.015] [PMID: 21036388]

[32] Kim BE, Leung DYM, Boguniewicz M, Howell MD. Loricrin and involucrin expression is down-regulated by Th2 cytokines through STAT-6. Clin Immunol 2008; 126(3): 332-7.

[http://dx.doi.org/10.1016/j.clim.2007.11.006] [PMID: 18166499]

[33]   Gruber R, Elias PM, Crumrine D, *et al.* Filaggrin genotype in ichthyosis vulgaris predicts abnormalities in epidermal structure and function. Am J Pathol 2011; 178(5): 2252-63.
[http://dx.doi.org/10.1016/j.ajpath.2011.01.053] [PMID: 21514438]

[34]   Boguniewicz M, Leung DYM. Recent insights into atopic dermatitis and implications for management of infectious complications. J Allergy Clin Immunol 2010; 125(1): 4-13.
[http://dx.doi.org/10.1016/j.jaci.2009.11.027] [PMID: 20109729]

[35]   Rippke F, Schreiner V, Schwanitz HJ. The acidic milieu of the horny layer: new findings on the physiology and pathophysiology of skin pH. Am J Clin Dermatol 2002; 3(4): 261-72.
[http://dx.doi.org/10.2165/00128071-200203040-00004] [PMID: 12010071]

[36]   Howell M, Wollenberg A, Gallo R, *et al.* Cathelicidin deficiency predisposes to eczema herpeticum. J Allergy Clin Immunol 2006; 117(4): 836-41.
[http://dx.doi.org/10.1016/j.jaci.2005.12.1345] [PMID: 16630942]

[37]   Gruber R, Börnchen C, Rose K, *et al.* Diverse regulation of claudin-1 and claudin-4 in atopic dermatitis. Am J Pathol 2015; 185(10): 2777-89.
[http://dx.doi.org/10.1016/j.ajpath.2015.06.021] [PMID: 26319240]

[38]   Byrd AL, Deming C, Cassidy SKB, *et al. Staphylococcus aureus* and *Staphylococcus epidermidis* strain diversity underlying pediatric atopic dermatitis. Sci Transl Med 2017; 9(397): eaal4651.
[http://dx.doi.org/10.1126/scitranslmed.aal4651] [PMID: 28679656]

[39]   Nowicka D, Grywalska E. The role of immune defects and colonization of *Staphylococcus aureus* in the pathogenesis of atopic dermatitis. Anal Cell Pathol (Amst) 2018; 2018: 1-7.
[http://dx.doi.org/10.1155/2018/1956403] [PMID: 29854575]

[40]   Tsakok T, Woolf R, Smith CH, Weidinger S, Flohr C. Atopic dermatitis: the skin barrier and beyond. Br J Dermatol 2019; 180(3): 464-74.
[http://dx.doi.org/10.1111/bjd.16934] [PMID: 29969827]

[41]   Brodská P, Panzner P, Pizinger K, Schmid-Grendelmeier P. IgE-mediated sensitization to malassezia in atopic dermatitis: more common in male patients and in head and neck type. Dermatitis 2014; 25(3): 120-6.
[http://dx.doi.org/10.1097/DER.0000000000000040] [PMID: 24819285]

[42]   Cookson W. The immunogenetics of asthma and eczema: a new focus on the epithelium. Nat Rev Immunol 2004; 4(12): 978-88.
[http://dx.doi.org/10.1038/nri1500] [PMID: 15573132]

[43]   Paton DM. Crisaborole: Phosphodiesterase inhibitor for treatment of atopic dermatitis. Drugs Today (Barc) 2017; 53(4): 239-45.
[http://dx.doi.org/10.1358/dot.2017.53.4.2604174] [PMID: 28492291]

[44]   Leung DYM, Boguniewicz M, Howell MD, Nomura I, Hamid QA. New insights into atopic dermatitis. J Clin Invest 2004; 113(5): 651-7.
[http://dx.doi.org/10.1172/JCI21060] [PMID: 14991059]

[45]   Zedan K. Immunoglobulin E, Interleukin-18 and Interleukin-12 in Patients with Atopic Dermatitis: Correlation with Disease Activity. J Clin Diagn Res 2015; 9(4): WC01-5.
[http://dx.doi.org/10.7860/JCDR/2015/12261.5742]

[46]   Sonkoly E, Muller A, Lauerma AI, *et al.* IL-31: A new link between T cells and pruritus in atopic skin inflammation. J Allergy Clin Immunol 2006; 117(2): 411-7.
[http://dx.doi.org/10.1016/j.jaci.2005.10.033] [PMID: 16461142]

[47]   Mansouri Y, Guttman-Yassky E. Immune pathways in atopic dermatitis, and definition of biomarkers through broad and targeted therapeutics. J Clin Med 2015; 4(5): 858-73.
[http://dx.doi.org/10.3390/jcm4050858] [PMID: 26239452]

[48]   Hori S, Nomura T, Sakaguchi S. Control of regulatory T cell development by the transcription factor *Foxp3*. Science 2003; 299(5609): 1057-61.
[http://dx.doi.org/10.1126/science.1079490] [PMID: 12522256]

[49]   Mack MR, Brestoff JR, Berrien-Elliott MM, *et al*. Blood natural killer cell deficiency reveals an immunotherapy strategy for atopic dermatitis. Sci Transl Med 2020; 12(532): eaay1005.
[http://dx.doi.org/10.1126/scitranslmed.aay1005] [PMID: 32102931]

[50]   Kim J, Kim BE, Leung DYM. Pathophysiology of atopic dermatitis: Clinical implications. Allergy Asthma Proc 2019; 40(2): 84-92.
[http://dx.doi.org/10.2500/aap.2019.40.4202] [PMID: 30819278]

[51]   Danso M, Boiten W, van Drongelen V, *et al*. Altered expression of epidermal lipid bio-synthesis enzymes in atopic dermatitis skin is accompanied by changes in stratum corneum lipid composition. J Dermatol Sci 2017; 88(1): 57-66.
[http://dx.doi.org/10.1016/j.jdermsci.2017.05.005] [PMID: 28571749]

[52]   Li S, Villarreal M, Stewart S, *et al*. Altered composition of epidermal lipids correlates with *Staphylococcus aureus* colonization status in atopic dermatitis. Br J Dermatol 2017; 177(4): e125-7.
[http://dx.doi.org/10.1111/bjd.15409] [PMID: 28244066]

[53]   Kim K. Neuroimmunological mechanism of pruritus in atopic dermatitis focused on the role of serotonin. Biomol Ther (Seoul) 2012; 20(6): 506-12.
[http://dx.doi.org/10.4062/biomolther.2012.20.6.506] [PMID: 24009842]

[54]   Feld M, Garcia R, Buddenkotte J, *et al*. The pruritus- and TH2-associated cytokine IL-31 promotes growth of sensory nerves. J Allergy Clin Immunol 2016; 138(2): 500-508.e24.
[http://dx.doi.org/10.1016/j.jaci.2016.02.020] [PMID: 27212086]

[55]   Shiratori-Hayashi M, Koga K, Tozaki-Saitoh H, *et al*. STAT3-dependent reactive astrogliosis in the spinal dorsal horn underlies chronic itch. Nat Med 2015; 21(8): 927-31.
[http://dx.doi.org/10.1038/nm.3912] [PMID: 26193341]

[56]   Helm RM, Burks AW. Mechanisms of food allergy. Curr Opin Immunol 2000; 12(6): 647-53.
[http://dx.doi.org/10.1016/S0952-7915(00)00157-6] [PMID: 11102767]

[57]   Tham EH, Leung DYM. Mechanisms by which atopic dermatitis predisposes to food allergy and the atopic march. Allergy Asthma Immunol Res 2019; 11(1): 4-15.
[http://dx.doi.org/10.4168/aair.2019.11.1.4] [PMID: 30479073]

[58]   Kantor R, Silverberg JI. Environmental risk factors and their role in the management of atopic dermatitis. Expert Rev Clin Immunol 2017; 13(1): 15-26.
[http://dx.doi.org/10.1080/1744666X.2016.1212660] [PMID: 27417220]

[59]   Simpson EL, Chalmers JR, Hanifin JM, *et al*. Emollient enhancement of the skin barrier from birth offers effective atopic dermatitis prevention. J Allergy Clin Immunol 2014; 134(4): 818-23.
[http://dx.doi.org/10.1016/j.jaci.2014.08.005] [PMID: 25282563]

[60]   Ahluwalia A. Topical glucocorticoids and the skin-mechanisms of action: an update. Mediators Inflamm 1998; 7(3): 183-93.
[http://dx.doi.org/10.1080/09629359891126] [PMID: 9705606]

[61]   Stuetz A, Baumann K, Grassberger M, Wolff K, Meingassner JG. Discovery of topical calcineurin inhibitors and pharmacological profile of pimecrolimus. Int Arch Allergy Immunol 2006; 141(3): 199-212.
[http://dx.doi.org/10.1159/000095289] [PMID: 16926539]

[62]   Jeziorkowska R, Sysa-Jędrzejowska A, Samochocki Z. Topical steroid therapy in atopic dermatitis in theory and practice. Postepy Dermatol Alergol 2015; 3(3): 162-6.
[http://dx.doi.org/10.5114/pdia.2014.40962] [PMID: 26161055]

[63]   Chia BKY, Tey HL. Systematic review on the efficacy, safety, and cost-effectiveness of topical

calcineurin inhibitors in atopic dermatitis. Dermatitis 2015; 26(3): 122-32.
[http://dx.doi.org/10.1097/DER.0000000000000118] [PMID: 25984688]

[64]   Zebda R, Paller AS. Phosphodiesterase 4 inhibitors. J Am Acad Dermatol 2018; 78(3) (Suppl. 1): S43-52.
[http://dx.doi.org/10.1016/j.jaad.2017.11.056] [PMID: 29248522]

[65]   Faergemann J, Larkö O. The effect of UV-light on human skin microorganisms. Acta Derm Venereol 1987; 67(1): 69-72.
[PMID: 2436418]

[66]   Pérez Ferriols A, Aguilera J, Aguilera P, *et al.* Determination of minimal erythema dose and anomalous reactions to UVA radiation by skin phototype. Actas Dermo-Sifiliográficas (English Edition) 2014; 105(8): 780-8.
[http://dx.doi.org/10.1016/j.adengl.2014.05.020] [PMID: 24996228]

[67]   Tintle S, Shemer A, Suárez-Fariñas M, *et al.* Reversal of atopic dermatitis with narrow-band UVB phototherapy and biomarkers for therapeutic response. J Allergy Clin Immunol 2011; 128(3): 583-593.e4, 4.
[http://dx.doi.org/10.1016/j.jaci.2011.05.042] [PMID: 21762976]

[68]   Ortiz-Salvador JM, Pérez-Ferriols A. Phototherapy in Atopic Dermatitis. In: Ahmad S, Ed. Ultraviolet Light in Human Health, Diseases and Environment Advances in Experimental Medicine and Biology, Springer, Cham,. 2017; Vol. 996: pp. 279–286.
[http://dx.doi.org/10.1007/978-3-319-56017-5_23]

[69]   Rodenbeck DL, Silverberg JI, Silverberg NB. Phototherapy for atopic dermatitis. Clin Dermatol 2016; 34(5): 607-13.
[http://dx.doi.org/10.1016/j.clindermatol.2016.05.011] [PMID: 27638440]

[70]   Brazzelli V, Prestinari F, Chiesa MG, Borroni RG, Ardigò M, Borroni G. Sequential treatment of severe atopic dermatitis with cyclosporin A and low-dose narrow-band UVB phototherapy. Dermatology 2002; 204(3): 252-4.
[http://dx.doi.org/10.1159/000057893] [PMID: 12037459]

[71]   Bogaczewicz J, Malinowska K, Sysa-Jedrzejowska A, Wozniacka A. Medium-dose ultraviolet A1 phototherapy and mRNA expression of TSLP, TARC, IL-5, and IL-13 in acute skin lesions in atopic dermatitis. Int J Dermatol 2016; 55(8): 856-63.
[http://dx.doi.org/10.1111/ijd.12992] [PMID: 26475182]

[72]   Tzaneva S, Seeber A, Schwaiger M, Hönigsmann H, Tanew A. High-dose *versus* medium-dose UVA1 phototherapy for patients with severe generalized atopic dermatitis. J Am Acad Dermatol 2001; 45(4): 503-7.
[http://dx.doi.org/10.1067/mjd.2001.114743] [PMID: 11568738]

[73]   Krutmann J. Phototherapy for atopic dermatitis. Clin Exp Dermatol 2000; 25(7): 552-8.
[http://dx.doi.org/10.1046/j.1365-2230.2000.00700.x] [PMID: 11122227]

[74]   Jekler J, Larkö O. Combined UVA-UVB *versus* UVB phototherapy for atopic dermatitis: A paired-comparison study. J Am Acad Dermatol 1990; 22(1): 49-53.
[http://dx.doi.org/10.1016/0190-9622(90)70006-4] [PMID: 2298965]

[75]   Valkova S, Velkova A. UVA/UVB phototherapy for atopic dermatitis revisited. J Dermatolog Treat 2004; 15(4): 239-44.
[http://dx.doi.org/10.1080/09546630410035338] [PMID: 15764039]

[76]   Carrascosa JM, Gardeazábal J, Pérez-Ferriols A, *et al.* Consensus document on phototherapy: PUVA therapy and narrow-band UVB therapy. Actas Dermosifiliogr 2005; 96(10): 635-58.
[http://dx.doi.org/10.1016/S0001-7310(05)73153-7] [PMID: 16476315]

[77]   Morison WL, Parrish JA, Fitzpatrick TB. Oral psoralen photochemotherapy of atopic eczema. Br J Dermatol 1978; 98(1): 25-30.

[http://dx.doi.org/10.1111/j.1365-2133.1978.tb07329.x] [PMID: 626712]

[78]   Stern RS, Nichols KT, Väkevä LH. Malignant melanoma in patients treated for psoriasis with methoxsalen (psoralen) and ultraviolet A radiation (PUVA). The PUVA Follow-Up Study. N Engl J Med 1997; 336(15): 1041-5.
[http://dx.doi.org/10.1056/NEJM199704103361501] [PMID: 9091799]

[79]   Der-Petrossian M, Seeber A, Hönigsmann H, Tanew A. Half-side comparison study on the efficacy of 8-methoxypsoralen bath-PUVA *versus* narrow-band ultraviolet B phototherapy in patients with severe chronic atopic dermatitis. Br J Dermatol 2000; 142(1): 39-43.
[http://dx.doi.org/10.1046/j.1365-2133.2000.03239.x] [PMID: 10651692]

[80]   Tzaneva S, Kittler H, Holzer G, *et al.* 5-Methoxypsoralen plus ultraviolet (UV) A is superior to medium-dose UVA1 in the treatment of severe atopic dermatitis: a randomized crossover trial. Br J Dermatol 2010; 162(3): 655-60.
[http://dx.doi.org/10.1111/j.1365-2133.2009.09514.x] [PMID: 19769631]

[81]   Becker D, Langer E, Seemann M, *et al.* Clinical efficacy of blue light full body irradiation as treatment option for severe atopic dermatitis. PLoS One 2011; 6(6): e20566.
[http://dx.doi.org/10.1371/journal.pone.0020566] [PMID: 21687679]

[82]   Kromer C, Nühnen VP, Pfützner W, *et al.* Treatment of Atopic Dermatitis Using a Full-Body Blue Light Device (AD-Blue): Protocol of a Randomized Controlled Trial. JMIR Res Protoc 2019; 8(1): e11911.
[http://dx.doi.org/10.2196/11911] [PMID: 30622089]

[83]   Galli E, Chini L, Moschese V, *et al.* Methylprednisolone bolus: a novel therapy for severe atopic dermatitis. Acta Paediatr 1994; 83(3): 315-7.
[http://dx.doi.org/10.1111/j.1651-2227.1994.tb18102.x] [PMID: 8038536]

[84]   Kim JE, Kim HJ, Lew BL, *et al.* Consensus guidelines for the treatment of atopic dermatitis in Korea (part II): systemic treatment. Ann Dermatol 2015; 27(5): 578-92.
[http://dx.doi.org/10.5021/ad.2015.27.5.578] [PMID: 26512172]

[85]   Haeck IM, Knol MJ, ten Berge O, van Velsen SGA, de Bruin-Weller MS, Bruijnzeel-Koomen CAFM. Enteric-coated mycophenolate sodium *versus* cyclosporin A as long-term treatment in adult patients with severe atopic dermatitis: A randomized controlled trial. J Am Acad Dermatol 2011; 64(6): 1074-84.
[http://dx.doi.org/10.1016/j.jaad.2010.04.027] [PMID: 21458107]

[86]   Roekevisch E, Spuls PI, Kuester D, Limpens J, Schmitt J. Efficacy and safety of systemic treatments for moderate-to-severe atopic dermatitis: a systematic review. J Allergy Clin Immunol 2014; 133(2): 429-38.
[http://dx.doi.org/10.1016/j.jaci.2013.07.049] [PMID: 24269258]

[87]   Laube S, Stephens M, Smith AG, Whittaker SJ, Tan BB. Lymphomatoid papulosis in a patient with atopic eczema on long-term ciclosporin therapy. Br J Dermatol 2005; 152(6): 1346-8.
[http://dx.doi.org/10.1111/j.1365-2133.2005.06548.x] [PMID: 15949007]

[88]   Badihi A, Frušić-Zlotkin M, Soroka Y, *et al.* Topical nano-encapsulated cyclosporine formulation for atopic dermatitis treatment. Nanomedicine 2020; 24: 102140.
[http://dx.doi.org/10.1016/j.nano.2019.102140] [PMID: 31830614]

[89]   Schram ME, Roekevisch E, Leeflang MMG, Bos JD, Schmitt J, Spuls PI. A randomized trial of methotrexate *versus* azathioprine for severe atopic eczema. J Allergy Clin Immunol 2011; 128(2): 353-9.
[http://dx.doi.org/10.1016/j.jaci.2011.03.024] [PMID: 21514637]

[90]   Meggitt SJ, Gray JC, Reynolds NJ. Azathioprine dosed by thiopurine methyltransferase activity for moderate-to-severe atopic eczema: a double-blind, randomised controlled trial. Lancet 2006; 367(9513): 839-46.
[http://dx.doi.org/10.1016/S0140-6736(06)68340-2] [PMID: 16530578]

[91] Weatherhead SC, Wahie S, Reynolds NJ, Meggitt SJ. An open-label, dose-ranging study of methotrexate for moderate-to-severe adult atopic eczema. Br J Dermatol 2007; 156(2): 346-51.
[http://dx.doi.org/10.1111/j.1365-2133.2006.07686.x] [PMID: 17223876]

[92] Goujon C, Viguier M, Staumont-Sallé D, *et al.* Methotrexate *versus* cyclosporine in adults with moderate-to-severe atopic dermatitis: a phase III randomized noninferiority trial. J Allergy Clin Immunol Pract 2018; 6(2): 562-569.e3.
[http://dx.doi.org/10.1016/j.jaip.2017.07.007] [PMID: 28967549]

[93] Ballester I, Silvestre JF, Pérez-Crespo M, Lucas A. Severe adult atopic dermatitis: treatment with mycophenolate mofetil in 8 patients. Actas Dermosifiliogr 2009; 100(10): 883-7.
[http://dx.doi.org/10.1016/S0001-7310(09)72917-5] [PMID: 20038365]

[94] Benez A, Fierlbeck G. Successful long-term treatment of severe atopic dermatitis with mycophenolate mofetil. Br J Dermatol 2001; 144(3): 638-9.
[http://dx.doi.org/10.1046/j.1365-2133.2001.04108.x] [PMID: 11260038]

[95] Simon D, Bieber T. Systemic therapy for atopic dermatitis. Allergy 2014; 69(1): 46-55.
[http://dx.doi.org/10.1111/all.12339] [PMID: 24354911]

[96] Thijs JL, Van Der Geest BAM, Van Der Schaft J, *et al.* Predicting therapy response to mycophenolic acid using UGT1A9 genotyping: towards personalized medicine in atopic dermatitis. J Dermatolog Treat 2017; 28(3): 242-5.
[http://dx.doi.org/10.1080/09546634.2016.1227420] [PMID: 27549213]

[97] Ring J, Alomar A, Bieber T, *et al.* Guidelines for treatment of atopic eczema (atopic dermatitis) Part I. J Eur Acad Dermatol Venereol 2012; 26(8): 1045-60.
[http://dx.doi.org/10.1111/j.1468-3083.2012.04635.x] [PMID: 22805051]

[98] Grahovac M, Molin S, Prinz JC, Ruzicka T, Wollenberg A. Treatment of atopic eczema with oral alitretinoin. Br J Dermatol 2010; 162(1): 217-8.
[http://dx.doi.org/10.1111/j.1365-2133.2009.09522.x] [PMID: 19886882]

[99] D'Erme AM, Milanesi N, Agnoletti AF, Maio V, Massi D, Gola M. Efficacy of treatment with oral alitretinoin in patient suffering from lichen simplex chronicus and severe atopic dermatitis of hands. Dermatol Ther 2014; 27(1): 21-3.
[http://dx.doi.org/10.1111/dth.12035] [PMID: 24502306]

[100] Ruzicka T, Lynde CW, Jemec GBE, *et al.* Efficacy and safety of oral alitretinoin (9-cis retinoic acid) in patients with severe chronic hand eczema refractory to topical corticosteroids: results of a randomized, double-blind, placebo-controlled, multicentre trial. Br J Dermatol 2008; 158(4): 808-17.
[http://dx.doi.org/10.1111/j.1365-2133.2008.08487.x] [PMID: 18294310]

[101] Hamilton JD, Suárez-Fariñas M, Dhingra N, *et al.* Dupilumab improves the molecular signature in skin of patients with moderate-to-severe atopic dermatitis. J Allergy Clin Immunol 2014; 134(6): 1293-300.
[http://dx.doi.org/10.1016/j.jaci.2014.10.013] [PMID: 25482871]

[102] Shroff A, Guttman-Yassky E. Successful use of ustekinumab therapy in refractory severe atopic dermatitis. JAAD Case Rep 2015; 1(1): 25-6.
[http://dx.doi.org/10.1016/j.jdcr.2014.10.007] [PMID: 27075132]

[103] Weiss D, Schaschinger M, Ristl R, *et al.* Ustekinumab treatment in severe atopic dermatitis: Down-regulation of T-helper 2/22 expression. J Am Acad Dermatol 2017; 76(1): 91-97.e3.
[http://dx.doi.org/10.1016/j.jaad.2016.07.047] [PMID: 27745907]

[104] Puya R, Alvarez-López M, Velez A, Asuncion EC, Moreno JC. Treatment of severe refractory adult atopic dermatitis with ustekinumab. Int J Dermatol 2012; 51(1): 115-6.
[http://dx.doi.org/10.1111/j.1365-4632.2011.05195.x] [PMID: 22182388]

[105] Samrao A, Berry TM, Goreshi R, Simpson EL. A pilot study of an oral phosphodiesterase inhibitor (apremilast) for atopic dermatitis in adults. Arch Dermatol 2012; 148(8): 890-7.

[http://dx.doi.org/10.1001/archdermatol.2012.812] [PMID: 22508772]

[106] Simpson EL, Imafuku S, Poulin Y, *et al.* A Phase 2 Randomized Trial of Apremilast in Patients with Atopic Dermatitis. J Invest Dermatol 2019; 139(5): 1063-72.
[http://dx.doi.org/10.1016/j.jid.2018.10.043] [PMID: 30528828]

[107] Nydegger UE, Sturzenegger M. Adverse effects of intravenous immunoglobulin therapy. Drug Saf 1999; 21(3): 171-85.
[http://dx.doi.org/10.2165/00002018-199921030-00003] [PMID: 10487396]

[108] Stevens SR, Hanifin JM, Hamilton T, Tofte SJ, Cooper KD. Long-term effectiveness and safety of recombinant human interferon gamma therapy for atopic dermatitis despite unchanged serum IgE levels. Arch Dermatol 1998; 134(7): 799-804.
[http://dx.doi.org/10.1001/archderm.134.7.799] [PMID: 9681342]

[109] Schneider LC, Baz Z, Zarcone C, Zurakowski D. Long-term therapy with recombinant interferon-γ (rIFN-γ) for atopic dermatitis. Ann Allergy Asthma Immunol 1998; 80(3): 263-8.
[http://dx.doi.org/10.1016/S1081-1206(10)62968-7] [PMID: 9532976]

[110] Lintu P, Savolainen J, Kortekangas-Savolainen O, Kalimo K. Systemic ketoconazole is an effective treatment of atopic dermatitis with IgE-mediated hypersensitivity to yeasts. Allergy 2001; 56(6): 512-7.
[http://dx.doi.org/10.1034/j.1398-9995.2001.056006512.x] [PMID: 11421895]

[111] Mayser P, Kupfer J, Nemetz D, *et al.* Treatment of head and neck dermatitis with ciclopiroxolamine cream—results of a double-blind, placebo-controlled study. Skin Pharmacol Physiol 2006; 19(3): 153-8.
[http://dx.doi.org/10.1159/000092596] [PMID: 16612143]

[112] Rusu E, Enache G, Cursaru R, *et al.* Prebiotics and probiotics in atopic dermatitis. Exp Ther Med 2019; 18(2): 926-31.
[http://dx.doi.org/10.3892/etm.2019.7678] [PMID: 31384325]

[113] Samochocki Z, Bogaczewicz J, Jeziorkowska R, *et al.* Vitamin D effects in atopic dermatitis. J Am Acad Dermatol 2013; 69(2): 238-44.
[http://dx.doi.org/10.1016/j.jaad.2013.03.014] [PMID: 23643343]

[114] Kim G, Bae JH. Vitamin D and atopic dermatitis: A systematic review and meta-analysis. Nutrition 2016; 32(9): 913-20.
[http://dx.doi.org/10.1016/j.nut.2016.01.023] [PMID: 27061361]

[115] Hattangdi-Haridas SR, Lanham-New SA, Wong WHS, Ho MHK, Darling AL. Vitamin D deficiency and effects of vitamin D supplementation on disease severity in patients with atopic dermatitis: a systematic review and meta-analysis in adults and children. Nutrients 2019; 11(8): 1854.
[http://dx.doi.org/10.3390/nu11081854] [PMID: 31405041]

[116] Chun PIF, Lehman H. Current and future monoclonal antibodies in the treatment of atopic dermatitis. Clin Rev Allergy Immunol 2020; 59(2): 208-19.
[http://dx.doi.org/10.1007/s12016-020-08802-9] [PMID: 32617839]

[117] Simpson EL, Flohr C, Eichenfield LF, *et al.* Efficacy and safety of lebrikizumab (an anti-IL-13 monoclonal antibody) in adults with moderate-to-severe atopic dermatitis inadequately controlled by topical corticosteroids: A randomized, placebo-controlled phase II trial (TREBLE). J Am Acad Dermatol 2018; 78(5): 863-871.e11.
[http://dx.doi.org/10.1016/j.jaad.2018.01.017] [PMID: 29353026]

[118] Wollenberg A, Howell MD, Guttman-Yassky E, *et al.* Treatment of atopic dermatitis with tralokinumab, an anti–IL-13 mAb. J Allergy Clin Immunol 2019; 143(1): 135-41.
[http://dx.doi.org/10.1016/j.jaci.2018.05.029] [PMID: 29906525]

[119] Kabashima K, Furue M, Hanifin JM, *et al.* Nemolizumab in patients with moderate-to-severe atopic dermatitis: Randomized, phase II, long-term extension study. J Allergy Clin Immunol 2018; 142(4):

1121-1130.e7.
[http://dx.doi.org/10.1016/j.jaci.2018.03.018] [PMID: 29753033]

[120] Richards C, Gandhi R, Botelho F, Ho L, Paolini J. Oncostatin M induction of monocyte chemoattractant protein 1 is inhibited by anti-oncostatin M receptor beta monoclonal antibody KPL-716. Acta Derm Venereol 2020; 100(14): adv00197.
[http://dx.doi.org/10.2340/00015555-3505] [PMID: 32374409]

[121] Fraser KA. American Academy of Dermatology Annual Meeting: San Diego, CA, USA, 16–20 Feb 2018. Am J Clin Dermatol 2018; 19(2): 287-90.
[http://dx.doi.org/10.1007/s40257-018-0351-z] [PMID: 29525933]

[122] Guttman-Yassky E, Brunner PM, Neumann AU, *et al.* Efficacy and safety of fezakinumab (an IL-22 monoclonal antibody) in adults with moderate-to-severe atopic dermatitis inadequately controlled by conventional treatments: A randomized, double-blind, phase 2a trial. J Am Acad Dermatol 2018; 78(5): 872-881.e6.
[http://dx.doi.org/10.1016/j.jaad.2018.01.016] [PMID: 29353025]

[123] Guttman-Yassky E, Pavel AB, Zhou L, *et al.* GBR 830, an anti-OX40, improves skin gene signatures and clinical scores in patients with atopic dermatitis. J Allergy Clin Immunol 2019; 144(2): 482-493.e7.
[http://dx.doi.org/10.1016/j.jaci.2018.11.053] [PMID: 30738171]

[124] Simpson EL, Parnes JR, She D, *et al.* Tezepelumab, an anti–thymic stromal lymphopoietin monoclonal antibody, in the treatment of moderate to severe atopic dermatitis: A randomized phase 2a clinical trial. J Am Acad Dermatol 2019; 80(4): 1013-21.
[http://dx.doi.org/10.1016/j.jaad.2018.11.059] [PMID: 30550828]

[125] Szalus K, Trzeciak M, Nowicki RJ. JAK-STAT inhibitors in atopic dermatitis from pathogenesis to clinical trials results. Microorganisms 2020; 8(11): 1743.
[http://dx.doi.org/10.3390/microorganisms8111743] [PMID: 33172122]

[126] Bissonnette R, Papp KA, Poulin Y, *et al.* Topical tofacitinib for atopic dermatitis: a phase II a randomized trial. Br J Dermatol 2016; 175(5): 902-11.
[http://dx.doi.org/10.1111/bjd.14871] [PMID: 27423107]

[127] Kim BS, Howell MD, Sun K, Papp K, Nasir A, Kuligowski ME. Treatment of atopic dermatitis with ruxolitinib cream (JAK1/JAK2 inhibitor) or triamcinolone cream. J Allergy Clin Immunol 2020; 145(2): 572-82.
[http://dx.doi.org/10.1016/j.jaci.2019.08.042] [PMID: 31629805]

[128] Simpson EL, Lacour JP, Spelman L, *et al.* Baricitinib in patients with moderate-to-severe atopic dermatitis and inadequate response to topical corticosteroids: results from two randomized monotherapy phase III trials. Br J Dermatol 2020; 183(2): 242-55.
[http://dx.doi.org/10.1111/bjd.18898] [PMID: 31995838]

[129] Nakagawa H, Nemoto O, Igarashi A, Saeki H, Kaino H, Nagata T. Delgocitinib ointment, a topical Janus kinase inhibitor, in adult patients with moderate to severe atopic dermatitis: A phase 3, randomized, double-blind, vehicle-controlled study and an open-label, long-term extension study. J Am Acad Dermatol 2020; 82(4): 823-31.
[http://dx.doi.org/10.1016/j.jaad.2019.12.015] [PMID: 32029304]

[130] Nakagawa H, Nemoto O, Igarashi A, *et al.* Phase 2 clinical study of delgocitinib ointment in pediatric patients with atopic dermatitis. J Allergy Clin Immunol 2019; 144(6): 1575-83.
[http://dx.doi.org/10.1016/j.jaci.2019.08.004] [PMID: 31425780]

[131] Guttman-Yassky E, Thaçi D, Pangan AL, *et al.* Upadacitinib in adults with moderate to severe atopic dermatitis: 16-week results from a randomized, placebo-controlled trial. J Allergy Clin Immunol 2020; 145(3): 877-84.
[http://dx.doi.org/10.1016/j.jaci.2019.11.025] [PMID: 31786154]

[132] Silverberg JI, Simpson EL, Thyssen JP, *et al.* Efficacy and safety of abrocitinib in patients with

moderate-to-severe atopic dermatitis. JAMA Dermatol 2020; 156(8): 863-73.
[http://dx.doi.org/10.1001/jamadermatol.2020.1406] [PMID: 32492087]

[133]   Piscitelli S, Lee J, McHale K, *et al.* Cerdulatinib (DMVT-502), a novel, topical, dual Janus kinase/spleen tyrosine kinase inhibitor, improves the cellular and molecular cutaneous signature in patients with atopic dermatitis. Exp Dermatol 2018; 27: 44-5.

[134]   Bissonnette R, Maari C, Forman S, *et al.* The oral Janus kinase/spleen tyrosine kinase inhibitor ASN 002 demonstrates efficacy and improves associated systemic inflammation in patients with moderate-to-severe atopic dermatitis: results from a randomized double-blind placebo-controlled study. Br J Dermatol 2019; 181(4): 733-42.
[http://dx.doi.org/10.1111/bjd.17932] [PMID: 30919407]

[135]   Werfel T, Layton G, Yeadon M, *et al.* Efficacy and safety of the histamine H_4 receptor antagonist ZPL-3893787 in patients with atopic dermatitis. J Allergy Clin Immunol 2019; 143(5): 1830-1837.e4.
[http://dx.doi.org/10.1016/j.jaci.2018.07.047] [PMID: 30414855]

[136]   Hanifin JM, Ellis CN, Frieden IJ, *et al.* OPA-15406, a novel, topical, nonsteroidal, selective phosphodiesterase-4 (PDE4) inhibitor, in the treatment of adult and adolescent patients with mild to moderate atopic dermatitis (AD): A phase-II randomized, double-blind, placebo-controlled study. J Am Acad Dermatol 2016; 75(2): 297-305.
[http://dx.doi.org/10.1016/j.jaad.2016.04.001] [PMID: 27189825]

[137]   Saeki H, Baba N, Oshiden K, Abe Y, Tsubouchi H. Phase 2, randomized, double-blind, placebo-controlled, 4-week study to evaluate the safety and efficacy of OPA- 15406 (difamilast), a new topical selective phosphodiesterase type-4 inhibitor, in Japanese pediatric patients aged 2–14 years with atopic dermatitis. J Dermatol 2020; 47(1): 17-24.
[http://dx.doi.org/10.1111/1346-8138.15137] [PMID: 31713267]

[138]   Ohba F, Matsuki S, Imayama S, *et al.* Efficacy of a novel phosphodiesterase inhibitor, E6005, in patients with atopic dermatitis: An investigator-blinded, vehicle-controlled study. J Dermatolog Treat 2016; 27(5): 467-72.
[http://dx.doi.org/10.3109/09546634.2016.1157257] [PMID: 27080209]

[139]   Paller AS, Stein Gold L, Soung J, Tallman AM, Rubenstein DS, Gooderham M. Efficacy and patient-reported outcomes from a phase 2b, randomized clinical trial of tapinarof cream for the treatment of adolescents and adults with atopic dermatitis. J Am Acad Dermatol 2021; 84(3): 632-8.
[http://dx.doi.org/10.1016/j.jaad.2020.05.135] [PMID: 32502588]

[140]   Lee YW, Won C-H, Jung K, *et al.* Efficacy and safety of PAC-14028 cream - a novel, topical, nonsteroidal, selective TRPV1 antagonist in patients with mild-to-moderate atopic dermatitis: a phase IIb randomized trial. Br J Dermatol 2019; 180: 1030-8.
[http://dx.doi.org/10.1111/bjd.17455] [PMID: 30623408]

[141]   Crosby CM, Komori HK, Adams JW. 030 Etrasimod, an oral, selective sphingosine 1-phosphate receptor modulator improves skin inflammation in a contact hypersensitivity dermatitis model. J Invest Dermatol 2019; 139(9): S219.
[http://dx.doi.org/10.1016/j.jid.2019.07.033]

[142]   Rani S, Khan SA, Ali M. Phytochemical investigation of the seeds of *Althea officinalis* L. Nat Prod Res 2010; 24(14): 1358-64.
[http://dx.doi.org/10.1080/14786411003650777] [PMID: 20803381]

[143]   Naseri V, Chavoshzadeh Z, Mizani A, *et al.* Effect of topical marshmallow (*Althaea officinalis*) on atopic dermatitis in children: A pilot double-blind active-controlled clinical trial of an *in-silico* - analyzed phytomedicine. Phytother Res 2021; 35(3): 1389-98.
[http://dx.doi.org/10.1002/ptr.6899] [PMID: 33034099]

[144]   Blumenthal M, Goldberg A, Brinckmann J. Herbal medicine: expanded commission E monographs. Integrative Medicine Communications. 2000.
[http://dx.doi.org/10.7326/0003-4819-133-6-200009190-00031]

[145] Lyss G, Schmidt TJ, Merfort I, Pahl HL. Helenalin, an anti-inflammatory sesquiterpene lactone from Arnica, selectively inhibits transcription factor NF-kappaB. Biol Chem 1997; 378(9): 951-61.
[http://dx.doi.org/10.1515/bchm.1997.378.9.951] [PMID: 9348104]

[146] Nebus J, Nollent V, Wallo W. New Learnings on the Clinical Benefits of Colloidal Oatmeal in Atopic Dermatitis. Supplement to the October 2012.

[147] Aries MF, Vaissiere C, Fabre B, Charveron M, Gall Y. Avena rhealba inhibits arachidonic acid cascade, CPLA2 and COX expression in human keratinocytes. Interest in cutaneous inflammatory disorders. J Invest Dermatol 2003; 121.

[148] Paolini M, Pozzetti L, Sapone A, Cantelli-Forti G. Effect of licorice and glycyrrhizin on murine liver CYP-dependent monooxygenases. Life Sci 1998; 62(6): 571-82.
[http://dx.doi.org/10.1016/S0024-3205(97)01154-5] [PMID: 9464470]

[149] Blumenthal M, Goldberg A, Brinckmann J. Herbal medicine. Integrative Medicine Communications. Integrative Medicine Communications 2000.

[150] Kim J, Kim BE, Leung DYM. Pathophysiology of atopic dermatitis: Clinical implications. Allergy Asthma Proc 2019; 40(2): 84-92.
[http://dx.doi.org/10.2500/aap.2019.40.4202] [PMID: 30819278] [PMCID: PMC6399565]

[151] Bisset NG, Wichtl M. Herbal Drugs and Phytopharmaceuticals. Medpharm GmbH Scientific Publishers 1994; pp. 91-5.

[152] Brown DJ, Dattner AM. Phytotherapeutic approaches to common dermatologic conditions. Arch Dermatol 1998; 134(11): 1401-4.
[http://dx.doi.org/10.1001/archderm.134.11.1401] [PMID: 9828875]

[153] Monographs ESCOP. Matricariae flos—Matricaria flower. Thieme 2003.

[154] Alamgir ANM. Pharmacopoeia and Herbal Monograph, the Aim and Use of WHO's Herbal Monograph, WHO's Guide Lines for Herbal Monograph, Pharmacognostical Research and Monographs of Organized, Unorganized Drugs and Drugs from Animal Sources Therapeutic Use of Medicinal Plants and Their Extracts. Springer 2017; Vol. 1: pp. 295-353.
[http://dx.doi.org/10.1007/978-3-319-63862-1_7]

[155] Pytkowska K. Effect of lipids on epidermal barrier function. Wiadomości PTK 2003; 2: 7-10.

[156] Van Gool CJAW, Zeegers MPA, Thijs C. Oral essential fatty acid supplementation in atopic dermatitis-a meta-analysis of placebo-controlled trials. Br J Dermatol 2004; 150(4): 728-40.
[http://dx.doi.org/10.1111/j.0007-0963.2004.05851.x] [PMID: 15099370]

[157] Ganzera M, Schneider P, Stuppner H. Inhibitory effects of the essential oil of chamomile (Matricaria recutita L.) and its major constituents on human cytochrome P450 enzymes. Life Sci 2006; 78(8): 856-61.
[http://dx.doi.org/10.1016/j.lfs.2005.05.095] [PMID: 16137701]

[158] Oladeji OS, Oyebamiji AK. *Stellaria media* (L.) Vill.- A plant with immense therapeutic potentials: phytochemistry and pharmacology. Heliyon 2020; 6(6): e04150.
[http://dx.doi.org/10.1016/j.heliyon.2020.e04150] [PMID: 32548330]

[159] Peirce A. American pharmaceutical association practical guide to natural medicines. Morrow 1999.

[160] Botanical Safety Handbook - Google Books. CRC press 1997.

[161] Liu J, Mo X, Wu D, *et al.* Efficacy of a Chinese herbal medicine for the treatment of atopic dermatitis: A randomised controlled study. Complement Ther Med 2015; 23(5): 644-51.
[http://dx.doi.org/10.1016/j.ctim.2015.07.006] [PMID: 26365443]

[162] Yen CY, Hsieh CL. Therapeutic Effect of *Tzu-Yun* Ointment on Patients with Atopic Dermatitis: A Preliminary, Randomized, Controlled, Open-Label Study. J Altern Complement Med 2016; 22(3): 237-43.

[http://dx.doi.org/10.1089/acm.2015.0324] [PMID: 26914336]

[163] Hadjiminaglou F, Bolcato O. The potential role of specific essential oils in the replacement of dermacorticoid drugs (strong, medium and weak) in the treatment of acute dry or weeping dermatitis. Int J Aromather 2005; 15(2): 66-73.
[http://dx.doi.org/10.1016/j.ijat.2005.03.013]

[164] Lim GS, Kim R, Cho H, Moon YS, Choi CN. Comparison of volatile compounds of chamaecyparis obtusa essential oil and its application on the improvement of atopic dermatitis. KSBB J 2013; 28(2): 115-22.
[http://dx.doi.org/10.7841/ksbbj.2013.28.2.115]

CHAPTER 2

Superficial Mycoses as a Challenging Skin Disorder

Wiwit Suttithumsatid[1] and **Pharkphoom Panichayupakaranant**[1,*]

[1] *Department of Pharmacognosy and Pharmaceutical Botany, Faculty of Pharmaceutical Sciences, Prince of Songkla University, Hat-Yai 90112, Thailand*

Abstract: Superficial mycoses of the skin, nails and hair caused by dermatophytes, non-dermatophyte molds, yeasts and yeast-like fungi are among the most common morbidity of the skin, especially in tropical regions of the world. Various antifungal agents, including polyenes, fluoropyrimidines, echinocandins, and azoles, have been commonly used, topically and/or orally, for the treatment of superficial mycoses. Nevertheless, the conventional treatment guideline is not always successful due to drug resistance as well as the possibility of drug interactions and side effects. Recently, the search for new antifungal compounds, such as naphthoquinones, anthraquinones, terpenoids, saponins and flavonoids from medicinal plants toward novel drug development, has attracted a lot of attention. This chapter describes the common superficial mycoses as well as their pathophysiology, epidemiology and current treatment options. Promising herbal extracts or phytochemicals and their products used as therapeutic alternatives for combating superficial mycosis are also highlighted.

Keywords: Antifungal, Candidiasis, Dermatophytes, Phytochemicals, Superficial mycoses, Tinea versicolor.

INTRODUCTION

Fungi are microorganisms in a group of eukaryotes characterized by a complex cellular organization. Notable examples of fungi include organisms such as yeasts, rusts, smuts, mildews, molds, and mushrooms [1, 2]. Fungi can infect and are capable of causing diseases in plants, animals and humans. More than 100,000 species of fungi have been identified as the cause of various diseases [3]. Superficial fungal infections or superficial mycoses is a common skin, nail, and hair diseases caused by pathogenic fungi. The major pathogenic agents of superficial fungal infections consist of dermatophytes, non-dermatophyte molds,

* **Corresponding author Pharkphoom Panichayupakaranant:** Department of Pharmacognosy and Pharmaceutical Botany, Faculty of Pharmaceutical Sciences, Prince of Songkla University, Hat-Yai 90112, Thailand; Tel: +66-74-288980; E-mail: pharkphoom.p@psu.ac.th

Heba Abd El-Sattar El-Nashar, Mohamed El-Shazly & Nouran Mohammed Fahmy (Eds.)

yeasts, and yeast-like fungi [4]. Dermatophytes are fungi that use keratin for growth. Three genera of dermatophytes, namely *Trichophyton*, *Microsporum*, and *Epidermophyton,* are commonly found to be the major cause of superficial fungal infections. Less commonly found in superficial mycoses are the non-dermatophyte fungi, including *Cladosporium* spp., *Neoscytalidim dimidatum*, and *Alternaria* spp. Additionally, yeasts and yeast-like fungi are accounted as a cause of superficial mycoses. Among the yeasts, *Candida* spp. and *Malassezia* spp. are considered to be the most common fungal infectious diseases in humans. Yeast-like fungi such as *Kodamaea ohmeri*, *Geotrichum* spp. and *Cryptococcus* spp. have also been reported as another common cause of superficial mycoses [5, 6].

Superficial mycoses do not only cause cosmetic disfigurement, but also affect the function of infected organ systems. Although superficial mycoses rarely induce life-threatening symptoms, they are still a major problem globally due to their high worldwide incidence rate, particularly in tropical countries [6]. Generally, topical and systemic antifungal agents, including polyenes, fluoropyrimidines, echinocandins, and azoles along with good personal hygiene practices, are commonly recommended as standard treatment guidelines for superficial mycoses [7]. However, these treatment guidelines are not always successful, because of the increasing incidence of anti-fungal drug resistance as well as the possibility of side effects and drug interactions [8]. Recently, the use of natural compounds, particularly phytochemicals, has attracted intense research interest and proposed as pragmatic alternative antifungal agents due to their unique and diverse mechanisms of action along with lower adverse effects. Various phytochemicals, including naphthoquinones, anthraquinones, terpenoids, saponins and flavonoids, have been reported for their anti-fungal potential in drug development [9].

This chapter aims to describe the common characteristics of superficial mycoses as well as their pathophysiology, epidemiology, and current treatment options. Furthermore, the recent targeted drug development from herbal extracts and the promising phytochemicals as well as their innovative products potentially used as alternative therapeutic agents for superficial mycoses treatment, are also highlighted.

SUPERFICIAL MYCOSES AND PATHOPHYSIOLOGY

Superficial mycoses are conditions of fungal infections of the skin, hair, and nail that are usually limited to the stratum corneum and the superficial layers of the skin, and infrequently invade the dermis. It can be classified into two main groups according to its pathogenesis, *viz*: non-inflammatory infections (pityriasis versicolor, tinea nigra, piedras) and inflammatory infections (dermatophytosis, tinea capitis, tinea corporis, tinea cruris, tinea pedis, tinea unguium, tinea barbae, tinea imbricata, and candidiasis) [6, 10]. Generally, superficial mycoses are not life-threatening diseases. However, it may affect internal organs in exceedingly rare cases. Pathophysiology of the most common superficial mycoses, including pityriasis versicolor, dermatophytosis, and candidiasis, is summarized as follows.

Pityriasis Versicolor

Pityriasis versicolor is mainly caused by *Malassezia*, a genus of yeast that is normally found on the superficial area of humans. Recently, more than ten species of *Malassezia* have been reported as the main cause of most cases of pityriasis versicolor, particularly *Malassezia furfur*, *M. globosa*, and *M. sympodialis*. Transformation of *Malassezia* from normal skin flora to its pathogenic counterpart is a key pathway toward the development of superficial mycoses [11, 12].

Due to the general lipophilic properties of *Malassezia*, the seborrheic areas of the body, such as the upper back and chest, face and forehead, are usually colonized by the yeasts [13]. Overgrowth of the yeasts, particularly in hot, humid conditions, hyperhidrosis, and the use of topical skin oils, promote the production of dicarboxylic acids such as azelaic acid. This suppresses the activity of the tyrosinase enzyme, thereby causing depigmentation [14]. Pityriasis versicolor occurs more commonly in immunocompromised hosts, indicating that a patient's immune system may be another important factor in the pathogenesis of this disease [15].

Dermatophytosis

Dermatophytosis is a fungal infection of the cutaneous area that is normally caused by a dermatophyte. The categorization of dermatophytes is dependent on their normal habitat, including human (anthropophilic species) animals (zoophilic species) or soil (geophilic species), and site of infection, for example, scalp hair (tinea capitis), beard hair (tinea barbae) and nails (tinea unguium or dermatophyte onychomycosis). Three main genera of dermatophytes, *i.e.*, *Trichophyton*, *Epidermophyton* and *Microsporum*, commonly invade human keratin and cause dermatophytosis [6, 16].

The process of dermatophyte infection in humans consists of three major steps, namely adherence, invasion, and development of a host response, respectively. In the beginning, dermatophytes contact and adhere to keratinized tissue, then degrade keratin and penetrate into the stratum corneum area by producing a variety of virulence factors. After the invasion step, antigenic compounds such as chitin and glucan, as well as the metabolites produced by dermatophytes-induced host cells, *e.g.*, glycopeptides, peptides and carbohydrates, stimulate the response of the host immune system, which subsequently produce the clinical manifestations of dermatophytosis, such as erythema, raised patches, or pustule formation as well as an itchy sensation [17, 18].

Candidiasis

Candidiasis is a fungal infection caused by yeasts from the genus *Candida*, especially *Candida albicans*. Various immune responses of the host cells and fungal factors play an important role in candidiasis. Early in the pathogenesis, *Candida* cells adhere to host epithelial cells. Invasion of the pathogen is then initiated *via* two mechanisms, including inductions of endocytosis and active penetration. This is followed by multiplication and filamentation processes that cause clinical manifestations, including inflammatory lesions, itching, irritation, and chafing [19, 20].

EPIDEMIOLOGY OF SUPERFICIAL MYCOSES

Superficial mycoses are a global infectious disease. It is commonly found in warm and humid tropical countries, particularly in America and Southeast Asia, because of the optimum temperature and environment for the growth of most fungi. The incidence rate of infection is increasing year by year, and this trend is expected to continue into the future. It has been reported that one out of four of the world's population is affected with superficial mycoses, with the sites of most frequent infections involving the nail (49.7%), skin (43%), and head (6.26%) [21]. Individuals between the ages of 21 to 30 are more likely to have superficial mycoses than other age ranges [22, 23]. The details of epidemiology for each type of superficial mycosis are discussed below.

Tinea versicolor exhibited the highest incidence in tropical wet and dry climates, with a prevalence of up to 50% in tropical countries. On the other hand, in cold climates like Scandinavia, the prevalence has been estimated as low as 1% [24, 25]. Tinea versicolor can be found in males and females equally. Teenagers and young adults are a more at-risk population to be affected with tinea versicolor because their sebaceous glands are most active and most favorable for *Malassezia* growth [26]. Besides, tinea versicolor is also found in infants and children.

The distribution of the dermatophytosis is related to their growth rate, in which 25° to 28°C are excellent for the dermatophyte's growth conditions [27]. Therefore, warm and humid countries usually show a higher incidence. Among cutaneous diseases, the prevalence of dermatophytosis ranges from 18.2% to 23.2% [28]. *Trichophyton rubrum* was found to be the predominant clinical isolate in Europe, whereas *T. mentagrophyte* was reported to have the highest incidence in Asia [29]. Furthermore, males were found to have a higher incidence than females, with a ratio of 1.7:1, and most patients were in the age ranges of 21 to 30 years old [30].

The incidence of superficial candidiasis has increased in recent years, especially in immunocompromised patients. Around 45% to 58% of candidiasis was caused by *Candida albicans*, followed by *C. glabrata* and *C. parapsilosis*, respectively [31]. Similar to most fungal infections, candidiasis is also more likely to be found in a tropical climate where environmental conditions are most favorable to the adaptability of *Candida*. No gender or racial predilection was found to be associated with candidiasis [32]. On the other hand, *Candida* infection is common in childhood, elderly, hospitalized and immunocompromised patients [33].

CURRENT TREATMENTS FOR SUPERFICIAL MYCOSES

Antifungal drugs, including topical and systemic dosage forms, are fundamental treatment options for superficial mycoses. However, the optimal treatment depends on the type of pathogenic fungus as well as the site and severity of the infection. Categories of antifungal medications are predominantly divided into five groups based on their mechanism of action as follows [34]:

1. Inhibition of RNA and/or DNA synthesis, *e.g.*, fluorinated pyrimidine analogs 5-FC.
2. Alteration of the membrane function, *e.g.*, nystatin and amphotericin B.
3. Alteration of cell wall biosynthesis by inhibition of β (1,3)-glucan synthase, *e.g.*, caspofungin and micafungin.
4. Inhibition of ergosterol biosynthesis by inhibition of squalene epoxidase and/or accumulation of toxic sterol intermediates, *e.g.*, naftifine and terbinafine.
5. Inhibition of lanosterol demethylase in ergosterol biosynthesis, *e.g.*, imidazole, ketoconazole, fluconazole, and itraconazole.

First-line therapy for pityriasis versicolor is mostly composed of topical selenium sulfide and zinc pyrithione as well as topical azoles (*e.g.*, ketoconazole, clotrimazole, and econazole), terbinafine, and ciclopirox [35, 36]. Oral therapy (fluconazole and itraconazole) is restricted for patients with refractory disease, widespread disease, or those untreatable with topical regimens. Generally, the duration of effective treatment ranges from a few days to a few weeks [35, 37].

Principal treatment of dermatophytosis aims to relieve clinical symptoms, reduce the opportunity for secondary bacterial infection, and inhibit the expansion of the infection to other areas. Dermatophytosis treatment normally begins with topical therapy using azoles, allylamines, butenafine, ciclopirox, tolnaftate, or amorolfine for topical infection. However, patients with widespread infection are required to start treatment with oral antifungal therapy using terbinafine, itraconazole, fluconazole, or griseofulvin [38, 39].

Candida infections are normally treated with antifungal agents in four classes, including flucytosine, azoles (fluconazole, itraconazole, voriconazole, and posaconazole), echinocandins (caspofungin, anidulafungin, and micafungin), and polyenes (amphotericin B). For skin infection and paronychia, topical azole and polyene are the drugs of choice. In the treatment of onychomycosis, oral treatment with itraconazole or terbinafine is preferred as the first-line drug, and griseofulvin is also used as an alternative antifungal drug [40 - 42].

TARGETING FOR NOVEL DRUG THERAPY AGAINST SUPERFICIAL MYCOSES

Treatment of superficial mycoses with antifungal medications has been developed since the 1960s [7]. Although several antifungal agents for superficial mycoses, particularly topical agents, have been discovered, there is still a limited amount of efficacious antifungal agents due to mutation and the emergence of a pathogenic fungus with antifungal resistance. Novel antifungal agents that act on different targets other than those of the conventional natural products, historically and at the moment, continues to play an important role in drug discovery due to their unique and special features when compared to conventional synthetic drugs. Several natural products have exhibited excellent antifungal activity, *in vitro* and *in vivo*. According to recent studies on fungal architecture, genomics, as well as life cycles, the targets of novel antifungal agents may involve disturbing fungal cellular integrity (*e.g.*, cell wall and cell membrane), metabolic pathways (*e.g.*, glyoxylate cycle, pyrimidine biosynthesis, and acetate metabolism), signal transduction pathways (*e.g.*, MAP kinase, PDK1, and calcium signaling), and gene expression (*e.g.*, transcription factors). These promising targets may open up new opportunities for developing novel antifungal drugs with better efficacy for the treatment of superficial mycoses [43 - 45].

HERBAL PRODUCTS WITH ANTIFUNGAL EFFECTS

Currently, herbal products in the form of crude extracts, active compounds enriched fractions, or pure phytochemicals have been increasingly studied for antifungal activity, *in vitro* and *in vivo*. Also, various evaluation methods have been developed for the determination of antifungal activity. Assessment of antifungal activity can be performed using an approach as simple as adding the samples to come into direct contact with pathogenic fungi. The popular methods are agar dilution, disk diffusion, bio-autography, and dilution tests as well as evaluation of efficacy in animal models [46, 47]. Examples of herbal products with antifungal effects are summarized in Table **1**. Some highlighted information about each herbal product is provided in alphabetical order below.

Table 1. Plant extracts and phytochemicals potentially used for the treatment of superficial mycoses.

Plant Name	Family	Tested Compounds	Expected Active Compounds	Activity/Mechanism of Action
Allium sativum	Amaryllidaceae	Bulb extract	Allicin	Effective against *M. furfur*, *Candida* spp., and dermatophyte by damaging organelles and disruption of genes expression
Aloe vera	Asphodelaceae (Liliaceae)	Leaf, root, and fruit extract	Polysaccharides, glycoproteins, phenolic compounds, salicylic acid, lignin, hormones, amino acids, vitamins, and saponins	Effective against *A. niger, C. albicans, F. oxysporum,* and clotrimazole-resistant *M. furfur*
		Aloin and aloe-emodin	-	Effective against *C. gloeosporioides* and *C. cucumerinum*
Alpinia galanga	Zingiberaceae	Rhizome extract	(2,6-dimethylphenyl) borate	Effective against *M. furfur*, *Candida* spp., and dermatophyte by induced to alter morphological of fungal cell size and shape, exerted massive vacuoles in yeast form, and suppressed the development of hyphae
Annona squamosa	Annonaceae	Leaf extract	Ephedradine A, ergosine, Ia, mudanpioside H, and trichosanic acid	Effective against *A. alternata, C. albicans, F. solani, M. canis,* and *A. niger*
Camellia sinensis	Theaceae	Extract	Catechins	Effective against *Candida* spp., *M. persicolor, T. mentagrophytes* by damaging cell membrane and inducing rapid leakage of small molecules entrapped in the intra liposomal space and aggregation of the liposomes

(Table 1) cont.....

Plant Name	Family	Tested Compounds	Expected Active Compounds	Activity/Mechanism of Action
Cinnamomum cassia	Lauraceae	Essential oil	Cinnamaldehyde	Effective against *M. pachydermatis, Candida* spp., *R. mucilaginosa,* and dermatophyte by disruption of plasma membrane ATPase as well as sterol synthesis as well as inhibition of H$^+$-ATPase
Citrus bergamia	Rutaceae	Essential oil	Terpenes and phenolic compounds	Effective against *C. albicans* and dermatophyte by to degrading of the cell wall, disrupt the microbial cytoplasmic membrane
Curcuma longa	Zingiberaceae	Rhizome extract	Curcumin	Effective against *Candida* spp. by decrease activity of $\Delta^{5,6}$ desaturase (ERG3) enzyme that inducing reduction in ergosterol synthesis, production ROS, reduce proteinase secretion, disruption of membrane, and induction of intracellular acidification and inhibition of hyphae
		Curcuminoid extract	Curcumin	Effective against *Candida* spp., especially *C. albicans* and *C. dubliniensis*
		Essential oil	Turmerone, atlantone, and zingiberone	Effective against dermatophyte
		Curcumin	-	Effective against *Candida* spp. especially *P. brasilensis*

(Table 1) cont.....

Plant Name	Family	Tested Compounds	Expected Active Compounds	Activity/Mechanism of Action
Cymbopogon citratus	Poaceae	Essential oil	Citral	Effective against *Candida* spp. and dermatophyte by disrupting fungal cell membrane, transforming its fluidity and permeability, interruption of ergosterol, DNA, and RNA synthesis or interfering with cellular respiration
Impatiens balsamina	Balsaminaceae	Stem and leaf extract	Lawsone, lawsone methyl ether, and methylene-3,3′-bilawsone	Effective against *P. italicum, P. digitatum, A. niger, A. oryzae, C. utilis* and dermatophyte by disintegration of cell wall, increase cell membrane permeability, promotes ROS production, inhibit ATG1 and ATG8 genes
Jasminum sambac	Oleaceae	Flower and leaf extract and	Sambacin, saponin, flavanoid and tanin	Effective against *Malassezia* spp. and *Candida* spp. damage to the microbial cell wall and flavonoid may link with denaturation of microbial cell proteins that can cause cell death
Rhinacanthus nasutus	Acanthaceae	Leaf extract	Rhinacanthins-C, -D, and -N	Effective against dermatophyte and *Malassezia* spp. by disruption intracellular signaling through G-proteins signaling and cell wall integrity pathway
		Rhinacanthins-C, -D, and -N	-	Effective against dermatophyte

(Table 1) cont.....

Plant Name	Family	Tested Compounds	Expected Active Compounds	Activity/Mechanism of Action
Sapindus emarginatus	Sapindaceae	Pericarp extract	3-O-(4-acetyl-β-D-xylopyranosyl)-(1→3)-α-L-rhamnopyranosyl-(1→2)-α-L-arabinopyranosyl-hederagenin and 3-O-(3,4-di-acet-1-β-D-xylopyranosyl)-(1→3)-α-L-rhamnopyranosyl-(1→2)-α- L-arabynopyranosyl-hederagenin	Effective against *Candida* spp. and dermatophyte by destroying the structural of fungal cell membrane and showed anti-biofilm forming activity
Senna alata	Fabaceae (Leguminosae)	Flower and leaf extract	Anthraquinone	Effective against *A. niger, G. candidum, C. utilis, A. brevipes, Penicillium* spp., dermatophyte by damaging cell membrane and cell wall as well as inhibit hyphae and macroconidia growth
		Anthraquinone-rich *S. alata*, aloe-emodin, rhein, emodin, chrysophanol	-	Effective against dermatophyte including *T. rubrum, T. mentagrophytes* and *M. gypseum*
Zingiber officinale	Zingiberaceae	Rhizome extract	Phenolic compounds such as gingerols, shogaols, and paradols	Effective against *Candida spp.* and dermatophyte
		Essential oil	Monoterpenes and sesquiterpenes, *e.g.,* eudesmol, γ-terpinene, and ar-curcumene	Effective against *Malassezia* spp. and some yeast molds by alter the permeability and fluidity of fungal plasma

Allium Sativum

Allium sativum or garlic, a bulbous perennial of the Amaryllidaceae family, is consumed worldwide as food and traditional medicine, especially for antimicrobial purposes. Based on antifungal screening using the disc diffusion method, fresh garlic juice (15 µl/disc) exhibited antifungal activity against *Aspergillus niger* and *Candida albicans*, with the inhibition zones of 41 and 28 mm, respectively [48]. The alcoholic extract inhibited dermatophytes, namely *Trichophyton mentagrophytes, T. rubrum, T. verrucosum, Microsporum gypseum* and *Epidermophyton floccosum*, with the inhibition zones of between 4.5-30.7 mm [49]. In addition, aqueous extracts of *A. sativum* exhibited potent antifungal activities against *Malassezia furfur, C. albicans*, and other *Candida* spp. (*C. glabrata, C. tropicalis, C. parapsilosis*), and dermatophyte species (*T. mentagrophytes, T. rubrum, M. gypseum, M. canis,* and *E. floccosum*) with the MIC values of 0.004-0.5, 0.016-2.0, 0.016-1.0, and 0.002-0.5 µg/ml, respectively

[50]. A study on mechanism of action found that garlic oil might have the ability to penetrate through cellular and organelle membranes and then damage organelles, which causes cell death. Garlic oil also links with the disruption of gene expression, mainly in 19KEGG pathways, crucial pathways that involve cell viability [51].

Allicin (Fig. **1**), a major sulfur-containing constituent of garlic, has been demonstrated as a key active compound contributing to the antifungal activity of garlic by drown regulation of gene expression for proteins involved in DNA replication, mitochondrial translation and chromatids cohesion, which results in interruption of cell cycle, growth and viability of yeast cells and lead to cell death [52].

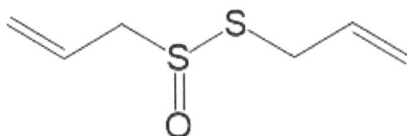

Fig. (1). Chemical structure of allicin.

Aloe Vera

Aloe vera (*A. barbadensis*) belongs to the Asphodelaceae (Liliaceae) family. *A. vera* grows in the dry regions of the world, including Asia, Africa, Europe, and America. Based on a well-diffusion assay, antifungal effect of the alcoholic extract of *A. vera* leaf was demonstrated against *Aspergillus niger*, but without any effect against *C. albicans* [53]. In contrast, some studies showed that *A. vera* gel exhibited antifungal activity against *C. albicans* as well as anti-biofilm forming activity at high concentrations [54]. According to data from disc diffusion assay, ethanol extract of *A. vera* leaves and roots (25-30 µl/disc) exhibited antifungal effects against *Fusarium oxysporum* and *A. niger* [55], while *A. vera* leaf extract (1 mg/disc) showed an inhibitory effect against *C. albicans* [56]. *A. vera* leaf extract also showed a notable effect toward clotrimazole-resistant *M. furfur*, with an MIC of 512 µl/ml [57]. Two anthraquinones, namely aloin and aloe-emodin, were identified as active principles against *Colletotrichum gloeosporioides* and *Cladosporium cucumerinum* [58].

Most antifungal investigations of *A. vera* were screening studies. Therefore, it is necessary to perform further studies to clarify its potency, active constituents, and mechanism of action before its clinical applications.

Alpinia Galanga

Alpinia galanga, an herbal plant in the Zingiberaceae family, was reported for its antifungal property. *A. galanga* alcoholic extract exhibited good anti-*Candida* activity against *C. glabrata* and *C. tropicalis*, with the same MIC of 64 µg/ml [59]. The ethanolic extract also inhibited the growth of *C. albicans*, *T. mentagrophytes*, *M. gypseum*, and *M. canis*, with IC_{50} values of 53.3, 45.3, 32.0, and 26.0 mg/ml, respectively [60]. In addition, hexane extract of *A. galanga* inhibited *M. furfur* with the MIC values of 40-80 µg/ml and MFC values of 40-160 µg/ml [61]. Based on GC-MS analysis, the major component of the active fraction obtained from the hexane extract was identified as (2,6-dimethylphenyl) borate (Fig. **2**) with a trace amount of 1,8-cineol and hydrocarbons. The antifungal mechanisms of *A. galanga* extract may involve alteration of fungal cell morphology (size and shape), exertion of massive vacuoles in yeast form, and suppression of hyphae development [61].

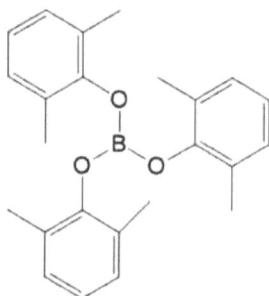

Fig. (2). Chemical structure of (2,6-dimethylphenyl)borate.

Annona Squamosa

Annona squamosa or custard apple, is a shrub or small tree from the Annonaceae family that is commonly found in tropical areas worldwide. The extracts from *A. squamosa* leaves have been reported to possess antifungal activity. The chloroform extract exhibited a strong antifungal effect against *Alternaria alternata*, *C. albicans*, and *Fusarium solani*, with the MIC values of 200, 600, and 300 µg/ml, respectively. Meanwhile, the methanol extract exhibited the most potent activity against *M. canis* and *A. niger*, with the same MIC of 400 µg/ml. In contrast, the aqueous extract did not show any antifungal effect [62]. Therefore, the documented reports implied that the antifungal active component of *A. squamosa* leaves is mostly hydrophobic compounds.

Recently, it has been reported that *A. niger* was identified as an endophytic fungus from *A. squamosa* leaves, and five antibacterial compounds, namely ephedradine A, ergosine, Ia, mudanpioside H, and trichosanic acid, were identified from the endophyte by GC-MS/MS method [63]. This implies that secondary metabolites produced from endophytic fungi may play an important role in the antibacterial effect of *A. squamosa* leaves.

Camellia Sinensis

Camellia sinensis, generally known as tea, is a member of the Theaceae family. Tea plant contains several biologically active polyphenols, and has been reported to possess antifungal effect against pathogenic yeast and dermatophytes. Crude acetone extract of *C. sinensis* was active against *C. albicans, C. glabrata, C. tropicalis, C. krusei*, and *Microsporum persicolor*, with the MIC values of 5, 10, 45, 50, and 20 µg/ml, respectively, and also effective against *C. albicans, C. glabrata* and *C. tropicalis* as well as *M. persicolor, in vivo* [64]. In addition, *the aqueous extract of tea was active against T. mentagrophytes*, with an MIC of 3.1 mg/ml. It has been reported that catechins, a major polyphenol found in tea, contributed to its antimicrobial activity. Catechins (Fig. **3**) play an important role in antifungal activity by inducing rapid leakage of small molecules entrapped in the intra-liposomal space and aggregation of the liposomes. Furthermore, catechins also damage the cell membrane resulting in the destruction of conidia and hyphae of dermatophyte. Other than catechins, theaflavins, dimeric catechins and their gallates have been reported to possess antifungal effects that can alter fungal cell membranes [65].

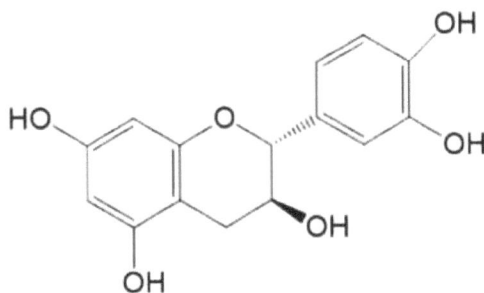

Fig. (3). Chemical structure of catechins.

Cinnamomum Cassia

Cinnamomum cassia, also called Chinese cassia or Chinese cinnamon, is an evergreen aromatic tree in the Lauraceae family. The plant originated in southern China and is currently widely distributed in many parts of South and Southeast Asia. Essential oil from *C. cassia* bark contains cinnamaldehyde (Fig. **4**) as a major active compound. Cinnamaldehyde has been reported to exhibit good antifungal activity against *Malassezia pachydermatis*, with an MIC of 2.5 µg/ml [66], and also inhibited fluconazole-resistant *Candida* spp. (*C. albicans, C.*

tropicalis, C. glabrata, C. krusei, and *C. guilliermodii*), with the MIC_{90} values of 100-500 µg/ml [67]. The essential oil of Chinese cinnamon with high content of cinnamaldehyde also showed a potent inhibitory effect against *Rhodotorula mucilaginosa,* displaying the MIC values of 8-125 µg/ml [68]. Cinnamaldehyde and the essential oil also inhibited *M. gypseum, T. rubrum,* and *T. mentagrophytes* with the MIC values of 19-28 and 25-38 µg/ml, respectively [69]. The antifungal mechanism of cinnamaldehyde may relate to the disruption of plasma membrane ATPase and sterol synthesis as well as inhibition of H^+-ATPase, leading to intracellular acidification [67].

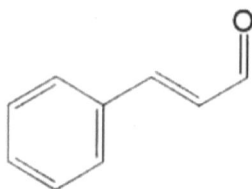

Fig. (4). Chemical structure of cinnamaldehyde.

Citrus Bergamia

Citrus bergamia or the bergamot orange, is a shrub from the Rutaceae family commercially grown in Europe. Its fruits and leaves contain many phytochemicals, including flavonoids and alkaloids. *C. bergamia* oil is a potent antifungal agent due to its great antifungal activity against dermatophytes and yeasts. Bergamot oil inhibited *T. mentagrophytes* (MIC of 0.08-0.16% v/v), *T. rubrum* (MIC of 0.16-0.62% v/v), *T. interdigitale* (MIC of 0.08-0.31% v/v), *T. tonsurans* (MIC of 1.25% v/v), *M. canis* (MIC of 0.08-0.62% v/v), *M. gypseum* (MIC of 1.25% v/v), and *E. floccosum* (MIC of 1.25% v/v) [70], and also inhibited *Candida* spp., including *C. albicans, C. glabrata, C. krusei, C. tropicalis, and C. parapsllosis* with the MIC values of 0.31-2.5%v/v. Normally, citrus essential oil consists of many volatile compounds. It has been suggested that terpenes and phenolic compounds are able to degrade the cell wall and disrupt the microbial cytoplasmic membrane resulting in loss of the membrane impermeability and cell death [71].

Curcuma Longa

Curcuma longa, commonly known as turmeric, is a perennial herb belonging to the Zingiberaceae family. *C. longa* extract composed of three major active compounds, including curcumin, demethoxycurcumin and bisdemeth oxycurcumin. Methanol extract of turmeric has been reported to inhibit the growth of *Cryptococcus neoformans* and *C. albicans,* with the MIC values of 128 and 256 µg/ml, respectively [72], while turmeric oil containing turmerone, atlantone, and zingiberone inhibited dermatophytes, including *M. gypseum, E. flocćosum, T. mentagrophyte*, and *T. rubrum*, with the MIC values of 460, 230, 230-919, and 230-919 µg/ml, respectively. In contrast, crude curcumin extract was not active against dermatophytes [73]. However, it has been reported that curcumin exhibited potent antifungal activity against *Candida* species, especially *C. albicans* and *C. dubliniensis*, with the MIC values of 32-64 µg/ml [74]. *In vivo* study using guinea pigs indicated that turmeric oil greatly improved lesions, including erythema and scale caused by *T. rubrum*, and the lesion disappeared within 6-7 days [72].

The antifungal mechanism of curcumin (Fig. **5**) was found to be *via* the suppression of $\Delta^{5,6}$ desaturase (ERG3) enzyme activity, which inhibits the synthesis of ergosterol required for the accumulation of biosynthetic precursors of ergosterol and production ROS that led to cell death in last step [75]. Another possible pathway of curcumin is a reduction of proteinase secretion and disruption of membrane-associated properties of ATPase activity [76]. In addition, induction of intracellular acidification and inhibition of hyphae *via* the global suppressor thymidine uptake 1 (TUP1) are possible processes involved in its antifungal activity [72].

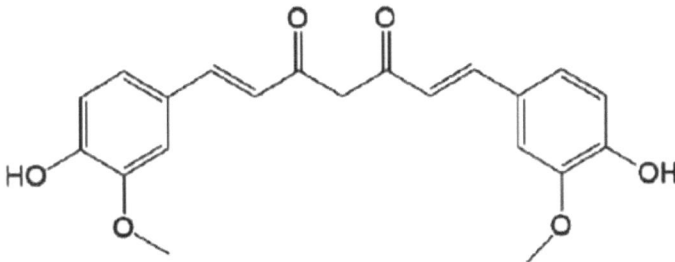

Fig. (5). Chemical structure of curcumin.

Cymbopogon Citratus

Cymbopogon citratus or lemon grass, is a perennial grass in the Poaceae family, which is distributed in many tropical countries, especially in Southeast Asia. Essential oil of lemon grass mainly contains geranial (*trans*-citral, citral A), neral (*cis*-citral, citral B), *cis*-geraniol, lavandulyl acetate, and caryophyllene. Citral (Fig. **6**), a mixture of geranial and neral, is a notable promising antifungal agent. The essential oil exhibited antifungal activity against *C. tropicalis*, with the MICs and MFCs of 1-4 µl/ml. The essential oil at sub-MIC values (0.125-0.25 MIC) also inhibited the biofilm formation of *C. tropicalis* [77]. Based on the disc diffusion method, citral (2 µl) showed a great inhibitory effect against *C. albicans, C. glabrata, C. krusei*, and *C. parapsilosis* [78]. *In vivo* study using guinea pigs indicated that the essential oil effectively cured ringworm caused by *T. rubrum* and *M. gypseum* [79]. Generally, the antifungal mechanism of most essential oils is related to disrupting fungal cell membranes, transforming their fluidity and permeability, interrupting ergosterol, DNA, and RNA synthesis, or interfering with cellular respiration [44].

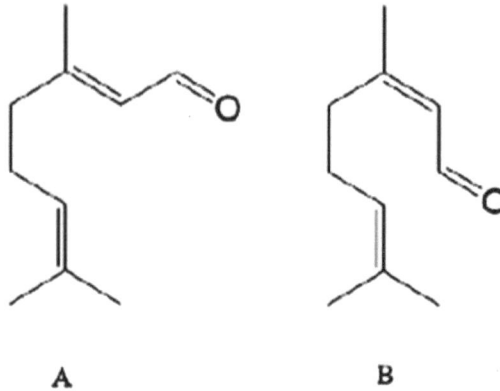

A   **B**

Fig. (6). Chemical structures of citral: geranial (**A**) and neral (**B**).

Impatiens Balsamina

Impatiens balsamina, also known as rose balsam or garden balsam, is an annual herb in the Balsaminaceae family. Several parts of this plant, including the leaf, flower, and stem, are used as traditional therapies for skin infectious diseases. The stem extract of *I. balsamina* containing high concentrations of phenolic and flavonoid compounds exhibited antifungal activity against various molds (*Penicillium italicum, P. digitatum, Aspergillus niger, A. oryzae*) and yeast, with the MIC values of 250-500 and 500 μg/ml, respectively [80]. Similarly, the leaf extracts of *I. balsamina* exhibited potent antifungal activity against dermatophytes and yeasts. Three naphthoquinones, namely lawsone, lawsone methyl ether, and methylene-3,3'-bilawsone (Fig. **7**) have been identified as the major bioactive compounds in the leaves. However, only lawsone and lawsone methyl ether exhibited antifungal activity against *T. rubrum, T. mentagrophytes*, and *M. gypseum* and *C. albicans*. Comparatively, lawsone methyl ether was the more potent antifungal agent against dermatophytes and yeasts, with the MIC and MFC values of 4-23 and 8-23 μg/ml, respectively, while lawsone was only active against dermatophytes with the MICs and MFCs of 62-250 and 125-250 μg/ml, respectively [81].

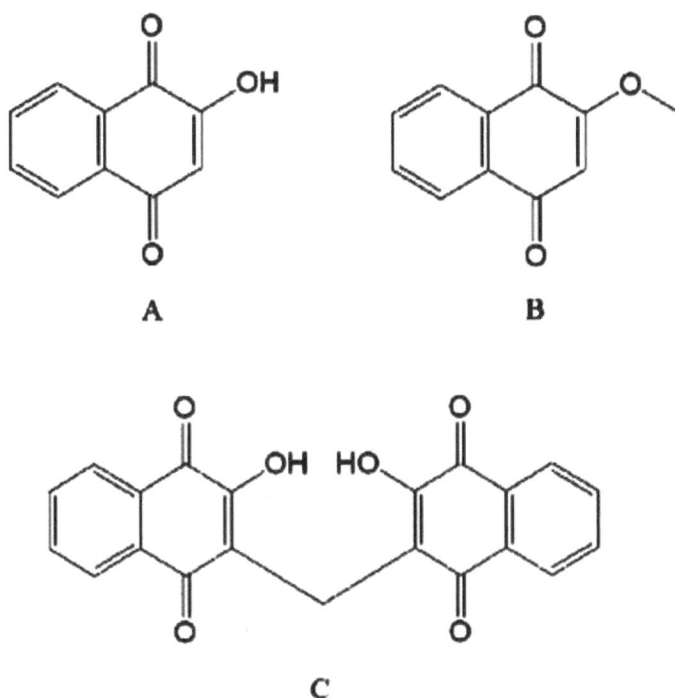

Fig. (7). Chemical structures of lawsone (**A**), lawsone methyl ether (**B**), and methylene-3,3'-bilawsone (**C**).

The antifungal mechanisms of lawsone were related to the disintegration of the cell wall and increased cell membrane permeability, leading to cell death. In addition, lawsone enhanced ROS production and induced the loss of viability and germination capacity of fungi. Lawsone also induced ATG1 and ATG8 gene expression, which are important for autophagy induction and autophagosome assembly. This implied that lawsone may inhibit the expression of some vital proteins leading to cell death through autophagy-related pathways [82].

Jasminum Sambac

Jasminum sambac, a small shrub belonging to the Oleaceae family, is native to tropical Asia. The most outstanding part of *J. sambac* is its attractive fragrant flowers. The flower and leaf extracts of *J. sambac* have been reported to possess antifungal activity. Methanol extract and essential oil from the flowers of *J. sambac* exhibited antifungal effect against *Malassezia* spp., including *M. sympodialis*, *M. dermatitis*, *M. furfur* and non-*Malassezia* species with the MIC values of 80-160 mg/ml for the methanol extract and 50-75% for the essential oil. The promising antifungal constituents in the methanol extract are mainly related to tannin and sambacin (Fig. **8**). In addition, α-farnesene, benzyl acetate, and linalool (Fig. **8**) may play an important role in the antifungal activity of *J. sambac* essential oil [83]. Furthermore, the methanol extract of *J. sambac* leaves exhibited inhibitory effect against *C. albicans*, with an MIC value of 25 mg/ml. Phytochemical screening of the methanol extract revealed the presence of alkaloids, flavonoids, glycosides, steroids, tannins, terpenoids and saponins [84]. Regarding the mechanism of action of *J. sambac*, saponin and tannin may damage the fungal cell wall, while flavonoid may act on denaturation of microbial cell proteins diminishing the cell viability [85].

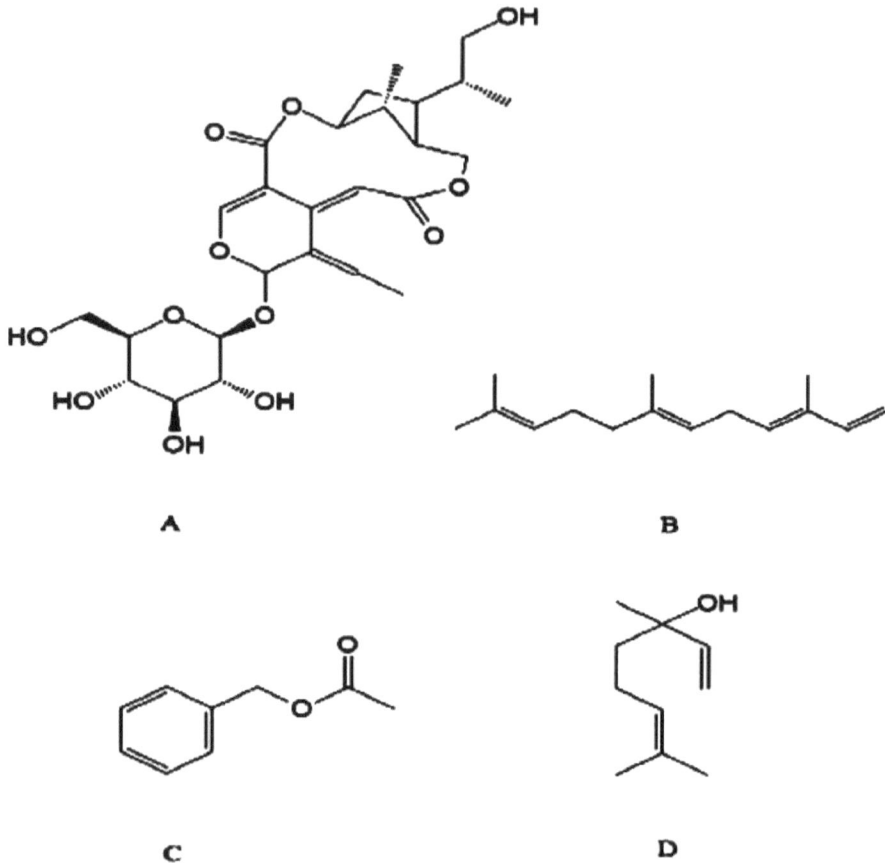

Fig. (8). Chemical structures of sambacin (**A**), α-farnesene (**B**), benzyl acetate (**C**), and linalool (**D**).

Rhinacanthus Nasutus

Rhinacanthus nasutus, a medical herb from the Acanthaceae family, is native to Southeast Asia. The plant has been used as traditional medicine for the treatment of skin diseases, including superficial mycoses. It has been reported that the naphthoquinone ester, namely rhinacanthin-C, -D and -N (Fig. **9**), mostly found in leaves and roots of *R. nasutus*, exhibited potent antifungal activity. In addition, rhinacanthin-rich extract that was prepared by fractionation of crude ethyl acetate extract of *R. nasutus* leaves using an anion exchange chromatography exhibited equivalent antifungal activity as the pure rhinacanthins against *T. rubrum, T. mentagrophytes*, and *M. gypseum* with the MIC values of 7.5, 31.2, and 125.0 µg/ml, respectively [86]. This may be due to synergistic effect of rhinacanthins in the rhinacanthins-rich extract. *R. nasutus* leaf extract prepared by extraction with a solution of 50% v/v propylene glycol in DMSO exhibited excellent antifungal activity against *M. furfur* and *M. globose* with an MIC of 25 µg/ml [87]. However, *R. nasutus* leaf extract containing rhinacanthin-C, -D and -N (71.1, 8.8 and 2.6% w/w) was not active against *C. albicans* at concentrations as high as 2,000 µg/ml [88].

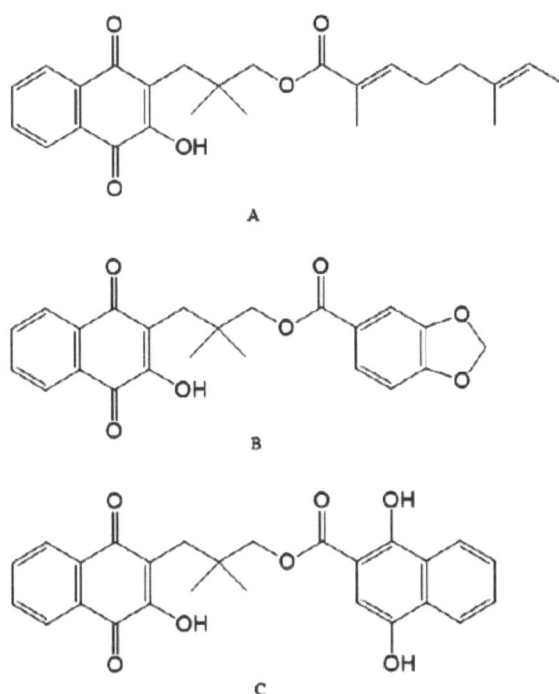

Fig. (9). Chemical structures of rhinacanthin C (**A**), rhinacanthin D (**B**), and rhinacanthin N (**C**).

Recently, three protein fractions (≤10, 10-30, and ≥30 kDa fractions) obtained from *R. nasutus* have been reported to inhibit *Talaromyces marneffei*, with the MIC values of 32-128 µg/ml. Regarding the mechanism of inhibition, the antifungal activity of the 10-30 kDa fraction was related to its effect on the G-proteins signaling pathway. Antifungal proteins from *R. nasutus* might be a source for novel antifungal drug development [89].

Sapindus Emarginatus

Sapindus emarginatus, an evergreen tree in the Sapindaceae family, is commonly known as a source of saponins used for medicinal purposes. A saponin-rich extract prepared from *S. emarginatus* pericarps has been demonstrated to inhibit *C. albicans*, *T. rubrum*, and *E. floccosum* with the MIC values of 7.8, 15.6, and 62.5 mg/ml, respectively [90]. In addition, *n*-butanol extract of *S. emarginatus* pericarps inhibited *C. albicans*, *C. glabrata*, *C. parapsilosis*, *C. tropicalis* with the MIC and MFC values of 300-600 µg/ml. Two saponins isolated from *S. emarginatus*, namely pyranosyl-(1→2)-α-L-arabinopyranosyl-hederagenin and 3-O-(3,4-di-acetyl-β-D-xylopyranosyl) -(1→3)-α-L-rhamnopyranosyl-(1→2)-α-L-arabynopyranosyl-hederagenin (Fig. **10**) inhibited *C. parapsilosis* with the MIC values of 70 and 250 µg/ml, respectively [91]. Although the exact antifungal mechanisms of *S. emarginatus* have not been clearly identified yet, some studies have shown that the fungicidal effect of plant saponin may relate to fungal cell membrane alteration and anti-biofilm forming activity [92, 93].

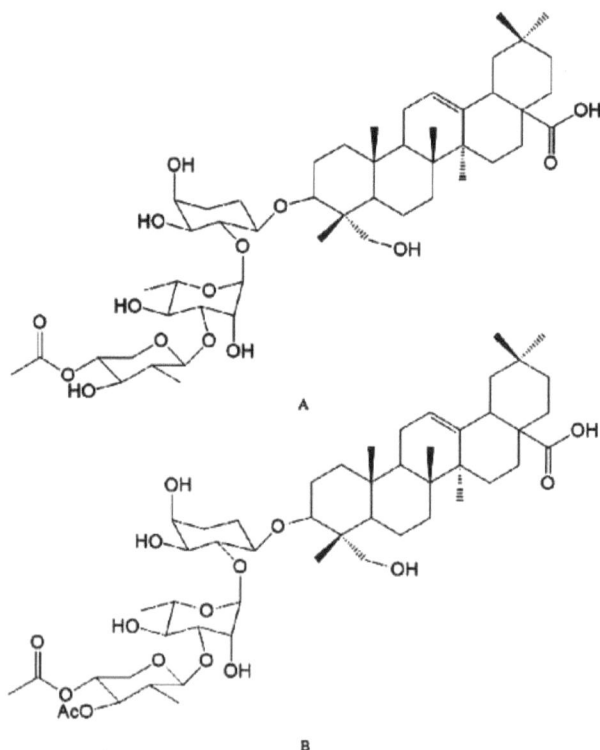

Fig. (10). Chemical structures of 3-O-(4-acetyl-β-D-xylopyranosyl)-(1→3)-α-Lrhamnopyrano-yl-(1→2)-α-L-arabinopyranosyl-hederagenin (**A**) and 3-O-(3,4-di-acetyl-β -D-xylopyranosyl)-(1→3)-α- L-rhamnopyranosyl -(1→2)-α-L-arabynopyranosyl -hederagenin (**B**).

Senna Alata

Senna alata is a shrub to small tree of the Fabaceae or Leguminosae family, and is normally found in tropical and humid regions. Ringworm bush is another name for *S. alata* due to its traditional use for treating ringworm. An extract from *S. alata* flowers exhibited antifungal effect against *Aspergillus niger* (MIC; 1.25-5 mg/ml), *A. brevipes* (MIC; 1.25-2.5 mg/ml), *Geotricum candidum* (MIC; 1.25-2.5 mg/ml), *Candida utilis* (MIC; 1.25-2.5 mg/ml), and *Penicillium* spp. (MIC; 0.31-2.5 mg/ml) [94]. Anthraquinone isolated from *S. alata*, including rhein, emodin, aloe-emodin and chrysophanol, has been reported to possess antimicrobial activity. Anthraquinone fraction obtained from *S. alata* leaf extract also showed outstanding antifungal effect against clinical strains of dermatophytes, including *T. rubrum*, *T. mentagrophytes*, *E. floccosum*, and *M. gypseum*, with the MIC values of 0.2, 0.3, 0.1, 0.3 mg/ml, respectively [95].

To improve the potency of the antifungal activity of *S. alata* leaf extracts, the anthraquinone content of the extracts needs to be increased. An anthraquinone-rich *S. alata* extract was prepared and standardized to contain total anthraquinone content of 16% w/w. Antifungal activity evaluation of the anthraquinone-rich *S. alata* extracts and the standard anthraquinones, aloe-emodin, rhein, emodin, and chrysophanol (Fig. **11**) against *T. rubrum, T. mentagrophytes* and *M. gypseum* revealed that the extract inhibited the growth of all tested dermatophytes (MIC values of 15.6 - 250 µg/ml), with the highest antifungal effect against *T. rubrum* (MIC of 15.6 µg/ml). All tested dermatophytes were also completely inhibited by emodin and rhein at concentrations between 2-1000 and 31.2-1000 µg/ml, respectively. Aloe-emodin exhibited the strongest antifungal activity against *T. rubrum* with an MIC of 1.0 µg/ml, but was not active against *T. mentagrophytes* and *M. gypseum* at the concentration of 1,000 µg/ml. In contrast, chrysophanol was not active against all tested dermatophytes at concentrations up to 1,000 µg/ml. Although the antifungal activity of the anthraquinone-rich extract against *T. rubrum* was lower than that of aloe-emodin and emodin, its antifungal activities against *T. mentagrophytes* and *M. gypseum* were markedly higher than those of aloe-emodin and emodin. This is probably due to the synergistic effect of anthraquinones in the extract [96]. The putative antifungal mechanisms of *S. alata* extracts may be related to the induction of cell fluid leaks by damaging cell membrane and cell wall [97, 98]. In addition, inhibition of hyphae and macroconidia growth are other plausible mechanisms of action [98].

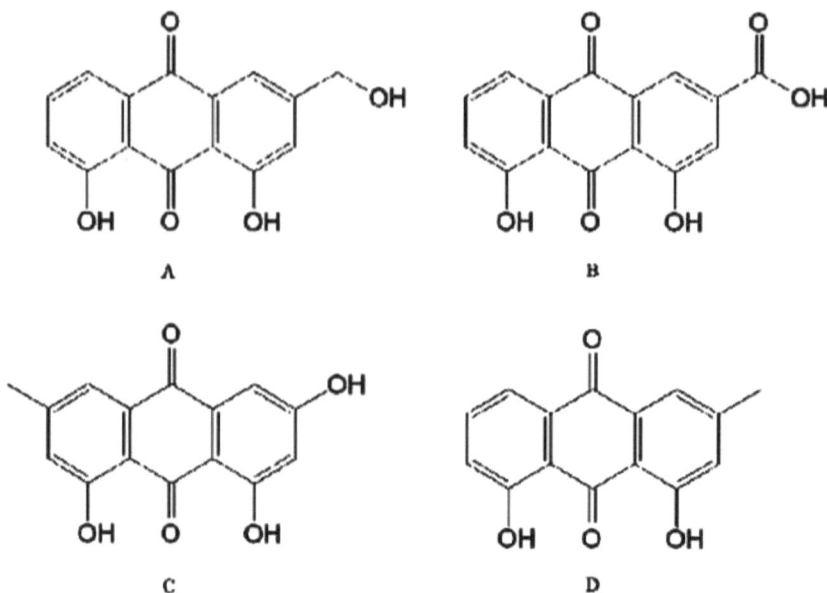

Fig. (11). Chemical structures of aloe-emodin (**A**), rhein (**B**), emodin (**C**), and chrysophanol (**D**).

Zingiber Officinale

Zingiber officinale or ginger, is a perennial herb and a member of the Zingiberaceae family. Rhizome of *Z. officinale* is widely used as a folk medicine due to its various bioactive compounds, including monoterpenes and sesquiterpenes, as well as phenolic compounds, such as gingerols, shogaols and paradols [99]. The ethanol extract of ginger rhizome was found to possess antifungal activity against *T. mentagrophytes* (MIC: 64 µg/ml; MFC: 512 µg/ml), *M. gypseum* (MIC: 128 µg/ml; MFC: 1024 µg/ml), *C. albicans* (MIC: 5 mg/ml) and *C. krusei* (MIC: 10 mg/ml) as well as anti-biofilm formation against *Candida* spp. [100]. Moreover, the essential oil of ginger strongly inhibited *M. furfur* growth, with an MIC of 0.03 µl/ml as well as some yeasts and molds [101, 102]. The antifungal effect of *Z. officinale* may be attributed to its phytochemical constituents, including monoterpenes and sesquiterpenes, of which the most abundant were identified as eudesmol, γ-terpinene, and ar-curcumene. These compounds may alter the permeability and fluidity of fungal plasma membrane [102].

PATENTS OF HERBAL AND PHYTOCHEMICAL PRODUCTS AGAINST SUPERFICIAL MYCOSES

Nowadays, many antifungal herbal products are popularly available in markets worldwide. As documented by the United States Patent and Trademark Office

(USPTO) and the Department of Intellectual Property (DIP) of Thailand, various innovative antifungal products made from herbal extracts have been patented, as shown in Table **2**.

Table **2**. Patents of herbal products for the treatment of superficial mycoses.

Patent No.	Description of Invention	References
10,406,193 (US patent)	A composition for topical application with antifungal activity, containing *Melaleuca alternifolia* essential oil, oregano essential oil, lime essential oil and an ester of vitamin E.	[103]
8,449,926 (US patent)	A composition made of selective mixtures of origanum oil, menthol, and Atlantic cedarwood oil, thuja oil, cedarwood oil, cinnamon oil, clove oil, cumin oil, fennel oil, peppermint oil, or rosemary oil, which provides antimicrobial activity for use as a topical anti-fungal agent.	[104]
10,646,525 (US patent)	Herbal composition consisted of *Curcuma longa* and other ingredient for treatment and management of infectious disease including fungal infection.	[105]
9,474,723 (US patent)	The invention pertains to an anti-microbial, in particular anti-fungal composition comprising cinnamaldehyde, *trans*-2-methoxy cinnamaldehyde, cinnamyl acetate and linalool.	[106]
11,116,813 (US patent)	The garlic extract comprises equal to or greater than 0.5% (w/w) polyphenol and/or 0.5% (w/w) allicin to be used as an antimicrobial agent.	[107]
2156 (Thai patent)	Herbal soap that consists of *Curcuma longa, Aloe vera, Senna alata,* other ingredient for treatment of tinea versicolor, dermatophytosis, and other skin diseases.	[108]
13324 (Thai patent)	Gel formulation of *Rhinacanthus nasutus* root extract for treatment of superficial mycoses.	[109]

CONCLUSION

Fungal infections of superficial areas are a common global problem. The availability of effective and safe medicinal treatment options has been limited due to the increasing incidence of resistance by pathogenic fungi to conventional medications. Therefore, alternative treatment options from herbal medicines present an attractive choice due to several beneficial therapeutic attributes. There are numerous herbal extracts and phytochemicals with demonstrable antifungal effectiveness against broad-spectrum pathogenic fungi causing superficial mycoses, including *Candida* spp., *Malassezia* spp., and dermatophytes. However, more comprehensive and thorough studies, including *in vitro*, *in vivo*, and most importantly, clinical trials, are needed to fully support the efficacy and safety of these herbal extracts and phytochemicals prior to their clinical application as practical alternatives for the treatment of superficial mycoses.

ACKNOWLEDGEMENTS

The authors wish to thank Dr. Fredrick Eze for assistance with English editing.

REFERENCES

[1]   Hernandez H, Martinez LR. Relationship of environmental disturbances and the infectious potential of fungi. Microbiology (Reading) 2018; 164(3): 233-41.
        [http://dx.doi.org/10.1099/mic.0.000620] [PMID: 29458659]

[2]   Chang CC, Levitz SM. Fungal immunology in clinical practice: Magical realism or practical reality? Med Mycol 2019; 57 (Suppl. 3): S294-306.
        [http://dx.doi.org/10.1093/mmy/myy165] [PMID: 31292656]

[3]   Goranov AI, Madhani HD. Functional profiling of human fungal pathogen genomes. Cold Spring Harb Perspect Med 2015; 5(3): a019596.
        [http://dx.doi.org/10.1101/cshperspect.a019596] [PMID: 25377143]

[4]   Bitew A. Dermatophytosis: prevalence of dermatophytes and non-dermatophyte fungi from patients attending Arsho advanced medical laboratory, Addis Ababa, Ethiopia. Dermatol Res Pract 2018; 2018: 1-6.
        [http://dx.doi.org/10.1155/2018/8164757] [PMID: 30402089]

[5]   Sharma B, Nonzom S. Superficial mycoses, a matter of concern: Global and Indian scenario-an updated analysis. Mycoses 2021; 64(8): 890-908.
        [http://dx.doi.org/10.1111/myc.13264] [PMID: 33665915]

[6]   Dias MFRG, Quaresma-Santos MVP, Bernardes-Filho F, Amorim AGF, Schechtman RC, Azulay DR. Update on therapy for superficial mycoses: review article part I. An Bras Dermatol 2013; 88(5): 764-74.
        [http://dx.doi.org/10.1590/abd1806-4841.20131996] [PMID: 24173183]

[7]   Dias MFRG, Bernardes-Filho F, Quaresma-Santos MVP, Amorim AGF, Schechtman RC, Azulay DR. Treatment of superficial mycoses: review - part II. An Bras Dermatol 2013; 88(6): 937-44.
        [http://dx.doi.org/10.1590/abd1806-4841.20132018] [PMID: 24474103]

[8]   Wiederhold N. Antifungal resistance: current trends and future strategies to combat. Infect Drug Resist 2017; 10: 249-59.
        [http://dx.doi.org/10.2147/IDR.S124918] [PMID: 28919789]

[9]   Rex J, Muthukumar N, Selvakumar P. Phytochemicals as a potential source for anti-microbial, anti-oxidant and wound healing-a review. MOJ Biorg Org Chem 2018; 2(2): 61-70.

[10]   Hay R. Superficial fungal infections. Medicine (Abingdon) 2013; 41(12): 716-8.
        [http://dx.doi.org/10.1016/j.mpmed.2013.09.011]

[11]   Gaitanis G, Magiatis P, Hantschke M, Bassukas ID, Velegraki A. The *Malassezia* genus in skin and systemic diseases. Clin Microbiol Rev 2012; 25(1): 106-41.
        [http://dx.doi.org/10.1128/CMR.00021-11] [PMID: 22232373]

[12]   Faergemann J. Pityriasis versicolor. Semin Dermatol 1993; 12(4): 276-9.
        [PMID: 8312142]

[13]   Saunte DML, Gaitanis G, Hay RJ. *Malassezia*-associated skin diseases, the use of diagnostics and treatment. Front Cell Infect Microbiol 2020; 10: 112.
        [http://dx.doi.org/10.3389/fcimb.2020.00112] [PMID: 32266163]

[14]   Cohen BA, Ed. Pediatric dermatology. 4th ed. Amsterdam: Elsevier Inc 2013; pp. 68-100.
        [http://dx.doi.org/10.1016/B978-0-7234-3655-3.00003-5]

[15]   Kundu R, Garg A. Yeast infections: candidiasis, tinea (pityriasis) versicolor, and *Malassezia* (*Pityrosporum*) folliculitis. In: Wolff KGL, Katz SI, Gilchrest BA, Paller AS, Leffell DJ, Eds.

Fitzpatrick's dermatology in general medicine. 8th ed. New York: McGraw-Hill 2012; pp. 2298-07.

[16]   Pires CAA, Cruz NFS, Lobato AM, Sousa PO, Carneiro FRO, Mendes AMD. Clinical, epidemiological, and therapeutic profile of dermatophytosis. An Bras Dermatol 2014; 89(2): 259-64.
[http://dx.doi.org/10.1590/abd1806-4841.20142569] [PMID: 24770502]

[17]   Tainwala R, Sharma YK. Pathogenesis of dermatophytoses. Indian J Dermatol 2011; 56(3): 259-61.
[http://dx.doi.org/10.4103/0019-5154.82476] [PMID: 21772583]

[18]   Burstein VL, Beccacece I, Guasconi L, Mena CJ, Cervi L, Chiapello LS. Skin immunity to dermatophytes: from experimental infection models to human disease. Front Immunol 2020; 11: 605644.
[http://dx.doi.org/10.3389/fimmu.2020.605644] [PMID: 33343578]

[19]   Maza PK, Bonfim-Melo A, Padovan ACB, *et al. Candida albicans*: The ability to invade epithelial cells and survive under oxidative stress is unlinked to hyphal length. Front Microbiol 2017; 8: 1235.
[http://dx.doi.org/10.3389/fmicb.2017.01235] [PMID: 28769876]

[20]   Sheppard DC, Filler SG. Host cell invasion by medically important fungi. Cold Spring Harb Perspect Med 2015; 5(1): a019687.
[http://dx.doi.org/10.1101/cshperspect.a019687] [PMID: 25367974]

[21]   Khodadadi H, Zomorodian K, Nouraei H, *et al.* Prevalence of superficial-cutaneous fungal infections in Shiraz, Iran: A five-year retrospective study (2015–2019). J Clin Lab Anal 2021; 35(7): e23850.
[http://dx.doi.org/10.1002/jcla.23850] [PMID: 34028857]

[22]   Khadka S, Sherchand JB, Pokharel DB, *et al.* Clinicomycological characterization of superficial mycoses from a tertiary care hospital in Nepal. Dermatol Res Pract 2016; 2016: 1-7.
[http://dx.doi.org/10.1155/2016/9509705] [PMID: 28003819]

[23]   Magdum RJ, Gadgil S, Kulkarni S, Rajmane V, Patil S. Clinico mycological study of superficial mycoses. J Krishna Inst Medical Sci 2016; 5: 37-44.

[24]   De Luca DA, Maianski Z, Averbukh M. A study of skin disease spectrum occurring in Angola phototype V-VI population in Luanda. Int J Dermatol 2018; 57(7): 849-55.
[http://dx.doi.org/10.1111/ijd.13958] [PMID: 29573271]

[25]   Alvarado Z, Pereira C. Fungal diseases in children and adolescents in a referral centre in Bogota, Colombia. Mycoses 2018; 61(8): 543-8.
[http://dx.doi.org/10.1111/myc.12774] [PMID: 29601109]

[26]   Raugi G, Nguyen TU. Superficial dermatophyte infections of the skin. In: Elaine CJ, Dennis LS, Eds. Netter's Infectious Diseases. Amsterdam: Elsevier Inc 2012; pp. 102-9.
[http://dx.doi.org/10.1016/B978-1-4377-0126-5.00022-7]

[27]   Nweze EI, Eke IE. Dermatophytes and dermatophytosis in the eastern and southern parts of Africa. Med Mycol 2018; 56(1): 13-28.
[http://dx.doi.org/10.1093/mmy/myx025] [PMID: 28419352]

[28]   Alshehri BA, Alamri AM, Rabaan AA, Al-Tawfiq JA. Epidemiology of dermatophytes isolated from clinical samples in a hospital in Eastern Saudi Arabia: a 20-year survey. J Epidemiol Glob Health 2021; 11(4): 405-12.
[http://dx.doi.org/10.1007/s44197-021-00005-5] [PMID: 34734382]

[29]   AL-Khikani F. Dermatophytosis a worldwide contiguous fungal infection: Growing challenge and few solutions. Biomed Biotechnol Res J 2020; 4: 117-22. [BBRJ].

[30]   Balamuruganvelu S, Reddy SV, Babu G. Age and genderwise seasonal distribution of dermatophytosis in a tertiary care hospital, Puducherry, India. J Clin Diagn Res 2019; 13(2): 6-10.
[http://dx.doi.org/10.7860/JCDR/2019/39515.12615]

[31]   Leeyaphan C, Bunyaratavej S, Foongladda S, *et al.* Epidemiology, clinical characteristics, sites of infection and treatment outcomes of mucocutaneous candidiasis caused by non-*Albicans* species of

Candida at a dermatologic clinic. J Med Assoc Thai 2016; 99(4): 406-11.
[PMID: 27396225]

[32] Bohner F, Gacser A, Toth R. Epidemiological attributes of *Candida* species in tropical regions. Curr Trop Med Rep 2021; 8(2): 59-68.
[http://dx.doi.org/10.1007/s40475-021-00226-5]

[33] Achkar JM, Fries BC. *Candida* infections of the genitourinary tract. Clin Microbiol Rev 2010; 23(2): 253-73.
[http://dx.doi.org/10.1128/CMR.00076-09] [PMID: 20375352]

[34] Bondaryk M, Kurzątkowski W, Staniszewska M. Antifungal agents commonly used in the superficial and mucosal candidiasis treatment: mode of action and resistance development. Postepy Dermatol Alergol 2013; 5(5): 293-301.
[http://dx.doi.org/10.5114/pdia.2013.38358] [PMID: 24353489]

[35] Gupta A, Foley K. Antifungal treatment for pityriasis versicolor. J Fungi (Basel) 2015; 1(1): 13-29.
[http://dx.doi.org/10.3390/jof1010013] [PMID: 29376896]

[36] Hu SW, Bigby M. Pityriasis versicolor. Arch Dermatol 2010; 146(10): 1132-40.
[http://dx.doi.org/10.1001/archdermatol.2010.259] [PMID: 20956647]

[37] Hay R. Therapy of skin, hair and nail fungal infections. J Fungi (Basel) 2018; 4(3): 99.
[http://dx.doi.org/10.3390/jof4030099] [PMID: 30127244]

[38] Gupta AK, Renaud HJ, Quinlan EM, Shear NH, Piguet V. The growing problem of antifungal resistance in onychomycosis and other superficial mycoses. Am J Clin Dermatol 2021; 22(2): 149-57.
[http://dx.doi.org/10.1007/s40257-020-00580-6] [PMID: 33354740]

[39] El-Gohary M, van Zuuren EJ, Fedorowicz Z, *et al.* Topical antifungal treatments for tinea cruris and tinea corporis. Cochrane Libr 2014; 4(8): CD009992.
[http://dx.doi.org/10.1002/14651858.CD009992.pub2] [PMID: 25090020]

[40] Johnson MD, Perfect JR. Use of antifungal combination therapy: agents, order, and timing. Curr Fungal Infect Rep 2010; 4(2): 87-95.
[http://dx.doi.org/10.1007/s12281-010-0018-6] [PMID: 20574543]

[41] Pappas PG, Rex JH, Sobel JD, *et al.* Guidelines for treatment of candidiasis. Clin Infect Dis 2004; 38(2): 161-89.
[http://dx.doi.org/10.1086/380796] [PMID: 14699449]

[42] Shirwaikar AA, Thomas T, Shirwaikar A, Lobo R, Prabhu KS. Treatment of onychomycosis: An update. Indian J Pharm Sci 2008; 70(6): 710-4.
[http://dx.doi.org/10.4103/0250-474X.49088] [PMID: 21369429]

[43] McCarthy MW, Kontoyiannis DP, Cornely OA, Perfect JR, Walsh TJ. Novel agents and drug targets to meet the challenges of resistant fungi. J Infect Dis 2017; 216 (Suppl. 3): S474-83.
[http://dx.doi.org/10.1093/infdis/jix130] [PMID: 28911042]

[44] Harris R. Progress with superficial mycoses using essential oils. Int J Aromath 2002; 12(2): 83-91.
[http://dx.doi.org/10.1016/S0962-4562(02)00032-2]

[45] Atanasov AG, Zotchev SB, Dirsch VM, Supuran CT. Natural products in drug discovery: advances and opportunities. Nat Rev Drug Discov 2021; 20(3): 200-16.
[http://dx.doi.org/10.1038/s41573-020-00114-z] [PMID: 33510482]

[46] Scorzoni L, Benaducci T, Almeida AMF, Silva DHS, Bolzani VS, Gianinni MJSM. The use of standard methodology for determination of antifungal activity of natural products against medical yeasts *Candida* sp and *Cryptococcus* sp. Braz J Microbiol 2007; 38(3): 391-7.
[http://dx.doi.org/10.1590/S1517-83822007000300001]

[47] Cantón E, Espinel-Ingroff A, Pemán J. Trends in antifungal susceptibility testing using CLSI reference and commercial methods. Expert Rev Anti Infect Ther 2009; 7(1): 107-19.

[http://dx.doi.org/10.1586/14787210.7.1.107] [PMID: 19622060]

[48] Abdallah EM. Potential antifungal activity of fresh garlic cloves (*Allium sativum* L.) from Sudan. J Biotech Res 2017; 3(11): 106-9.

[49] Mercy KA, Ijeoma I, Emmanuel KJ. Anti-dermatophytic activity of garlic (*Allium sativum*) extracts on some dermatophytic fungi. Int Lett Nat Sci 2014; 24: 34-40.
[http://dx.doi.org/10.56431/p-2o985a]

[50] Shams-Ghahfarokhi M, Shokoohamiri MR, Amirrajab N, *et al. In vitro* antifungal activities of *Allium cepa, Allium sativum* and ketoconazole against some pathogenic yeasts and dermatophytes. Fitoterapia 2006; 77(4): 321-3.
[http://dx.doi.org/10.1016/j.fitote.2006.03.014] [PMID: 16690223]

[51] Li WR, Shi QS, Dai HQ, *et al.* Antifungal activity, kinetics and molecular mechanism of action of garlic oil against *Candida albicans*. Sci Rep 2016; 6(1): 22805.
[http://dx.doi.org/10.1038/srep22805] [PMID: 26948845]

[52] Sarfraz M, Nasim MJ, Jacob C, Gruhlke MCH. Efficacy of allicin against plant pathogenic fungi and unveiling the underlying mode of action employing yeast based chemogenetic profiling approach. Appl Sci (Basel) 2020; 10(7): 2563.
[http://dx.doi.org/10.3390/app10072563]

[53] Saniasiay J, Salim R, Mohamad I, Harun A. Antifungal effect of Malaysian *Aloe vera* leaf extract on selected fungal species of pathogenic otomycosis species in *in vitro* culture medium. Oman Med J 2017; 32(1): 41-6.
[http://dx.doi.org/10.5001/omj.2017.08] [PMID: 28042402]

[54] Nazar KA, Meidyawati R. Antifungal effects of *aloe vera* irrigant on *Candida albicans* biofilm. Int J App Pharm 2019; 11(1): 10-2.

[55] Danish P, Ali Q, Hafeez MM, Malik A. Antifungal and antibacterial activity of *Aloe vera* plant extract. Biologic Clin Sci Res J 2020; 2020(1): 4.
[http://dx.doi.org/10.54112/bcsrj.v2020i1.4]

[56] Manipal S, Shireen F, Prabu D. Anti-fungal activity of Aloe vera: *In vitro* study. SRM J Res Dent Sci 2015; 16(2): 92-5.
[http://dx.doi.org/10.4103/0976-433X.155464]

[57] Fozouni L, Taghizadeh F, Kiaei E. Anti-microbial effect of *Aloe vera* extract on clotrimazole-resistant *Malassezia Furfur* strains isolated from patients with seborrheic dermatitis in the city of Sari. Ann Mil Health Sci Res 2018; 16(2): e82841.
[http://dx.doi.org/10.5812/amh.82841]

[58] Sebastian E, Ganeshan G, Lokesha AN. Antifungal activity of some extractives and constituents of *Aloe vera*. Res J Med Plant 2011; 5(2): 196-200.
[http://dx.doi.org/10.3923/rjmp.2011.196.200]

[59] Khodavandi A, Tahzir NAB, Cheng PW, *et al.* Antifungal activity of rhizome coptidis and *Alpinia galangal* against *Candida* species. J Pure Appl Microbiol 2013; 7(3): 1725-30.

[60] Trakranrungsie N, Chatchawanchonteera A, Khunkitti W. Ethnoveterinary study for antidermatophytic activity of *Piper betle, Alpinia galanga* and *Allium ascalonicum* extracts *in vitro*. Res Vet Sci 2008; 84(1): 80-4.
[http://dx.doi.org/10.1016/j.rvsc.2007.03.006] [PMID: 17482221]

[61] Laokor N, Juntachai W. Exploring the antifungal activity and mechanism of action of *Zingiberaceae rhizome* extracts against *Malassezia furfur*. J Ethnopharmacol 2021; 279: 114354.
[http://dx.doi.org/10.1016/j.jep.2021.114354] [PMID: 34157325]

[62] Kalidindi N, Thimmaiah NV, Jagadeesh NV, Nandeep R, Swetha S, Kalidindi B. Antifungal and antioxidant activities of organic and aqueous extracts of *Annona squamosa* Linn. leaves. Yao Wu Shi Pin Fen Xi 2015; 23(4): 795-802.

[PMID: 28911497]

[63]   Ola AR, Sugi Y, Lay CS. Isolation, identification and antimicrobial activity of secondary metabolites of endophytic fungi from annona leaves (*Annona squamosa* L.) growing in dry land. IOP Conf Ser: Mater Sci Eng. Eng 2020; 823(1): 012039.
[http://dx.doi.org/10.1088/1757-899X/823/1/012039]

[64]   Akroum S. Antifungal activity of *Camellia sinensis* crude extracts against four species of *Candida* and *Microsporum persicolor*. J Mycol Med 2018; 28(3): 424-7.
[http://dx.doi.org/10.1016/j.mycmed.2018.06.003] [PMID: 29960870]

[65]   Erolls CS, Margret M, Christine B. Antifungal activities of *Camellia sinensis* crude extract, mixture with milk, on selected pathogenic and mycotoxic fungi. J Med Plants Res 2015; 9(42): 1070-80.
[http://dx.doi.org/10.5897/JMPR2015.5939]

[66]   Schlemmer KB, Jesus FPK, Tondolo JSM, *et al. In vitro* activity of carvacrol, cinnamaldehyde and thymol combined with antifungals against *Malassezia pachydermatis*. J Mycol Med 2019; 29(4): 375-7.
[http://dx.doi.org/10.1016/j.mycmed.2019.08.003] [PMID: 31455580]

[67]   Shreaz S, Bhatia R, Khan N, *et al.* Spice oil cinnamaldehyde exhibits potent anticandidal activity against fluconazole resistant clinical isolates. Fitoterapia 2011; 82(7): 1012-20.
[http://dx.doi.org/10.1016/j.fitote.2011.06.004] [PMID: 21708228]

[68]   Butzge JC, Ferrão SK, Mezzomo L, *et al.* Antifungal activity of essential oils from *Cinnamomum cassia, Myristica fragrans* and *Syzygium aromaticum* against *Rhodotorula mucilaginosa*. Drug Anal Res 2020; 4(2): 3-11.
[http://dx.doi.org/10.22456/2527-2616.104615]

[69]   Ooi LSM, Li Y, Kam SL, Wang H, Wong EYL, Ooi VEC. Antimicrobial activities of cinnamon oil and cinnamaldehyde from the Chinese medicinal herb *Cinnamomum cassia* Blume. Am J Chin Med 2006; 34(3): 511-22.
[http://dx.doi.org/10.1142/S0192415X06004041] [PMID: 16710900]

[70]   Sanguinetti M, Posteraro B, Romano L, *et al. In vitro* activity of *Citrus bergamia* (bergamot) oil against clinical isolates of dermatophytes. J Antimicrob Chemother 2006; 59(2): 305-8.
[http://dx.doi.org/10.1093/jac/dkl473] [PMID: 17118937]

[71]   Jing L, Lei Z, Li L, *et al.* Antifungal activity of citrus essential oils. J Agric Food Chem 2014; 62(14): 3011-33.
[http://dx.doi.org/10.1021/jf5006148] [PMID: 24628448]

[72]   Moghadamtousi SZ, Kadir HA, Hassandarvish P, Tajik H, Abubakar S, Zandi K. A review on antibacterial, antiviral, and antifungal activity of curcumin. Biomed Res Int 2014; 2014: 186864.
[PMID: 24877064]

[73]   Apisariyakul A, Vanittanakom N, Buddhasukh D. Antifungal activity of turmeric oil extracted from *Curcuma longa* (Zingiberaceae). J Ethnopharmacol 1995; 49(3): 163-9.
[http://dx.doi.org/10.1016/0378-8741(95)01320-2] [PMID: 8824742]

[74]   Martins CVB, da Silva DL, Neres ATM, *et al.* Curcumin as a promising antifungal of clinical interest. J Antimicrob Chemother 2008; 63(2): 337-9.
[http://dx.doi.org/10.1093/jac/dkn488] [PMID: 19038979]

[75]   Sharma M, Manoharlal R, Puri N, Prasad R. Antifungal curcumin induces reactive oxygen species and triggers an early apoptosis but prevents hyphae development by targeting the global repressor *TUP1* in *Candida albicans*. Biosci Rep 2010; 30(6): 391-404.
[http://dx.doi.org/10.1042/BSR20090151] [PMID: 20017731]

[76]   Neelofar K, Shreaz S, Rimple B, Muralidhar S, Nikhat M, Khan LA. Curcumin as a promising anticandidal of clinical interest. Can J Microbiol 2011; 57(3): 204-10.
[http://dx.doi.org/10.1139/W10-117] [PMID: 21358761]

[77] Sahal G, Woerdenbag HJ, Hinrichs WLJ, *et al.* Antifungal and biofilm inhibitory effect of *Cymbopogon citratus* (lemongrass) essential oil on biofilm forming by *Candida tropicalis* isolates; an *in vitro* study. J Ethnopharmacol 2020; 246: 112188.
[http://dx.doi.org/10.1016/j.jep.2019.112188] [PMID: 31470085]

[78] Silva CdeB, Guterres SS, Weisheimer V, Schapoval EE. Antifungal activity of the lemongrass oil and citral against *Candida* spp. Braz J Infect Dis 2008; 12(1): 63-6.
[PMID: 18553017]

[79] Kishore N, Mishra AK, Chansouria JPN. Fungitoxicity of essential oils against dermatophytes. Mycoses 1993; 36(5-6): 211-5.
[http://dx.doi.org/10.1111/j.1439-0507.1993.tb00753.x] [PMID: 8264720]

[80] Su BL, Zeng R, Chen JY, Chen CY, Guo JH, Huang CG. Antioxidant and antimicrobial properties of various solvent extracts from *Impatiens balsamina* L. stems. J Food Sci 2012; 77(6): C614-9.
[http://dx.doi.org/10.1111/j.1750-3841.2012.02709.x] [PMID: 22582943]

[81] Sakunphueak A, Panichayupakaranant P. Comparison of antimicrobial activities of naphthoquinones from *Impatiens balsamina*. Nat Prod Res 2012; 26(12): 1119-24.
[http://dx.doi.org/10.1080/14786419.2010.551297] [PMID: 21895457]

[82] Dananjaya SHS, Udayangani RMC, Shin SY, *et al. In vitro* and *in vivo* antifungal efficacy of plant based lawsone against *Fusarium oxysporum* species complex. Microbiol Res 2017; 201: 21-9.
[http://dx.doi.org/10.1016/j.micres.2017.04.011] [PMID: 28602398]

[83] Santhanam J, Abd Ghani FN, Basri DF. Antifungal activity of *Jasminum sambac* against *Malassezia* sp. and non-*Malassezia* sp. isolated from human skin samples. J Mycol 2014; 2014: 1-7.
[http://dx.doi.org/10.1155/2014/359630]

[84] Kumar S, Navneet GS, Gautam SS. Screening of antimicrobial properties of *Jasminum sambac* Linn. leaf extracts against dental pathogens. Res J Phytochem 2015; 9(4): 195-200.
[http://dx.doi.org/10.3923/rjphyto.2015.195.200]

[85] Sihite NW, Rusmarilin H, Suryanto D, Sihombing DR. Utilization of jasmine flower extract as antimicrobial in tempeh sausage. IOP Conf Ser Earth Environ Sci 2018; 205: 012037.
[http://dx.doi.org/10.1088/1755-1315/205/1/012037]

[86] Panichayupakaranant P, Charoonratana T, Sirikatitham A. RP-HPLC analysis of rhinacanthins in *Rhinacanthus nasutus*: validation and application for the preparation of rhinacanthin high-yielding extract. J Chromatogr Sci 2009; 47(8): 705-8.
[http://dx.doi.org/10.1093/chromsci/47.8.705] [PMID: 19772749]

[87] Wisuitiprot W. Antifungal activity of *Rhinacantus nasutus* extract against *Malassezia* sp. J Health Sci (Sarajevo) 2012; 31(3): 521-8.

[88] Puttarak P, Charoonratana T, Panichayupakaranant P. Antimicrobial activity and stability of rhinacanthins-rich *Rhinacanthus nasutus* extract. Phytomedicine 2010; 17(5): 323-7.
[http://dx.doi.org/10.1016/j.phymed.2009.08.014] [PMID: 19879741]

[89] Jeenkeawpieam J, Yodkeeree S, Andrianopoulos A, Roytrakul S, Pongpom M. Antifungal activity and molecular mechanisms of partial purified antifungal proteins from *Rhinacanthus nasutus* against *Talaromyces marneffei*. J Fungi (Basel) 2020; 6(4): 333.
[http://dx.doi.org/10.3390/jof6040333] [PMID: 33287246]

[90] Manjulatha K, Jaishree B, Purohit M. Antimicrobial activity of fruits of *Sapindus emarginatus.* J Pharmacogn 2012; 3(2): 55-8.

[91] Tsuzuki JK, Svidzinski TIE, Shinobu CS, *et al.* Antifungal activity of the extracts and saponins from *Sapindus saponaria* L. An Acad Bras Cienc 2007; 79(4): 577-83.
[http://dx.doi.org/10.1590/S0001-37652007000400002] [PMID: 18066429]

[92] Zhang JD, Xu Z, Cao YB, *et al.* Antifungal activities and action mechanisms of compounds from

Tribulus terrestris L. J Ethnopharmacol 2006; 103(1): 76-84.
[http://dx.doi.org/10.1016/j.jep.2005.07.006] [PMID: 16169173]

[93] Barros Cota B, Batista Carneiro de Oliveira D, Carla Borges T, *et al.* Antifungal activity of extracts and purified saponins from the rhizomes of *Chamaecostus cuspidatus* against *Candida* and *Trichophyton* species. J Appl Microbiol 2021; 130(1): 61-75.
[http://dx.doi.org/10.1111/jam.14783] [PMID: 32654270]

[94] Adedayo O, Anderson WA, Moo-Young M, Kolawole DO. Antifungal properties of some components of *Senna alata* flower. Pharm Biol 1999; 37(5): 369-74.
[http://dx.doi.org/10.1076/phbi.37.5.369.6061]

[95] Wuthi-udomlert M, Kupittayanant P, Gritsanapan W. *In vitro* evaluation of antifungal activity of anthraquinone derivatives of *Senna alata*. J Health Res 2010; 24(3): 117-22.

[96] Sakunpak A, Sirikatitham A, Panichayupakaranant P. Preparation of anthraquinone high-yielding *Senna alata* extract and its stability. Pharm Biol 2009; 47(3): 236-41.
[http://dx.doi.org/10.1080/13880200802434757]

[97] Phongpaichit S, Pujenjob N, Rukachaisirikul V, Ongsakul M. Antifungal activity from leaf extracts of *Cassia alata* L., *Cassia fistula* L. and *Cassia tora* L. Songklanakarin J Sci Technol 2004; 26(5): 741-8.

[98] Legaspi CLB, Maramba-Lazarte CC. The phytochemical content and the *in vitro* antifungal properties of *Senna alata* (Linn.) Roxb.: a review. Acta Med Philipp 2020; 54(1): 86-93.
[http://dx.doi.org/10.47895/amp.v54i1.1111]

[99] Mao QQ, Xu XY, Cao SY, *et al.* Bioactive compounds and bioactivities of ginger (*Zingiber officinale* Roscoe). Foods 2019; 8(6): 185.
[http://dx.doi.org/10.3390/foods8060185] [PMID: 31151279]

[100] Aghazadeh M, Zahedi Bialvaei A, Aghazadeh M, *et al.* Survey of the antibiofilm and antimicrobial effects of *Zingiber officinale* (*in vitro* study). Jundishapur J Microbiol 2016; 9(2): e30167.
[http://dx.doi.org/10.5812/jjm.30167] [PMID: 27127591]

[101] Richa Sharma , Sharma M. Additive and inhibitory effect of antifungal activity of *Curcuma longa* (Turmeric) and *Zingiber officinale* (Ginger) essential oils against Pityriasis versicolor infections. J Med Plants Res 2011; 5(32): 6987-90.
[http://dx.doi.org/10.5897/JMPR11.1032]

[102] López EIC, Balcázar MFH, Mendoza JMR, *et al.* Antimicrobial activity of essential oil of *Zingiber officinale* Roscoe (Zingiberaceae). Am J Plant Sci 2017; 8(7): 1511-24.
[http://dx.doi.org/10.4236/ajps.2017.87104]

[103] Panin G. Composition for topical application with antifungal activity. US Patent No. US20190224263A1, 2019.

[104] Boegli CJ. Topical antifungal composition. US Patent No. US20110008474A1, 2013.

[105] Shetty MV. Herbal composition for treatment and management of infectious diseases and method of preparation thereof. US Patent No. US20190134124A1, 2020.

[106] Tesse N. Anti-microbial composition. US Patent No. US20130289103A1, 2016.

[107] Peng LV, Lim KT, Costa PD. Antimicrobial garlic compositions. US Patent No. US11116813B2, 2021.

[108] Saengnaleang S. Liquid herbal soap. Thai Patent No.: 2156, 2005.

[109] Patamaporn P, Chttaporn PPJ, Panadda T, Nattawan M. Rinlapus A. inventors.Gel formulation of Rhinacanthus nasutus root extract for treatment of superficial mycoses. Thai Patent No. 13324, 2017.

CHAPTER 3

Acne and Current Possible Treatments

Yaseen Hussain[1,*] and **Haroon Khan**[2]

[1] *College of Pharmaceutical Sciences, Soochow University, Suzhou, Jiangsu, China*

[2] *Department of Pharmacy, Abdul Wali Khan University, Mardan, Pakistan*

Abstract: Acne vulgaris is one of the most skin diseases related to the sebaceous gland, characterized by multiple pathogenic factors. The treatment strategies involve the blockage of these pathological factors. Conventional therapies for the treatment of Acne vulgaris in controlling its pathological factors are still inadequate in providing therapeutic effectiveness and exhibit remarkable side effects. New therapeutic agent development for acne treatment is still stagnant. Recently, researchers have been focusing and seeking great interest in the treatment of acne through natural products – as a new therapeutic option. In this regard, multiple natural products have been evaluated for their potential to treat acne, including berberine, α-mangostin, curcumin, ampelopsin, fustin, ellagic acid, gallic acid, myricetin, lupeol and many more. These natural products have been reported as suitable candidates for blocking multiple pathogenic factors associated with acne. In addition, the nanotechnology-based delivery of natural products is a new platform and treatment option for Acne vulgaris. Natural products nano-based delivery resolves many other issues concerned with natural products apart from treatment aid. Natural products, therefore, pose a precious source in determining new agents for the treatment of acne. However, reported studies are preclinical, and to obtain reliable and conclusive results, further clinical studies are required to uplift natural products from bench top to clinical setup in treating the worst consequences of Acne vulgaris.

Keywords: Acne, Pathological factors, Treatment, Natural products, Nano-delivery.

INTRODUCTION

Acne vulgaris is a disease of pilo-sebaceous follicles characterized by chronic inflammation. It's a multi factorial and most prevalent skin disorder affecting people of all ages and ethnic [1, 2]. Acne vulgaris, irrespective of nationality, sex and socioeconomic status, is mostly concerned with adolescence, which is attribu-

---

Corresponding author Yaseen Hussain: College of Pharmaceutical Sciences, Soochow University, Suzhou, Jiangsu, China; E-mail: pharmycc@gmail.com

Heba Abd El-Sattar El-Nashar, Mohamed El-Shazly & Nouran Mohammed Fahmy (Eds.)

ted to androgen production during puberty [3]. Acne incidence is greater in women (12%) than in men, and in the US, the cost of acne treatment is about 3 billion dollars per year [4, 5]. However, acne vulgaris is not a life-threatening complication since it leads to normal activities disturbances like anxiety and lack of self-confidence [6].

Multiple pathological factors are involved in the development of acne, including colonization and proliferation of Propionibacterium acnes, excessive production of sebum, acquired and innate immunity and abnormal hyperkeratinization of follicles [7]. In addition, acne lesions are developed and affected by family history and diet as well [8]. It is very necessary to develop a new pharmacological intervention for the management of acne to cope with current related problems like lack of confidence, to improve quality of life, to boost the lack-response, and more specifically, to bypass the problems and complications associated with drug therapy [9].

Among conventional therapies, hormonal therapy is one of them. Spironolactone, flutamide and cyproterone acetate were used as androgen receptor blockers for the treatment of acne [10]. Laser and light-based therapies have been explored for acne treatment along with pharmacological measures to synergize the effect [11]. Topical, systemic and antibacterial conventional therapies were carried out for the treatment of acne; however, age, site of acne lesion and types as well are risk factors for consideration. In addition, different barriers in conventional therapies have made it quite challenging, and failure of therapy has been observed [12]. Thus there is a need to select alternate therapy choices for acne treatment that might be effective with clinical significance and reduced side effects.

It is obvious that phytochemicals used for the treatment of acne are hydrophobic, and mostly that exhibit low penetration as well as reduced bioavailability or/and low availability at the target side [13]. Some of them are concerned with worse adverse effects. All these barriers are associated with conventional therapy for acne as well. To overwhelm these problems, nanotechnology is an effective platform that deals effectively with them [14]. In acne treatment, topical formulations from nanoplatforms were evaluated mostly, showing clinical significance with reduced side effects. Nano gels and emulsions have shown optimal therapeutic outcomes topically with efficient penetration. Phytochemical nanoparticles have also shown remarkable outputs in the form of nano structure lipid carriers and niosomes as well [15, 16]. Therefore in recent research, nanoformulations for phytochemicals were extensively carried out and evaluated.

In addition to nano-based formulations, phytochemicals were directly employed for the treatment of acne. Different classes of phytochemicals, mostly in topical gels and cream form, showed desired therapeutic outcomes. This book chapter highlights the role of phytochemicals as a source of current possible treatments for acne. Apart from it, phytochemicals in nano form also act as a newer approach for the treatment of acne that covers prominent problems associated with phytochemical therapy and provides certain effective outcomes to phytochemical-based therapy that pave the way for acne treatment.

Conventional Therapies for Acne

Focusing lesions associated with acne vulgaris were treated in women with oral contraceptives containing a combination of progestin and estrogen. Results of a meta–analysis study revealed that using combination hormonal therapy for acne lesions, a 62% reduction in inflammation related to acne was observed [17]. Due to optimal therapeutic outcome, FDA has approved combination hormonal therapy for acne treatment, *i.e.*, ethinyl estradiol– drospirenone, ethinyl estradiol–norgestimate, ethinyl estradiol–norethindrone [18]. Spironolactone, due to its antiandrogen activity, has been evaluated for anti-acne potential. Observational and retrospective data showed that it is effective in the treatment of acne, particularly in females [19].

In case of moderate to severe acne problems, oral antibiotics were used to deal with the concerned inflammation however, due to increased oral antibiotic resistance, the therapy was switched to systemic therapy [20]. The systemic administration of antibiotics for acne treatment was favored by using benzoyl peroxide and retinoids as a part of combination therapy. Such a combination therapy in clinical trials was assessed and resulted in a 60% reduction in acne lesion inflammation within a time period of three months [21]. The concentration of Cutibacterium acne was effectively reduced after treatment with tetracycline. So tetracycline is another alternative and can be prescribed for acne treatment [22]. However, it needs to be taken on an empty stomach and inconsistent bioavailability limit its use in acne treatment. In addition to tetracycline, other antibiotics used for the treatment of acne include macrolide, penicillin, cephalosporin, and trimethoprim–sulfamethoxazole [23].

Topical retinoid is another choice for the treatment of acne vulgaris however, it still has taken the tag of underprescribing by dermatologists and health care providers. Topical retinoid can be used in combination with isotretinoin and tazarotene. Such a combination exhibit photosensitizing activity, however, it can be overcome by the use of sunscreen [24]. In addition to topical retinoids, topical antimicrobial agents are also used for the treatment of acne vulgaris [25]. Clindamycin and erythromycin are effective as topical antimicrobial agents. However, its worth to mention that individual antibiotics face the problem of resistance therefore, combination antimicrobial therapy is carried out to cope with microbial resistance and ensure optimal antibiotic therapeutic outcomes [26, 27]. Studies have shown that combination antimicrobial therapy in topical application exhibit maximum potential for reduction in the concentration of Cutibacterium acne. All these conventional therapies are efficient in acne therapy however, some of them face certain barriers and problems in their way. In recent years, phytochemicals have been explored for their anti-acne potential. Most of them overcome the concerned problems.

Pharmacological Targets for Phytochemicals Targeting Acne

Phytochemicals are recently explored for the management of Acne vulgaris. The management of acne through phytochemicals follows certain pharmacological targets. Among these, follicular hyperkeratinization (FH) is the main target for retinoids [28]. FH in sebaceous glands and follicular infundibulum (factors for acne pathogenesis) shed the skin cells. Ductal hyper cornification and retention hyperkeratosis are various terms used for hyperkeratinization [29]. An epithelial function is disturbed by fatty acid deficiency, which is mainly attributed to the induction of follicular hyperkeratinization [30]. Similarly, oxidative stress is also involved as phytochemical pharmacological target. Sebaceous glands produce sebum with reactive oxygen species and other free radicals. Such free radicals are either directly or indirectly responsible for the irritation of the skin in Acne vulgaris [31]. So, oxidative stress is another pharmacological target for phytochemicals used in the management of acne.

Androgen motivates the production of sebum and thus acts as a key factor in acne development [32]. Testosterone is converted to its more active form (5α-DHT) *via* 5α – reductase [33]. This is another target for phytochemicals targeting acne. In addition, sebum is considered as a best substrate for the proliferation of Propionibacterium acnes. Also during the pathogenesis of acne, lipid squalene is a key factor following squalene oxidation activity during the colonization of Propionibacterium acnes [34]. Thus, microbial proliferation and colonization can be targeted *via* phytochemicals during acne management.

CURRENT POSSIBLE TREATMENTS USING PHYTOCHEMICALS

Phytochemicals

Acne vulgaris is extensively studied through conventional therapies, however, using natural products for acne treatment is still challenging and less explored. Following is literature that studied phytochemicals used in the treatment of acne.

Overall, extracts from medicinal plants exhibit anti-acne activity. Some of them are shown in Table **1**.

Table 1. Medicinal plant extracts used in the treatment of acne.

Specie	Part Used	Medicinal Use	References
Aloe ferox	Roots and leaves	Acne, eczema and dermatitis treatment	[35]
Bulbine frutescens	Juice from leaves	Acne wounds treatment	[36]
Aloe vera	Gel from leaves	Acne treatment	[37]
Aspalathus linearis	Extract from leaves	Acne and nappy rash treatment	[38]
Harpephyllum caffrum Bernh	Bark	Acne and eczema treatment	[39]
Centella asiatica	Root and leaves	Acne and leprosy management	[40]
Berberis aristata	Roots	Acne treatment	[41]
Glycyrrhiza glabra	Roots	Acne and pruritis treatment	[42]

Cryptomeria japonica is a specie that contains γ-eudesmol and sabinene as their active constituents. Its active compounds were evaluated against *Propionibacterium acnes*. Results of the study suggested that both compounds showed antibacterial action against *Propionibacterium acnes* at an inhibitory concentration of 0.156μL/mL [43]. Mentioned active compounds from *Cryptomeria japonica* have the potential to treat *Acne vulgaris*. Similarly, γ-terpinene isolated from *Eucalyptus globulus Labill* showed anti-*Propionibacterium acnesi* activity at an inhibitory concentration of 9.38mg/mL [44]. *Berberis vulgaris* constitutes berberine that kills bacteria through inflammasome activation, inhibition of TNF-α protein release, and reduction of reactive oxygen species in mitochondrion [45 - 47]. Apart from its antibacterial action against *Propionibacterium acnes*, its anti-acne activity is attributed to androgen synthesis inhibition and reduction in sebum production in sebaceous glands through lipogenesis suppression [48]. It shows that plant constituents from different sources hit various targets like androgens, inflammatory pathways and reactive oxygen species. All these are factors involved in the pathogenesis of acne.

A recent research study was conducted against *Placacnes places* and *staphylococcus epidermidis,* which are responsible for acne induction. An extract from *Morus nigra* (black mulberry) was evaluated for its antibacterial action against these species. The results of the study suggested an impressive antibacterial action against these acne-causing bacteria [49]. In another study, the crude extract of *Lagerstroemia Indica* leaf was evaluated against *Acne vulgaris*. Results of the study showed an effective anti-bacterial action against *Propionibacterium acnes* [50]. Similarly, terpinen-4-ol is a major isolated constituent from *Zingiber cassumunar* that has the potential to treat acne. The active constituent showed an antibacterial action against *Propionibacterium acnes* in a minimal bactericidal concentration of 2.5 volume % [51]. It is concluded that various constituents of phytochemicals have the potential to eradicate acne bacteria through their bactericidal action.

Tea tree oil extracted from *Melaleuca alternifolia* leaves. It is used in the form of topical gel, lotion, cream and ointment. It is used in the treatment of acne and its related wounds as well. Its anti-acne activity was confirmed by two clinical trials [52]. In one clinical trial, its efficacy against acne was carried out in 124 patients where 5% tea tree oil significantly reduced lesions associated with acne. Similarly, another clinical trial conducted on 60 patients reduced the acne wounds within 45 days with effective anti-acne activity [53]. Quercetin and iso-quercetin isolated from *Fagopyrum tataricum* (buckwheat) were evaluated for their antibacterial potential against *Propionibacterium acnes*. The results of the study indicated an effective anti-acne activity at a minimum effective concentration of 512 µg/mL [54]. The current paragraph concludes that phytochemicals were also evaluated clinically, which gives awesome results against acne and can be uplifted from benchtop to commercial level.

Accumulation of excessive oils from the skin is removed by Witch hazel. In addition, it exhibits antibacterial activity. Its later function was evaluated against *Propionibacterium acnes* and showed an effective outcome. Its formulated cream for acne treatment is available in the market. Similarly, ethanolic extracts of walnut leaves were evaluated against *Propionibacterium acnes,* and it was found that at a bactericidal concentration of 15mg/mL and inhibitory concentration of 12mg/mL, walnut leaves extract showed effective antibacterial activity [55]. Rosemary extract was introduced in a mouse model *in vivo* to check its antibacterial and anti-inflammatory action against *Propionibacterium acnes*. Results of the study indicated that applied extract inhibited cytokine production, leading to the inhibition of inflammation associated with acne. Additionally, no reaction/irritation was observed at the injection site [56]. From all these findings, it can be concluded that phytochemicals, due to their anti-acne activity, must be evaluated for other external infections as an alternative choice of drugs.

Nano Phytochemicals

Conventionally, the role of phytochemicals was explored recently however, it faces certain problems in its way, *i.e.*, low solubility, less penetration, toxicity, *etc*. To cope with these problems and increase the circulation of phytochemicals for efficient therapy, it might be formulated in nano form. To triumph the limitations in acne treatment, recently, some phytochemicals were formulated from nano platform that is discussed here.

Among delivery systems for acne treatment, topical delivery provided efficient local effects with maximal clinical efficacy and reduced side effects. Isotretinoin-loaded nanoemulsion was applied topically to acne in a research study. Results indicated an effective anti-bacterial action against *Propionibacterium acnes* with reduced side effects [57]. Similarly, nicotinamide-loaded chitosan nanoparticles were optimized, characterized and clinically tested for their topical anti-acne potential. *Ex-vivo* studies showed effective penetration (68%) and adhesion as well to the skin layers. Clinical results showed a significant reduction in the lesions associated with *Acne vulgaris* [58]. A split-face, double-blinded, randomized control study was conducted on 28 patients with acne. An extract from mangosteen fruit loaded on nano-gel was applied. Results of the study displayed a 67% reduction in inflammatory lesions associated with *Acne vulgaris* within three months [59]. It shows that using nanoparticles for acne treatment might be a sounding option with optimal therapeutic outcomes.

Coconut oil-loaded chitosan nanoparticles were fabricated, and their antibacterial activity was evaluated in *Propionibacterium acnes*. The resultant nanoparticles showed the highest antibacterial action against *Propionibacterium acnes* with 9% viability and reduced toxicity [60]. An *in vitro* anti-acne activity was carried out on lime peel essential oil-loaded chitosan nanoparticles, and its zone of inhibition was measured. The efficacy of fabricated nano particles was compared with non-encapsulated lime peel extract. Results showed a greater inhibitory zone (20 – 61mm) for nano particles as compared to (10 – 20mm) of conventional extract [61]. It showed that nano particles based formulation of lime peel extract is effective as compared to its pure delivery against *Propionibacterium acnes*. In a recent research study, Thymol loaded biodegradable and surface-modified nano particles were fabricated and evaluated against *Cutibacterium acnes*. The penetration capacity of fabricated nano particles were assessed in skin using pig skin model. An improved anti bacterial action was observed against *Cutibacterium acnes* with efficient penetration of nano particles loaded with thymol [62]. So it is obvious now that nano particle is an efficient platform for the delivery of phytochemicals with enhanced penetration, proved efficacy and reduced side effects treating acne.

Curcumin-loaded niosomes were evaluated for antibacterial potential against *Propionibacterium acnes* using a pig skin model. Curcumin niosomes significantly reduced *Propionibacterium acnes* content at a concentration of 0.43 µg/mL [63]. Similarly, nano structured lipid carriers were fabricated for curcumin delivery focusing on skin permeation. A high skin permeation and deposition were observed for curcumin, along with minimal expulsion of the drug upon storage. This study suggests that curcumin nanoparticles can be effectively targeted for *Acne vulgaris* [64]. Combination therapy has always been shown to be more effective than individual therapy. In this regard, quercetin and Isotretinoin were loaded into self-nanoemulsion for their anti-acne potential. The aim of the study was also to boost the solubility, bioavailability and permeation of mentioned phytochemicals across the skin. The formulated self nanoemulsion showed that a combination of both natural products can be effectively used for the treatment of acne delivered in the form of self-nanoemulsion with maximum clinical efficacy and reduced side effects. An enhanced penetration and improved bioavailability were also observed [65]. It means that nano-based delivery of phytochemicals, either loaded alone or in combination, will be a breakthrough in the treatment of *Acne vulgaris*.

Conventional topical Isotretinoin exhibits side effects thus, stem cell membrane-coated Isotretinoin was fabricated into nanoparticles and applied for the treatment of acne. The model used was hyperkeratinization, and a significant outcome was achieved with Isotretinoin-stem cells-nano particles. The effect of tight junction protein and keratin was reduced through Isotretinoin increased transdermal efficacy encapsulated in nanoparticles. Nanoparticles also aid in the absorption of Isotretinoin through enhanced endocytosis [66]. Azelaic acid from a natural source is considered to be effective against acne. Azelaic acid loaded nanostructured lipid carriers were formulated and evaluated for their anti-acne potential. Topical formulation was applied to mice ear targeting *Propionibacterium acnes*. An improved anti-acne effect was observed using a nanostructured lipid carrier without compromising the therapeutic and safety profile. The low solubility of Azelaic acid was also enhanced through its fabrication from a nano platform [67].

To sum up, phytochemicals can be effectively fabricated into nano formulations for the treatment of *Acne vulgaris*. Nano platform is an efficient tool to boost the bioavailability of phytochemicals, mimic penetration across the skin and deliver the cargo at the desired site during acne treatment.

CONCLUSION

Acne vulgaris is a chronic inflammatory skin disorder characterized by multiple pathological factors. Controlling these factors provide a route for acne management and treatment. In addition to these multiple pathological factors, the existence of other pharmacological targets for treatment agents makes it easy to handle this worse ailment. Various conventional therapies have been explored for acne treatment that, includes hormone therapy and systemic and antibiotics therapy. However, these conventional therapies were limited by some barriers like reduced efficacy and increased side effects. To cope with it, phytochemicals were recently evaluated for its anti-acne potential, which has proven a remarkable treatment choice. Since, some phytochemicals pose the problem of low skin penetration and reduced target availability. These issues were overcome *via* the fabrication of phytochemicals into nano form. Nano-based formulations of phytochemicals pose an alternate and advanced current possible treatment option for *Acne vulgaris*. Nano phytochemicals provide enhanced clinical outcomes, and improved penetration with minimized side effects. Clinical trials were conducted for a couple of phytochemicals targeting acne however, more clinical studies are required to uplift phytochemicals from bench top to the market and make them a more sound option for the treatment of *Acne vulgaris*.

REFERENCES

[1]　Liu CH, Huang HY. *In vitro* anti-propionibacterium activity by curcumin containing vesicle system. Chem Pharm Bull (Tokyo) 2013; 61(4): 419-25.
[http://dx.doi.org/10.1248/cpb.c12-01043] [PMID: 23546001]

[2]　Zouboulis CC, Eady A, Philpott M, *et al.* What is the pathogenesis of acne? Exp Dermatol 2005; 14(2): 143-52.
[http://dx.doi.org/10.1111/j.0906-6705.2005.0285a.x] [PMID: 15679586]

[3]　March C, Witchel S. Acne, Hirsutism, and Other Signs of Increased Androgens Endocrine Conditions in Pediatrics. Springer 2021; pp. 85-94.

[4]　Bhate K, Williams HC. Epidemiology of acne vulgaris. Br J Dermatol 2013; 168(3): 474-85.
[http://dx.doi.org/10.1111/bjd.12149] [PMID: 23210645]

[5]　Perkins AC, Maglione J, Hillebrand GG, Miyamoto K, Kimball AB. Acne vulgaris in women: prevalence across the life span. J Womens Health (Larchmt) 2012; 21(2): 223-30.
[http://dx.doi.org/10.1089/jwh.2010.2722] [PMID: 22171979]

[6]　Marron SE, Chernyshov PV, Tomas-Aragones L. Quality-of-life research in acne vulgaris: current status and future directions. Am J Clin Dermatol 2019; 20(4): 527-38.
[http://dx.doi.org/10.1007/s40257-019-00438-6] [PMID: 30949881]

[7]　Cong TX, Hao D, Wen X, Li XH, He G, Jiang X. From pathogenesis of acne vulgaris to anti-acne agents. Arch Dermatol Res 2019; 311(5): 337-49.
[http://dx.doi.org/10.1007/s00403-019-01908-x] [PMID: 30859308]

[8]　Anaba EL, Oaku IR. Adult female acne: A cross-sectional study of diet, family history, body mass index, and premenstrual flare as risk factors and contributors to severity. Int J Womens Dermatol 2021; 7(3): 265-9.
[http://dx.doi.org/10.1016/j.ijwd.2020.11.008] [PMID: 34222581]

[9]　Anzengruber F, Ruhwinkel K, Ghosh A, Klaghofer R, Lang UE, Navarini AA. Wide range of age of onset and low referral rates to psychiatry in a large cohort of acne excoriée at a Swiss tertiary hospital. J Dermatolog Treat 2018; 29(3): 277-80.
[http://dx.doi.org/10.1080/09546634.2017.1364693] [PMID: 28784003]

[10]　Barros B, Thiboutot D. Hormonal therapies for acne. Clin Dermatol 2017; 35(2): 168-72.
[http://dx.doi.org/10.1016/j.clindermatol.2016.10.009] [PMID: 28274354]

[11]　Tsoukas MM, Pei S, Inamadar AC, Adya KA. Light-based therapies in acne treatment. Indian Dermatol Online J 2015; 6(3): 145-57.
[http://dx.doi.org/10.4103/2229-5178.156379] [PMID: 26009707]

[12]   Tan AU, Schlosser BJ, Paller AS. A review of diagnosis and treatment of acne in adult female patients. Int J Womens Dermatol 2018; 4(2): 56-71.
[http://dx.doi.org/10.1016/j.ijwd.2017.10.006] [PMID: 29872679]

[13]   Setiani NA, Aulifa DL, Septiningsih E, Eds. Phytochemical Screening and Antibacterial Activity of Flower, Stem, and Tuber of Polianthes tuberosa L. Against Acne-Inducing Bacteria. 2nd Bakti Tunas Husada-Health Science International Conference (BTH-HSIC 2019); 2020: Atlantis Press.
[http://dx.doi.org/10.2991/ahsr.k.200523.023]

[14]   Singh V, Redhu R, Verma R, Mittal V, Kaushik D. Anti-acne treatment using nanotechnology based on novel drug delivery system and Patents on acne formulations: a review. Recent Pat Nanotechnol 2021; 15(4): 331-50.
[http://dx.doi.org/10.2174/1872210514666200508121050] [PMID: 33302844]

[15]   Nawarathne NW, Wijesekera K, Wijayaratne WMDGB, Napagoda M. Development of novel topical cosmeceutical formulations from Nigella sativa L. with antimicrobial activity against acne-causing microorganisms. Sci World J 2019; 2019.

[16]   Romes NB, Abdul Wahab R, Abdul Hamid M. The role of bioactive phytoconstituents-loaded nanoemulsions for skin improvement: a review. Biotechnol Biotechnol Equip 2021; 35(1): 711-30.
[http://dx.doi.org/10.1080/13102818.2021.1915869]

[17]   Koo EB, Petersen TD, Kimball AB. Meta-analysis comparing efficacy of antibiotics *versus* oral contraceptives in acne vulgaris. J Am Acad Dermatol 2014; 71(3): 450-9.
[http://dx.doi.org/10.1016/j.jaad.2014.03.051] [PMID: 24880665]

[18]   Azarchi S, Bienenfeld A, Lo Sicco K, Marchbein S, Shapiro J, Nagler AR. Androgens in women. J Am Acad Dermatol 2019; 80(6): 1509-21.
[http://dx.doi.org/10.1016/j.jaad.2018.08.061] [PMID: 30312645]

[19]   Isvy-Joubert A, Nguyen JM, Gaultier A, *et al.* Adult female acne treated with spironolactone: a retrospective data review of 70 cases. Eur J Dermatol 2017; 27(4): 393-8.
[http://dx.doi.org/10.1684/ejd.2017.3062] [PMID: 28862134]

[20]   Bienenfeld A, Nagler AR, Orlow SJ. Oral antibacterial therapy for acne vulgaris: an evidence-based review. Am J Clin Dermatol 2017; 18(4): 469-90.
[http://dx.doi.org/10.1007/s40257-017-0267-z] [PMID: 28255924]

[21]   Zaenglein AL, Shamban A, Webster G, *et al.* A phase IV, open-label study evaluating the use of triple-combination therapy with minocycline HCl extended-release tablets, a topical antibiotic/retinoid preparation and benzoyl peroxide in patients with moderate to severe acne vulgaris. J Drugs Dermatol 2013; 12(6): 619-25.
[PMID: 23839176]

[22]   Moore AY, Charles JEM, Moore S. Sarecycline: a narrow spectrum tetracycline for the treatment of moderate-to-severe acne vulgaris. Future Microbiol 2019; 14(14): 1235-42.
[http://dx.doi.org/10.2217/fmb-2019-0199] [PMID: 31475868]

[23]   Patel DJ, Bhatia N. Oral Antibiotics for Acne. Am J Clin Dermatol 2021; 22(2): 193-204.
[http://dx.doi.org/10.1007/s40257-020-00560-w] [PMID: 32918267]

[24]   Zaenglein AL. Acne Vulgaris. N Engl J Med 2018; 379(14): 1343-52.
[http://dx.doi.org/10.1056/NEJMcp1702493] [PMID: 30281982]

[25]   Ogé' LK, Broussard A, Marshall MD. Acne vulgaris: diagnosis and treatment. Am Fam Physician 2019; 100(8): 475-84.
[PMID: 31613567]

[26]   Nenoff P, Koch D, Krüger C, *et al.* Activity of nadifloxacin and three other antimicrobial agents against *Cutibacterium acnes* isolated from patients with acne vulgaris. J Eur Acad Dermatol Venereol 2021; 35(10): e682-4.
[http://dx.doi.org/10.1111/jdv.17386] [PMID: 34018651]

[27] Karadag AS, Aslan Kayıran M, Wu CY, Chen W, Parish LC. Antibiotic resistance in acne: changes, consequences and concerns. J Eur Acad Dermatol Venereol 2021; 35(1): 73-8.
[http://dx.doi.org/10.1111/jdv.16686] [PMID: 32474948]

[28] Niculet E, Radaschin D, Nastase F, *et al.* Influence of phytochemicals in induced psoriasis. Exp Ther Med 2020; 20(4): 3421-4.
[http://dx.doi.org/10.3892/etm.2020.9013] [PMID: 32905089]

[29] Lambrechts IA, de Canha MN, Lall N. Exploiting medicinal plants as possible treatments for acne vulgaris Medicinal Plants for Holistic Health and Well-Being. Elsevier 2018; pp. 117-43.
[http://dx.doi.org/10.1016/B978-0-12-812475-8.00004-4]

[30] Dréno B. What is new in the pathophysiology of acne, an overview. J Eur Acad Dermatol Venereol 2017; 31 (Suppl. 5): 8-12.
[http://dx.doi.org/10.1111/jdv.14374] [PMID: 28805938]

[31] Kardeh S, Moein S, Namazi MR, Kardeh B. Evidence for the Important ¬role of oxidative stress in the pathogenesis of acne. Galen Med J 2019; 8: 1291.
[http://dx.doi.org/10.31661/gmj.v8i0.1291] [PMID: 34466486]

[32] Bienenfeld A, Azarchi S, Lo Sicco K, Marchbein S, Shapiro J, Nagler AR. Androgens in women. J Am Acad Dermatol 2019; 80(6): 1497-506.
[http://dx.doi.org/10.1016/j.jaad.2018.08.062] [PMID: 30312644]

[33] Motosko CC, Zakhem GA, Pomeranz MK, Hazen A. Acne: a side-effect of masculinizing hormonal therapy in transgender patients. Br J Dermatol 2019; 180(1): 26-30.
[http://dx.doi.org/10.1111/bjd.17083] [PMID: 30101531]

[34] Ma Z, Kochergin NG. Microbiome and acne vulgaris. Russ J Skin Vener Dis 2020; 23(6): 388-94.
[http://dx.doi.org/10.17816/dv60039]

[35] Jeong WY, Kim K. Anti- Propionibacterium acnes and the anti-inflammatory effect of Aloe ferox miller components. J Herb Med 2017; 9: 53-9.
[http://dx.doi.org/10.1016/j.hermed.2017.03.009]

[36] Bodede O, Prinsloo G. Ethnobotany, phytochemistry and pharmacological significance of the genus Bulbine (Asphodelaceae). J Ethnopharmacol 2020; 260: 112986.
[http://dx.doi.org/10.1016/j.jep.2020.112986] [PMID: 32492493]

[37] Arbab S, Ullah H, Weiwei W, *et al.* Comparative study of antimicrobial action of aloe vera and antibiotics against different bacterial isolates from skin infection. Vet Med Sci 2021; 7(5): 2061-7.
[http://dx.doi.org/10.1002/vms3.488] [PMID: 33949142]

[38] Van Wyk B-E, Wink M. Medicinal plants of the world: CABI 2018.

[39] Alfred Maroyi . Medicinal uses, biological and chemical properties of Wild Plum (Harpephyllum caffrum): An indigenous fruit plant of Southern Africa. J Pharm Nutr Sci 2019; 9(5): 258-68.
[http://dx.doi.org/10.29169/1927-5951.2019.09.05.4]

[40] Kuo CW, Chiu YF, Wu MH, *et al.* Gelatin/Chitosan Bilayer Patches Loaded with Cortex *Phellodendron amurense*/*Centella asiatica* Extracts for Anti-Acne Application. Polymers (Basel) 2021; 13(4): 579.
[http://dx.doi.org/10.3390/polym13040579] [PMID: 33671908]

[41] Prasad SB, Kaur D. *In vitro* anti acne activity of ethanolic extract of stem of berberis aristata. Int J Pharmacogn Phytochem Res 2017; 9(2): 190-2.
[http://dx.doi.org/10.25258/phyto.v9i2.8061]

[42] Raoufinejad K, Rajabi M. Licorice in the treatment of acne vulgaris and postinflammatory hyperpigmentation: A Review J Pharmaceuti Care 2020; 8(4).
[http://dx.doi.org/10.18502/jpc.v8i4.5242]

[43] Yoon W-J, Kim S-S, Oh T-H, Lee NH, Hyun C-G. Cryptomeria japonica essential oil inhibits the

growth of drug-resistant skin pathogens and LPS-induced nitric oxide and pro-inflammatory cytokine production. Pol J Microbiol 2009; 58(1): 61-8.
[PMID: 19469288]

[44] Sinha P, Srivastava S, Mishra N, Yadav NP. New perspectives on antiacne plant drugs: contribution to modern therapeutics. Biomed Res Int 2014; 2014.

[45] Li CG, Yan L, Jing YY, *et al.* Berberine augments ATP-induced inflammasome activation in macrophages by enhancing AMPK signaling. Oncotarget 2017; 8(1): 95-109.
[http://dx.doi.org/10.18632/oncotarget.13921] [PMID: 27980220]

[46] Zhang H, Shan Y, Wu Y, *et al.* Berberine suppresses LPS-induced inflammation through modulating Sirt1/NF-κB signaling pathway in RAW264.7 cells. Int Immunopharmacol 2017; 52: 93-100.
[http://dx.doi.org/10.1016/j.intimp.2017.08.032] [PMID: 28888780]

[47] Sun Y, Yuan X, Zhang F, *et al.* Berberine ameliorates fatty acid-induced oxidative stress in human hepatoma cells. Sci Rep 2017; 7(1): 11340.
[http://dx.doi.org/10.1038/s41598-017-11860-3] [PMID: 28900305]

[48] Li J, Tian Y, Zhao L, *et al.* Berberine inhibits androgen synthesis by interaction with aldo-keto reductase 1C3 in 22Rv1 prostate cancer cells. Asian J Androl 2016; 18(4): 607-12.
[http://dx.doi.org/10.4103/1008-682X.169997] [PMID: 26698234]

[49] Ramappa VK, Srivastava D, Singh P, *et al.* Mulberries: a promising fruit for phytochemicals, nutraceuticals, and biological activities. Int J Fruit Sci 2020; 20(3): S1254-79.

[50] Vishwakarma V, Patel N, Budholiya P. Phytochemical screening and antiacne activity of leaves extract of lagerstroemia indica. Int J Pharm Biol Sci Arch 2021; 9(2).
[http://dx.doi.org/10.32553/ijpba.v9i2.184]

[51] Han AR, Kim H, Piao D, Jung CH, Seo EK. Phytochemicals and bioactivities of *Zingiber cassumunar* Roxb. Molecules 2021; 26(8): 2377.
[http://dx.doi.org/10.3390/molecules26082377] [PMID: 33921835]

[52] Kokoska L, Kloucek P, Leuner O, Novy P. Plant-derived products as antibacterial and antifungal agents in human health care. Curr Med Chem 2019; 26(29): 5501-41.
[http://dx.doi.org/10.2174/0929867325666180831144344] [PMID: 30182844]

[53] Khameneh B, Eskin N, Iranshahy M, Fazly Bazzaz B. Phytochemicals: a promising weapon in the arsenal against antibiotic-resistant bacteria. Antibiotics (Basel) 2021; 10(9): 1044. PMCID: PMC8472480.
[http://dx.doi.org/10.3390/antibiotics10091044] [PMID: 34572626]

[54] Ho KV, Lei Z, Sumner L, *et al.* Identifying antibacterial compounds in black walnuts (*Juglans nigra*) using a metabolomics approach. Metabolites 2018; 8(4): 58.
[http://dx.doi.org/10.3390/metabo8040058] [PMID: 30274312]

[55] Shadab K, Aney J, Anjum P. Anti-acne herbs: a review. World J Pharm Res 2018; 7(9).

[56] Winkelman WJ. Aromatherapy, botanicals, and essential oils in acne. Clin Dermatol 2018; 36(3): 299-305.
[http://dx.doi.org/10.1016/j.clindermatol.2018.03.004] [PMID: 29908571]

[57] Yang JH, Yoon JY, Kwon HH, Min S, Moon J, Suh DH. Seeking new acne treatment from natural products, devices and synthetic drug discovery. Dermatoendocrinol 2017; 9(1): e1356520.
[http://dx.doi.org/10.1080/19381980.2017.1356520] [PMID: 29484092]

[58] Abd-Allah H, Abdel-Aziz RTA, Nasr M. Chitosan nanoparticles making their way to clinical practice: A feasibility study on their topical use for acne treatment. Int J Biol Macromol 2020; 156: 262-70.
[http://dx.doi.org/10.1016/j.ijbiomac.2020.04.040] [PMID: 32289418]

[59] Lueangarun S, Sriviriyakul K, Tempark T, Managit C, Sithisarn P. Clinical efficacy of 0.5% topical mangosteen extract in nanoparticle loaded gel in treatment of mild-to-moderate acne vulgaris: A 12-

week, split-face, double-blinded, randomized, controlled trial. J Cosmet Dermatol 2019; 18(5): 1395-403.
[http://dx.doi.org/10.1111/jocd.12856] [PMID: 30688020]

[60] Cakir-Koc R, Budama-Kilinc Y, Kaya Z, Orcen BB, Ucarkus E. Coconut oil-loaded chitosan nanoparticles for the treatment of acne vulgaris: cytotoxicity, antibacterial activity, and antibiofilm properties. Fresenius Environ Bull 2018; 27: 2642-8.

[61] Wijayadi LJ, Rusli TR, Eds. Encapsulated lime peel essential oil (Citrus hystrix) into chitosan nanoparticle: new entity to enhanced effectivity against propionilbacterium acne in vitro. IOP Conf Ser: Mater Sci Eng; IOP Publishing: 2020.

[62] Folle C, Díaz-Garrido N, Sánchez-López E, *et al.* Surface-modified multifunctional thymol-loaded biodegradable nanoparticles for topical acne treatment. Pharmaceutics 2021; 13(9): 1501.
[http://dx.doi.org/10.3390/pharmaceutics13091501] [PMID: 34575577]

[63] Paiva-Santos AC, Mascarenhas-Melo F, Coimbra SC, *et al.* Nanotechnology-based formulations toward the improved topical delivery of anti-acne active ingredients. Expert Opin Drug Deliv 2021; 18(10): 1435-54.
[http://dx.doi.org/10.1080/17425247.2021.1951218] [PMID: 34214003]

[64] Rapalli VK, Kaul V, Waghule T, *et al.* Curcumin loaded nanostructured lipid carriers for enhanced skin retained topical delivery: optimization, scale-up, *in-vitro* characterization and assessment of *ex-vivo* skin deposition. Eur J Pharm Sci 2020; 152: 105438.
[http://dx.doi.org/10.1016/j.ejps.2020.105438] [PMID: 32598913]

[65] Hosny KM, Al Nahyah KS, Alhakamy NA. Self-Nanoemulsion Loaded with a Combination of Isotretinoin, an Anti-Acne Drug, and Quercetin: Preparation, Optimization, and *In Vivo* Assessment. Pharmaceutics 2020; 13(1): 46.
[http://dx.doi.org/10.3390/pharmaceutics13010046] [PMID: 33396942]

[66] Wang S, Jiang R, Meng T, *et al.* Stem cell membrane-coated isotretinoin for acne treatment. J Nanobiotechnology 2020; 18(1): 106.
[http://dx.doi.org/10.1186/s12951-020-00664-9] [PMID: 32723398]

[67] Malik DS, Kaur G. Exploring therapeutic potential of azelaic acid loaded NLCs for the treatment of acne vulgaris. J Drug Deliv Sci Technol 2020; 55: 101418.
[http://dx.doi.org/10.1016/j.jddst.2019.101418]

Vitiligo and Treatment Protocols

Mehnaz Showkat[1], **Humaira Bilal**[1], **Bilquees Bhat**[1] and **Nahida Tabassum**[2,*]

[1]*Department of Pharmaceutical Sciences (Pharmacology Division), University of Kashmir, Hazratbal, Srinagar, Jammu and Kashmir, 190006, India*

[2] *Department of Pharmaceutical Sciences, Dean School of Applied Sciences and Technology, University of Kashmir, Hazratbal, Srinagar, Jammu and Kashmir, 190006, India*

Abstract: Vitiligo is an abiding acquired skin disorder caused by the epidermal disappearance of pigment cells of localized and general skin mucosa, characterized by the appearance of symmetrical patches on the skin. The exact cause of this disorder is unknown, but genetic susceptibility, melanocyte growth factor deficiency, autoimmunity, and some neurological and environmental factors are believed to play a triggering role. Although no drugs are completely successful in managing this disorder, many different approaches, such as topical corticosteroids, calcineurin inhibitors, transplantation, newly emerged phototherapy, or the combination approaches, however, have shown positive results and have helped to restore skin tone in people with small areas of depigmentation. The association of the adverse effects such as redness, itching, burning, pruritis, xerosis cutis, or potential risk of skin cancer and the high treatment cost with these therapies has necessitated the development of other newer treatment approaches such as phytotherapy for vitiligo. Also, novel drugs are being developed that either stimulate the melanocytes, like afamelanotide, or help control or protect the melanocytes. Many herbal drugs have been reported beneficial in the treatment of vitiligo, which has been shown to stimulate melanogenesis, proliferation or migration of melanocytes or have immunomodulatory properties. Further research on herbal drugs should be extended to develop safe, effective and affordable treatments for vitiligo.

Keywords: Afamelanotide, Corticosteroids, Depigmentation, Herbal drugs, Melanocyte growth factor, Phytotherapy, Skin patches, Vitiligo.

INTRODUCTION

Vitiligo is a progressive disorder of the skin characterized by delineated white lesions of inconstant size and shape. The appearance of these patches has been attributed to the selective loss of skin pigment cells (melanocytes), which in turn makes skin more prone to sunburn, aging and cancer. Although the exact etiology

* **Corresponding author Nahida Tabassum:** Department of Pharmaceutical Sciences, Dean School of Applied Sciences and Technology, University of Kashmir, Hazratbal, Srinagar, Jammu and Kashmir, 190006, India;
E-mail: n.tabassum.uk@gmail.com

Heba Abd El-Sattar El-Nashar, Mohamed El-Shazly & Nouran Mohammed Fahmy (Eds.)

of the disease is unknown, the progression of the disease might be due to some autoimmune, neural and biochemical mechanisms. It affects nearly 1-2% of the world population, mostly before adulthood, with high psychiatric morbidity and can be socially distressing for the affected individuals [1, 2]. The incidence of vitiligo in India has been reported between 0.25-4% in dermatology outpatients across India and up to 8.8% in Rajasthan and Gujarat [3]. With proper management and supervision, disease progression can be abated, and patients may attain repigmentation in order to restore the functional deficiencies and morphology of the depigmented areas [1]. Topical corticosteroids and calcineurin inhibitors have proved effective first-choice treatments for localized forms of this disease. However, in generalized form, phototherapy has revealed exceptional efficacy [4]. Light therapy (UVB) alone has shown better repigmentation rates and safety profiles in comparison to topical or oral psoralen and UVA combination (PUVA). Alternative treatment options include transplantation methods, depigmentation therapies, and other novel therapeutic approaches such as focused microphototherapy, systemic antioxidant therapy, *etc.* [1]. Many herbal drugs have been reported beneficial in the treatment of vitiligo, which has been shown to stimulate melanogenesis, proliferation or migration of melanocytes or have immunomodulatory properties [5]. In recent years, efforts to discover and develop new, safe, affordable, and effective vitiligo drugs from natural sources have gained much attention among researchers due to the recognition of the worldwide importance of fighting vitiligo disease.

ETIOLOGY

Despite the numerous efforts, the exact etiology underlying the disease is still unclear. However, several hypotheses regarding the loss of melanocytes have been put forth, but none of these hypotheses could clearly explain the complete spectrum of this disorder. The key factors that might play a triggering role in the progression of disease include genetic factors, neural factors, autoimmune factors, some self-destructing precursors of melanogenesis and defective melanocyte growth factor [1]. Nearly one-third of vitiligo-affected individuals have reported close family members affected by the disorder signifying that genetic factors have very important role in the pathogenesis of the disease [6]. Most recent theories in the pathophysiology of vitiligo include oxidative stress and accumulation of hydrogen peroxide (H_2O_2) in the epidermal layer of depigmented area. Oxidative stress theory states that oxygen radicals are the main reason for the apoptosis of melanocytes. Free radical levels may rise either due to an increase in the rate of their production or the reduced ability of cells to neutralize them [7]. In addition, accumulation of high levels of H_2O_2 in the epidermis is destructive for melanocytes, inhibits tyrosinase enzyme, and also disables catalase which is a peroxisomal enzyme catalyzing the reduction of H_2O_2 to water and oxygen. Such disparity between oxidative stress and antioxidant enzyme systems plays a significant role in the destruction of melanocytes [8, 9].

TYPES

The main types of vitiligo include [1, 10, 11]:

i. **Segmental/Localized Vitiligo:** It is the least common pattern, which mainly includes focal, segmental (limited to a particular section of the integument), and mucosal lesions often following the distribution of trigeminal nerve but do not progress to a generalized form.

ii. **Generalized/Non-Segmental Vitiligo:** It is the most common pattern which corresponds to all generalized symmetrical forms, including acrofacial, vulgaris and mixed acrofacialis and/or vulgaris and/or segmentalis form.

iii. **Universal Vitiligo:** It is a rare type of vitiligo, and comprises >80% depigmentation.

TREATMENT

Inspite of tremendous efforts, vitiligo treatment modalities are still derisory for the patients as most physicians contemplate it as a trivial form of the disease, which cannot be completely treated, and the patient has to live with it for a lifetime. This approach towards the disease makes the patient feel discouraged from seeking therapy. There must be a proper approach to explaining the disease and its treatment to the patient. Although there is no appropriate therapeutic cure for the disease, several conventional (Fig. **1**), novel treatment protocols (Fig. **2**) and herbal drugs which are being used for the treatment of vitiligo have revealed promising results in most patients.

Conventional Treatment Protocols

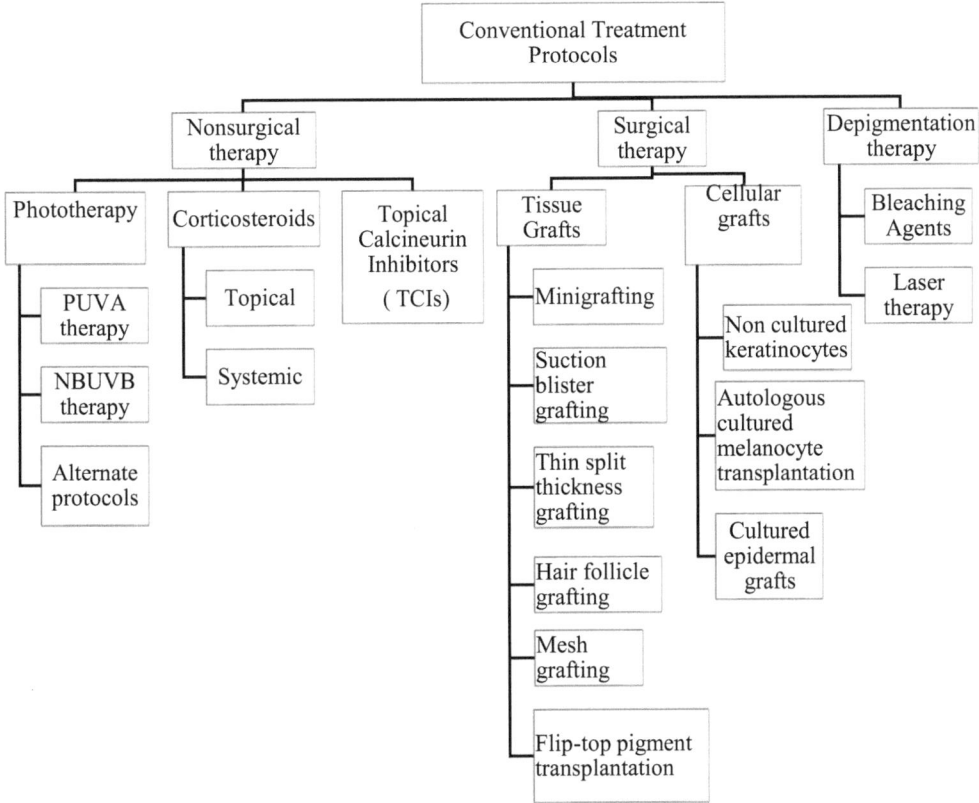

Fig. (1). Conventional treatment protocols.

Non Surgical Therapies

The nonsurgical therapies generally considered as first-line therapy mainly include:

- Phototherapy/Light therapy,
- Corticosteroids,
- Topical Calcineurin Inhibitors [12, 13].

Phototherapy/Light Therapy

This therapy is the most effective and harmless therapy among all the other therapies used to treat patients suffering from vitiligo, and it mainly includes:

- Psoralen plus Ultraviolet A (PUVA) therapy.
- Narrow Band Ultraviolet B (NBUVB) therapy.
- Other Alternative Protocols such as Broadband Ultraviolet B (BBUVB), Khellin plus UVA (KUVA) therapy, and Phenylalanine plus UVA (Phe-UVA) therapy.

Psoralen Plus UVA (PUVA) Therapy

It is the major therapy for generalized vitiligo and is quite a slow and tedious procedure, thus requiring highly motivated patients [14]. Nearly 60-80% of patients undergoing PUVA show effective repigmentation rates, the first evidence of which is generally seen after 1-4 months of treatment [14] or may occur as early as 3 weeks (Mild). This therapy uses a combination of ultraviolet (UV)A and photosensitizing compound psoralen (either topical PUVA or oral PUVA). The skin repigmenting use of psoralens in vitiligo has been reported in various Indian and Egyptians literatures. These are active furanocoumarin compounds capable of absorbing radiant energy [15]. Most often used agents used for the treatment of vitiligo include methoxsalen (8-methoxypsoralen or 8-MOP), 5-methoxypsoralen (bergapten or 5-MOP), trioxsalen (4,5′,8-trimethylpsoralen or TMP) [14]. These probably act synergistically with sunlight to stimulate melanogenesis [16].

This therapy mostly utilizes high-intensity UVA sources or UVA obtained from solar light natural sunlight (PUVASol) to activate chemicals known as Psoralens. It uses UVA radiation of 320-400nm wavelength. The preliminary UVA dose varies from 1-2J/cm^2 with maximum exposure of 8-12J/cm^2. Treatment on a daily basis is not mandatory, the recommended ideal frequency is one irradiation every third day to avoid any adverse phototoxic effect, and the risk of Koebner reaction due to overexposure and persistent erythema is apparent within 36-48 hours of exposure [14]. Psoralen derivatives are administered either systemically as microcrystalline tablets or capsules (8-MOP at doses varying from 0.3-0.6mg/kg, TMP at 0.6-1.2 mg/kg and 5-MOP either alone or in combination [17] or topically (8-MOP in the form of gel, cream soak or lotion) [18]. Oral psoralens should be ingested in a single dose 2 hours before exposure [14]. Exposure to sunlight must be avoided from the time of ingestion of psoralen and throughout the remainder of the day. UV-blocking sunglasses and broad-spectrum sunscreen must be used [19].

Mechanism of Action

PUVA is believed to act by stimulating melanogenesis which includes photoconjugation of psoralens or their derivatives in the melanocytes to DNA, subsequent mitosis followed by propagation of melanocytes which ultimately results in the repopulation of the epidermis, enhanced formation and melanization of melanosomes, greater transfer of melanosomes to keratinocytes, and increased synthesis of tyrosinase *via* stimulation of cAMP activity [20]. Repigmentation is therefore regarded as the result of the migration of these stimulated melanocytes into the depigmented skin areas [21]. Another study suggested that PUVA therapy may prompt the release of a certain melanocyte-stimulating growth factor that is capable of stimulating melanocyte proliferation in vitiligo [22].

Adverse Effects and Contraindications

Psoralens are generally well tolerated at therapeutic doses however, slight epigastric distress, nausea, insomnia, nervousness, fatigue, pruritus, and drowsiness has observed in some patients. Prolonged administration of 8-MOP mostly results in transient nausea for several hours, rarely occurs with TMP and 5-MOP, and can be minimised by taking them with food or milk or by splitting/ decreasing the psoralen dose [23]. Erythema is the most common adverse effect due to overexposure. It usually occurs within 24 hours and reaches a peak at 48-78 hours but occasionally occurs as late as 96 hours [24]. The other common side effect associated with psoralens is pruritus [25], the incidence of which is reported to be higher with 8-MOP than with 5-MOP [26]. Long-term side effects include carcinogenicity of skin (because of psoralen's ability to cause mutations in DNA *via* cross-link formation), alterations to the immune system, damage to eyes, cutaneous aging, pigmented lesions [24], aggravation of photodermatoses, potential drug interactions, induction of liver enzymes and hepatotoxicity [18]. PUVA therapy in not recommended for skin type I, skin malignancies, pregnant or lactating women (oral form), and is relatively contraindicated in patients younger than 12 years [23].

Narrow Band UVB (NBUVB) Therapy

NBUVB is an elementary form of phototherapy, as it refers to the use of artificial UVB radiation without any supplementary exogenous photosensitizers. Due to its higher efficacy and safety profile in comparison to PUVA therapy, it has gained much popularity and is preferred over PUVA for generalized vitiligo both in children and adults.

This therapy uses narrowband UV lamps (*e.g.*, Philips TL-01/100 W) with an emission spectrum of 310- modality 315nm and a maximum wavelength of 311nm [27, 28]. The preliminary dose is 0.25J/cm^2 (for all types of skin), and this is increased by 10- 20% until negligible erythema occurs in the depigmented areas. This regimen is given twice a week and at no time on 2 successive days. As certain regions of the body may reach minimal erythema faster, a differential dosage regimen per region of the body may be required [28]. NBUVB has gained more popularity as it offers various advantages in comparison to PUVA, such as shorter duration of treatment, cost-effectiveness, no systemic side effects, minimal incidents of burning, hyperkeratosis after prolonged irradiation, effective in children, pregnant and lactating women, no need for post-treatment eye protection [29].

Mechanism of Action

The exact mechanism underlying NBUVB therapy in vitiligo is still unknown. It is believed that it has some relation with the melanocyte reserve in the outer root sheath [30]. It has been proposed that NBUVB acts in two steps, the first step includes immunomodulation which down-regulates the attack against melanocytes, and the second step involves stimulation of melanocytes leading to their migration to the epidermis followed by synthesis of melanin [21]. This therapy also increases the synthesis of various cytokines, such as TNF-α, LTC-4 and IL-1, which induce the mitogenesis of melanocytes, melanin production and melanocyte migration. It has also been reported that TNF-α inhibits the expression of the enzyme tyrosinase, which is the chief enzyme involved in the synthesis of melanin. The inhibitory effect of TNF-α on melanin synthesis is dependent on the activation of nuclear factor kappa B (NFκB) [31]. It has been proposed that in human keratinocytes, enhanced expression of IL-1, endothelin-1, and tyrosinase after irradiation with UVB might be the possible mechanism of repigmentation [32]. Prostaglandins have also been shown to play a role in melanogenesis and proliferation of melanocytes. PGE2, which is synthesized in the skin, is believed to regulate melanocyte cell function, and promote melanocyte mitogenesis [33].

Adverse Effects and Contraindications

Adverse effects associated with NBUVB are less severe in comparison to PUVA, which mostly includes erythema, pruritus and xerosis cutis [34]. NBUVB may also cause a relapse of orolabial herpes [30]. It has also been observed in mice models that there is an increased risk of malignant skin cancers with NBUVB than Broad band UVB (BBUVB) *via* increased production of cyclobutane pyrimidine dimer (CPD), which confers high carcinogenic potential to NBUVB [35]. NBUVB should be given only to children who cannot be effectively managed with conservative protocols, who have a widespread form of disease or localized form associated with a substantial impact on quality of life (Mild).

Alternate Protocols

Broad Band UVB (BBUVB) Therapy

It offers various advantages in comparison to PUVA and is mostly effective in patients who cannot withstand PUVA therapy. This therapy utilizes broadband

UV lamps/ fluorescent tubes (*e.g.*, Philips TL-12, Westinghouse FS, Waldmann UV-6 or UV-21) with an emission spectrum of 290-320nm. The initial dose is 20mJ/cm^2 and can be increased to 20% until minimal erythema occurs, given twice to thrice weekly. It has been observed that BBUVB ceased the progression of vitiligo and induced repigmentation in 8-12 treatments. The side effects associated with BBUVB are minimal and mainly include erythema (mild), pruritus, folliculitis, and reactivation of the Herpes Simplex Virus (HSV) [36].

Khellin Plus UVA (KUVA) Therapy

It is an emerging alternative to PUVA. Khellin is furochromone derived from the plant *Ammi visnaga* and functions in the same way as psoralen but is less phototoxic and carcinogenic in comparison to PUVA because of its ability to form fever cross-links in DNA. Khellin, in combination with UVA or solar irradiation, has been reported to cause repigmentation in vitiligo patients as effectively as PUVA therapy [37]. In contrast to PUVA, it has been reported that this therapy does not induce hyperpigmentation of adjacent nonvitiliginous skin [38]. Khellin taken orally has been associated with fever and systemic side effects such as nausea and elevation of liver transaminases [39]. It has been observed that KUVA/khellin acts directly on isolated melanocytes to enhance the proliferation of melanocytes and melanogenesis. Melanogenesis in normal melanocytes was not stimulated by khellin or UVA alone, but together they enhanced the melanogenic process fourfold [37].

Phenylalanine Plus UVA (Phe-UVA) Therapy

L-Phenylalanine taken orally followed by UVA exposure, has revealed promising results in the treatment of vitiligo. Phenylalanine is an essential amino acid, which acts as a precursor of tyrosine in melanin synthesis. Most dietary phenylalanine undergoes hydroxylation into tyrosine which is then converted to melanin and fatty acids. Since it forms a part of daily dietary protein, serious side effects from the oral administration of Phe are unlikely. Effective repigmentation rates have been reported in about 50-90% of patients with mean phenylalanine. Blood levels range from 3.6 to 6.9 mg/dl and the mean total dosage of UVA is 352 ± 139 joules/cm^2. The major advantage associated with this therapy was an incidence of fewer or no side effects and thus represents an effective alternative therapy for childhood vitiligo [40]. Another study has reported gradual repigmentation rates mostly in adipose areas of skin after 4 months of treatment with various UVA doses ranging from 126.6-306.3 J according to the skin type and oral Phe in doses of 50 mg/kg body weight. The mechanism of repigmentation underlying this therapy has been attributed to the stimulatory effect of Phe or one of its metabolites in combination with UVA. So far, the results of Phe-UVA therapy are relatively promising. It is also worth mentioning that vitiliginous skin becomes less sensitive to sunlight and in addition, normal skin tans very well during Phe-UVA treatment [41].

Corticosteroids

Corticosteroids constitute an important modality for the treatment of vitiligo. They may arrest the progression of disease leading to repigmentation by suppressing the immune activity to reduce the inflammation [42] and can be administered *via* various routes such as topical, oral or intralesional [1], thus, proving their effectiveness in vitiligo treatment by suppressing the melanocyte cytotoxicity associated with autoantibodies [43].

Topical Corticosteroids

Topical corticosteroids are considered as first-line treatment for localized vitiligo both in children and adults [44]. Their cost-effectiveness, high compliance, and easy application are a few advantages of topical corticodteroids [45]. Most commonly used topical corticosteroids include Hydrocortisone, Betamethasone Valerate, Triamcinolone Acetonide, clobetasol, Methylprednisolone, Fluticasone, *etc*. [44]. Several studies have reported clobetasol- a topical corticosteroid that often produces pigmentation and is considered one of the most effective agents for treating vitiligo [46]. As the incidence of side effects associated with corticosteroids is higher in children, their recommended treatment regimens vary from that of adults [47]. It has been observed that topical application of Class II (high potency) corticosteroids have proven to be effective in about 56% of patients suffering from vitiligo with higher repigmentation rates, and likewise, application of Class III (medium to high potency) corticosteroids is effective in about 55% of total cases [48]. It has been postulated that Topical corticosteroids may either potentiate a melanocyte auto-destruction protective mechanism or locally suppress the immunological changes allowing inactive melanocytes to effect repigmentation [49]. The use of topical corticosteroids for generalized vitiligo is unreasonable because of associated side effects such as skin atrophy, telangiectasia, and striae distensae, hypopigmentation, and hypertrichosis [49 - 51]. Infancy, hepatic disease, kidney-associated diseases, underactive thyroid gland, overweightness, inefficient supervision, and quantity and strength of topical corticosteroids are a few of the risk factors that strengthen the chance of systemic side effects [43]. If there is no clinical improvement after 2 months of therapy, treatment must be withdrawn, and no repigmentation after 2 months necessitates a shift to alternative therapies [49].

Systemic Corticosteroids

Systemic corticosteroids may arrest the progression of vitiligo and lead to repigmentation by immunosuppression and may be given in case of progressing vitiligo but are usually not recommended due to high toxicity profile. Nearly 70.4% repigmentation rate has been observed with initially low-dose oral prednisolone (0.3mg/kg for 2 months and then half of the preliminary dose for subsequent three months) [42]. Effectiveness of i.v. methylprednisolone (8 mg/kg bodyweight) administrated on three successive days has been observed to induce

the termination of disease progression and repigmentation in 71% of cases, even though re-depigmentation was observed in 10–60% of the affected lesions [52].

It has also been reported that oral dexamethasone pulse treatment is effective in stopping disease progression yet fails to induce satisfactory repigmentation in a majority of vitiligo cases. Reported side effects are mild to moderate and mostly include acne, weight gain, insomnia, acne, anxiety, abnormalities in menstruation and hypertrichosis, however, continued suppression of endogenous cortisol production does not occur with the pulse regimen [53]. They are believed to act by reducing the complement-mediated cytotoxicity and antibody titer to surface antigens of melanocytes in the serum of users [50].

Topical Calcineurin Inhibitors (TCIs)/Topical Immunomodulators (TIMs)

Topical calcineurin inhibitors (TCIs), also called Topical immunomodulators (TIMs), are considered first-line treatments for localized forms of disease and have shown significant therapeutic effects [54] for the lesions on the neck and head and especially in long-lasting diseases [55]. The use of corticosteroids, along with TIMs such as tacrolimus and pimecrolimus, exerts immunosuppressive action hence, seems rational for the treatment of vitiligo [45]. Even though topical corticosteroids are preferred for localized vitiligo, they can be replaced by TIMs/TCIs, which display equivalent effectiveness and fewer side effects. The effectiveness of TCI monotherapy is often underrated. Topical tacrolimus offers the benefit of extended treatment without the adverse effects observed in the prolonged use of corticosteroids [56]. It has been observed that Tacrolimus is more effective than Pimecrolimus in localised stable vitiligo when treated and monitored for 6 months [57].

TCIs act *via* various mechanisms such as:

• They act on gene expression and block the transcription of proinflammatory cytokines (*e.g.*, interleukins, TNF-α and INFγ) [56].
• They also endorse the migration and propagation of melanocytes and

melanoblasts by increasing matrix metalloproteinase enzyme [58 - 61], and in addition to this, they also induce the expression of endothelin in melanoblasts [62].

- They act by inducing melanogenesis by increasing the expression of tyrosinase enzyme [58, 61, 63] and by enhancing dopa oxidase activity [58].
- It has been observed that topical tacrolimus (applied twice daily for 7 months) decreased oxidative stress and enhanced antioxidant activity in vitiligo patients [64].

A combination of TCIs with phototherapeutic modalities may represent a vital advancement in the treatment of disease. Tacrolimus, in combination with NB-UVB, showed synergistic effects [65, 66]. However, it has also been observed that the combination of NBUVB and 0.1% tacrolimus was not more efficacious than NB-UVB alone [67]. Combined therapy may also increase the risk of skin carcinogenesis [68]. Moreover, the use of tacrolimus may be beneficial in averting UVB-induced erythema by impeding initial events of the inflammatory process [50]. The adverse effects associated with TCIs are pruritus, burning sensation, and erythema [46]. Tacrolimus, in combination with 308-nm excimer, has shown potential for an even greater response rate [69]. Also, in infants under 2 years of age, pimecrolimus cream 1% or tacrolimus ointment 0.03% have proved to be good therapeutic option for treating vitiligo [70].

Surgical Therapies

Surgical therapies are considered in patients who do not adequately respond to nonsurgical therapies and in case of failure of medical therapies to cause repigmentation, particularly on lips, nipples, genitals and acral areas. These therapies are often used in segmental vitiligo cases, which show good response to the surgery and in the treatment of refractory stable lesions. The basic principle underlying these therapies is to attain repigmentation of vitiliginous skin by autologous melanocyte grafting from the unaffected area of a donor to vitiligo-affected areas of the recipient [71]. Several methods have been reported, which mainly include tissue and cellular grafts [72]. However, properly counseling the patient concerning the outcome is important prior to the procedure. These therapies can be used in combination with other medical and/or irradiation therapies. In addition, transplantation methods may also be considered as an option to treat segmental or stable forms of the disease. Even after effective grafting, disease progression cannot stop, and depigmentation of the grafts may still occur when recurrence of the disease takes place [71].

The choice of treatment depends on:

- Type of disease
- Affected area and location of the lesions
- Equipment availability
- Proficiency and expertise of the surgeon.

Surgery is contraindicated in patients with active unstable vitiligo, in patients with a history of Koebner phenomenon, bleeding disorders, and keloidal tendency [1, 73], and in children suffering from vitiligo because it is quite difficult to predict the disease progression in children, moreover medical therapy is quite effective in children than in adults. Also, the surgical procedure needs to be done under general anesthesia, which poses another risk in children [71].

Techniques of Grafting

Tissue Grafts

Tissue grafts mainly include minipunch grafting, suction blister grafting, thin split thickness grafting, hair follicle grafting, mesh grafting, and flip top pigment transplantation.

Minipunch Grafting

This technique involves harvesting punch grafts (2mm thick) from normally pigmented sites of the donor, such as hip, buttocks, *etc.* and subsequent transplantation of these to similar punched-out depigmented recipient sites. Grafts are placed 5-8mm apart from each other and the grafted area is then covered with adhesive tape [72, 74]. Subsequently, grafted areas are exposed to UVA ($10J/cm^2$) twice a week, which promotes the outgrowth of pigment cells from minigrafts. It is generally observed that pigment starts migrating concentrically migrating from the grafts into the depigmented skin, within 8 weeks following transplantation. Various complications that may occur at the donor site mainly include light scarring, postinflammatory hyper/hypopigmentation, and infection. However, at the recipient site, the cobblestone effect, the multicolored appearance of the grafts, sinking pits, and infection have been observed as adverse effects [75].

Suction Blister Grafting

This technique involves harvesting the grafts and subsequent removal of grafts with sharp scissors and forceps. The epidermal sheet is then grafted onto the stripped recipient site. The success rate of this technique is approximately 73-

88%. The spread of pigment after epidermal blister grafting can be improved by pre-operative therapy of the donor site using PUVA. However, temporary hyperpigmentation is observed in the grafted sites [76].

Thin Split Thickness Grafting

This technique involves procurement of a thin split-thickness graft using a dermatome and direct application of this to the derma braided recipient area. In the first few months, temporary small epithelial milia-like cysts are observed in the recipient area. Keloid formation at the donor site has also been observed in nearly 12% of patients. This technique has a high success rate of 78–91%, but more than one grafting session is necessary due to the limited availability of donor tissue [76].

Hair Follicle Grafting

This technique involves the replenishment of melanocytes using undifferentiated stem cells of the hair follicles by the follicular unit transplantation (FUT) technique. Minor and stable lesions affecting the hairy areas can be effortlessly and efficiently treated by this method. This technique reveals better results and minimal complications in comparison to other techniques. In this technique, donor follicles are extracted using a biopsy punch (follicular unit extraction/ FUE), usually from occipital or postauricular regions of the scalp. The hair follicles so removed are kept in normal cold saline and are transplanted intact as follicular units. Slits are created in the recipient area, and follicular units are gently introduced into these slits using forceps. To facilitate repigmentation, topical corticosteroid and tacrolimus or topical PUVAsol therapy is started after 10 days. FUE is quite a reasonable and harmless method of surgical repigmentation. It does not require any special apparatus or a classy theater setting. Leukotrichia was also found to improve with technique. This technique was also found to be effective in combination with other procedures [73].

Mesh Grafting

In this technique, the graft is extended by forming slits in it so that it looks like a mesh. The meshing of the graft allows coverage of large body areas even with a smaller graft due to graft expansion. Split thickness graft is obtained from the donor sit using a dermatome followed by meshing in an Ampligreffe or DiscardA-pad or manually using a sterile blade. The graft is then transferred to the cleaned and dermabraded recipient site, and bandaged with saline-soaked dressing which is then detached after a week. Light therapy follows up instantly or after one week [77].

Flip Top Pigment Transplantation

In this technique, the graft is kept in between a flap of dermis and epidermis at the recipient side. It mainly involves picking of thin split-thickness graft with the help of a sterile blade from either the upper portion of the arm or the lateral aspect of the thigh. The grafts are then kept in saline-soaked gauze so that they remain humid. The recipient site is thoroughly cleaned, and likewise, a flap of the epidermis is elevated using a sterile blade. The graft is reserved with the dermal side of the graft in contact with the dermis and subsequently, the flap is placed back in position to cover the graft. For securing the graft and flap, cyanoacrylate glue is used and subsequent dressing of both the donor and recipient area is done. Removal of dressing is done after a week and graft uptake is checked. The patient is subjected to phototherapy thereafter. The flap of the epidermis behaves as a biological dressing. The chances of falling off of the graft and secondary infection are less in this procedure. It is cheap, easy to perform, and a quick method [77].

Major disadvantages associated with tissue grafts include a large amount of donor skin which needs substantial skill and is not possible in patients having large lesions. Also, big donor grafts result in substantial morbidity to patients due to prolonged healing time of donor area, and infection, need for strict immobilization of grafted area, postoperative pain is other possible complications. These techniques are time-consuming, and problematic for minor lesions and areas which reveal disappointing results, such as earlobe, fingertips, *etc*. Common complications include perilesional halo, cobblestoning and hyperpigmentation of the recipient area [78]. These drawbacks can be overcome by cellular grafting techniques.

Cellular Grafts

Cellular grafts involve the following methods; noncultured keratinocyte and melanocyte transplantation, autologous cultured pure melanocyte suspension and cultured epidermal grafts [79]. Advantages of cellular grafts over tissue grafts include the need for a smaller amount of donor tissue for a large recipient area, reduction of postoperative morbidity and pain, application of cell suspension is easier in comparison to application of grafts, less immobilization needed, a postoperative amalgamation of grafted area with a pigmented area is better, more suitable for difficult areas for tissue grafts such as finger tips [80].

Non-Cultured Keratinocytes and Melanocytes Transplantation

This technique uses a suspension of non-cultured keratinocytes and melanocytes for the treatment of depigmented lesions in vitiligo. Generally, donor skin is harvested from the occipital area and subsequently immersed in a 0.25% solution of trypsin for 18hrs. On a subsequent day, using forceps the epidermis of donor skin *in vitro*. After numerous procedures, a cellular suspension is obtained [81]. For inducing blisters in the recipient's skin, liquid nitrogen is used, and cellular suspension from the donor site is injected into each blister at the recipient area after aspiration of the viscid blister fluid. The blister top is a natural dressing that holds the transplanted cells in place. It is essential not to separate keratinocytes from melanocytes before grafting because factors furnished by keratinocytes sustain melanocyte growth [76].

Autologous Cultured Melanocyte Transplantation

Use of cultured pure autologous human melanocytes was first described by Lerner *et al.* [82]. In this method *in vitro* cultured melanocytes are used for treatment of vitiligo. The donor skin is reaped from the gluteal region by shave excision and the separation of epidermis from the dermis is done by trypsinization. By forceful vortexing Melanocytes are separated from keratinocytes and are kept in an altered melanocyte medium containing several growth factors for 15-30 days. As soon as sufficient numbers are achieved, melanocytes are detached from culture plates. Technique such as Superficial dermabrasion or CO_2 laser ablation is used to prepare the recipient area and the suspension is then transplanted on this area in a density of $1000 - 2000$ melanocytes/mm^2. There are various ways by which pigment cells can be transplanted, such as in the form of free suspension or in combination with keratinocytes as a co-culture, or in combination with epidermal sheets. The site is then covered with gauze, saturated in a culture medium, and followed by an occlusive dressing. The immovability is recommended for 8-10 hrs and the dressing is changed after a gap of 1 week. This technique allows a large area to be treated in a single session and uses a larger donor-to-recipient ratio in comparison to the non-cultured technique. However, it requires a special laboratory [83, 84], and some safety concerns have been there regarding the use of cultured autografts in vitiligo. Other potential risks are mutagenicity and carcinogenicity. TPA (12- tetradecanoylphorbol 13-acetate), which was used as a constituent of culture medium, has the potential to promote tumors, hence, apprehensions about its long-term safety have been articulated. However, the current accessibility of serum- free media and TPA-free media is a probable resolution to overcome this problem. In addition, Beta fibroblast growth factor (bFGF), a substitute for TPA, is believed to offer pleasing results [83, 85].

Cultured Epidermal Grafts

The most common source for epidermal cell culture is the shave biopsy of normally pigmented skin. After proper separation of the epidermis from the dermis the cells are kept in a medium that permits co-cultivation of melanocytes and keratinocytes. A Cultured sheet is obtained after a week, released by treatment with enzyme dispase and attached to petrolatum gauze as support. Subsequently, the gauze to which the epithelium attaches is applied onto the derma braided recipient site and is covered with an occlusive dressing. The major advantage of this technique is the expansion of the cells in culture, which allows the treatment of a larger area of hypomelanosis with a small donor skin. Because only superficial dermabrasion is performed, the technique is non-scaring [86].

Depigmentation Therapy

Depigmentation of residual melanin is mostly considered in patients with either widespread depigmentation (>80%) or in patients having disfiguring lesions not responding to repigmentation therapies. Bleaching or removal of the remaining pigmentation is a permanent and irreversible process and during or even after completion of therapy, patients are at permanent risk of acquiring sunburn from solar irradiation, so patient should be well informed about this before seeking therapy and must therefore be advised to minimize sun exposure and to apply broad-spectrum sunscreens [1]. Various depigmenting agents include:

Bleaching Agents

Monobenzylether of Hydroquinone (MBEH)

Also known as monobenzone, is most frequently used in concentrations of 20-40% for the removal of residual melanin in patients with vitiligo universalis. It is a potent melanocytotoxic agent [87]. Depigmentation therapy using MBEH does not necessarily require frequent visits to the doctor and can be carried out at home as well. Prior to the application of cream, an open-use test is performed on the pigmented skin of the forearm to check for the development of contact dermatitis. If contact dermatitis does not develop, the cream can then be applied by the patient to the affected areas. Mostly patients prefer to treat the areas with residual pigment from highest to lowest priority. It is used in varying concentrations depending upon the area to be treated, *e.g.*, 10% on the face, 5% on the neck, and 20% on the arms and legs. However, the concentration of MBEH can be increased to 30% and 40% only if 20% MBEH is not effective and these concentrations are mostly recommended over extremities such as elbows and knees. Progressive lightening of the lesions occurs over 4-12 months [88]. It has been observed that tretinoin, in combination with MBEH, enhances the depigmentation of the skin [87]. In order to maintain the depigmentation, it may occasionally be used even beyond one year. It has been reported that all-trans retinoic acid (ATRA), when combined with MBEH, results in the enhancement of depigmenting and melanocytotoxic effects of MBEH. This can be used to overcome the problem of using 40% MBEH, which turns out to be harsh on the skin [89].

MBEH is believed to cause depigmentation in various ways, which are listed below [90]:

- It acts by reacting with tyrosinase, the main enzyme involved in melanogenesis, forming highly reactive quinone product, which in turn covalently binds to cysteine residues in tyrosinase protein, forming neo-antigens in the tyrosinase peptide chain, which stimulates melanocyte destructive, inflammatory response.
- It also acts by producing reactive oxygen species (ROS), such as peroxide, by inducing oxidative stress in exposed pigmented cells. ROS, in turn, induces lysosomal degradation of melanosomes, and disruption of melanosomal membranes and melanosome structure.
- Generation of ROS causes a release of tyrosinase and MART-1 antigen-containing exosomes, thus further contributing to immune response.
- It also causes the activation of rapid and persistent innate immunity. MBEH being a contact-sensitizer, acts by inducing type IV delayed-type hypersensitivity response against the reactive quinone hapten.

Adverse effects associated with MBEH mainly include irritation, contact dermatitis, in pigmented areas rather than vitiliginous skin [91]. Other possible side effects include xerosis, erythema, rash, edema, conjunctival melanosis, unmasking of telangiectasias, phlebectasias on the lower extremities, pruritus, and distant depigmentation and potential risk of carcinogenesis [88, 92].

Monomethyl Ether of Hydroquinone/4-0 Methoxyphenol (4-MP)

It is mostly used as an oil/water cream base in 20% concentration. An open-use test is done on the normal pigmented skin prior to application of cream to check for the development of any allergic reaction. Those with a negative allergic reaction are permitted to spread the cream on remaining pigmented areas twice a day till complete depigmentation is observed [93].

It acts in a similar way as MBEH. Melanocytes in the hair follicles are less susceptible to the 4-MP in comparison to epidermal melanocytes [87]. 4MP and ATRA combination have proven to be more effective in hyperactive melanocytes in UV irradiated skin as ATRA is more effective in inhibiting synthesis of melanin and tyrosinase activity in stimulated cells in contrast to that in non-stimulated cells [94]. It produces adverse effects similar to MBEH, like irregular leukoderma, contact dermatitis, ochronosis mild burning or itching, and mild risk of carcinogenesis.

Phenol

It is quite inexpensive and has been used mostly topically for chemical peelings. All phenolic compounds show toxicity towards melanocytes. A typical feature of phenol cauterizing is either temporary or definite hypopigmentation as a result of melanocytic inability, *i.e.*, it does not destroy melanocytes, rather, it negotiates its activity. Prior application of phenol, the skin is thoroughly cleaned with alcohol-soaked gauze. Then a swab dampened with phenol is used to treat the minor lesion, until cutaneous frosting occurs. A burning sensation may be felt for nearly 60 seconds, the intensity of which decreases progressively and can last from minutes to hours. Complete elimination of residual pigment is noticed nearly after two sessions. However, there are no signs of repigmentation till afterward one and a half years of the procedure. Various complications associated with phenol (88%) include dyschromia, formation of non-aesthetic scar, dyschromia, and development of herpetic eczema. High-doses of phenol should not be applied over larger areas as it is toxic. Phenol, on coming in contact with any tissue, exerts a corrosive action. Its Cellular uptake is fast and passive because of its lipophilic nature and soon after exposure to phenol, signs of systemic toxicity appear. Cardiovascular shock, abnormal rhythm, bradycardia, as well as metabolic acidosis have been reported within 6 hours of peeling procedures with phenol. Chances of repigmentation occur if patients do not safeguard themselves properly from ultraviolet radiation [95].

Laser Therapy

Depigmentation by lasers is reported to attain faster depigmentation in comparison to bleaching agents. Lasers are mostly used in case of failure of MBEH/other bleaching agents and for specific areas like the face where fast depigmentation is vital within days [93] The main advantages of laser therapy include safety, effectiveness, shorter duration of treatment, faster depigmentation rate, less risk of scar formation and its effectiveness in patients with a positive Koebner phenomenon [96]. Laser therapy also surmounts the disadvantages of topical therapies, *e.g.*, redness, burning and itching. With lasers, larger areas of skin can be depigmented in one sitting, in contrast to depigmentation performed using a bleaching agent [93].

Q-Switched Ruby (QSR) Laser (694nm)

Effective use of QSR laser for depigmentation of vitiligo lesions was first reported by Njoo *et al*. Larger merging areas of pigment on the extremes can first be treated with topical therapy. Combination therapy was seen to give better results than any methods alone. Depigmentation is fast and occurs within 1 to 2 weeks. QSR laser discharges pulses of 694nm wavelength and duration of pulse between 25-28 nanoseconds at a frequency of 1-1.2 Hz. A test spot of 5 cm^2 is first treated and subsequently assessed after 8 weeks to see whether there is any sign of clinical depigmentation. If depigmentation is apparent, then further treatment with a laser is done till full depigmentation occurs. If depigmentation does not occur, then additional treatment with a laser is not done. The procedure is performed under a eutectic mixture of lidocaine (EMLA) 25 mg/g or prilocaine 25 mg/g to avoid any pain. A maximum size of 80 cm^2 can be treated per session. The treated area is covered with sterile gauze and patients are recommended to avoid exposure to sunlight for 6 weeks. Multiple treatments are done at an interval of 2-4 weeks to bring about comprehensive depigmentation involving larger areas [93].

Lasers have demonstrated high effectiveness in selectively destroying melanin and melanin-containing structures in the skin, leading to depigmentation. QSR lasers have wavelengths between 600-800nm, which are absorbed easily by melanin, hence act by inducing selective photothermolysis of pigmented lesions. Also, there is minimal risk of scar formation with QSR therapy [87].

Q-Switched Alexandrite (QSA) Laser (755nm)

The use of QSA laser therapy was first reported in a woman aged 68years who showed a futile response to approximately 18 sessions of QSR laser over a period 5 years in combination with 20% MBEH, and repigmentation of the most treated areas occurred within 3 months after each session. Subsequent application of QSA laser (755nm, 50-100 nanosec) resulted in the complete disappearance of pigment within treated sites within 22 months. Topical MBEH therapy was withdrawn on laser-treated sites. The QSA laser offers various advantages over QSR laser since it has a quicker pulse frequency, resulting in rapid therapy. Furthermore, due to its higher wavelength (755nm), in comparison to the QSR laser (694nm), it easily penetrates the tissues showing improved results [97].

Several other Q-switched lasers that act by selectively destructing the melanocytes include frequency-doubled Nd:YAG laser (532nm) and neodymium: yttrium aluminium garnet (Nd: YAG) laser (1064nm) [87]. The disadvantages of laser therapy include requirement of local anesthesia as the procedure is painful, and it is quite costly. This therapy does not guarantee the complete exclusion of pigmented patches, and even after several months of therapy, and since the migration of perifollicular melanocytes to the epidermis occurs, there are fair chances of the appearance of follicular repigmentation. The depigmenting result of this laser therapy can be thought of as a Koebner phenomenon. Thus, laser therapy acts well in patients with active than in those with stable disease [93]. Another effective depigmentation therapy includes a single session of cryotherapy followed by topical 4-hydroxyanisole (4-HA) [98]. The use of sunscreens, concealment products, and proper guidance may assist the patient to deal better with the disease.

NOVEL TREATMENT PROTOCOLS

Various novel treatment protocols include:

NOVEL TREAMENT PROTOCOLS	Excimer Laser Therapy
	Topical Vitamin D3 Analogues
	Cryotherapy
	Depigmenting Agents
	Intradermal therapy/ Mesotherapy
	Inhibition of IL-15 Signalling with Anti-CD122 Antibody
	Janus Kinase (JAK) Inhibitors
	Alpha Melanocyte Stimulating Hormone Agonist- Afamelanotide
	Combination of Climatotherapy and Pseudocatalase cream (PC-KUS)
	Antioxidants
	Microneedling
	Prostaglandins

Fig. (2). Various novel treatment protocols.

Excimer Laser Therapy

The 308-nm excimer laser, formally referred to as xenon chloride (XeCl) excimer laser, is a relatively newer treatment protocol for vitiligo and works by delivering a monochromatic beam of NBUVB laser light of high energy that is distributed precisely in short pulses to the depigmented area [99, 100]. It has been hypothesized that this therapy works by inducing movement of reservoir melanocytes from the outer root sheath of hair follicles, resulting in repigmentation of the vitiliginous area. Moreover, the 308-nm wavelength is chiefly effective at inducing apoptosis of T-lymphocytes, requiring only 95 mJ/cm^2, which is far less than the requirement of traditional NbUVB therapy (320mJ/cm^2) [101]. This therapy is highly effective in vitiligo treatment even in the absence of any topical, resulting in a greater repigmentation rate, depending on dosage and location of treatment [102, 103]. Combination treatment using the 308-nm excimer laser and topical medications (tacrolimus), have shown potential for an even greater response rate [69]. This therapy involves application to clean, dry skin nearly one to three times weekly, for at least 25-30 treatments [104]. Early repigmentation generally occurs perifollicularly. The level of response to 308-nm excimer laser varies greatly based on the location of the skin, with UV-sensitive areas such as the face, neck, trunk, and proximal extremities responding best to therapy with a repigmentation rate of more than 75% reported in 15% to 50% of treated lesions [102]. Treatment is generally well tolerated, with only minimal side effects such as mild to moderate erythema, edema, burning, and stinging. Rarely, more-severe effects, including severe erythema or blister formation, may occur, requiring a reduction of the UV dose [102, 104]. A major limitation to the widespread use of 308-nm excimer laser therapy is the cost of treatments and equipment maintenance, as well as the difficulty in treating patients with large body surface area involvement (>20%) because of the 30-mm maximum size of the laser focus [100].

Topical Vitamin D3 Analogues

Topical vitamin D3 analogues are novel addition to the therapeutic modalities for vitiligo. Calcipotriol (calcipotriene), is a synthetic vitamin D3 analogue that has been used as a monotherapy, in combination with NB-UVB, PUVA, excimer laser or topical corticosteroids [105]. Calcipotriol inhibits the activation of T-cell, stimulates melanocyte and keratinocyte growth and differentiation and also induces synthesis of melanin by decreasing the altered calcium influx into melanocytes, thus, reinstating calcium homeostasis. It has been observed that Calcipotriol alone displayed slight or no response [56]. The exact mechanism of action is not clear, but numerous observations support a link between calcium metabolism and vitiligo [106, 107]. In addition to this, it has been seen that vitamin D shields the epidermal melanin and reestablishes melanocyte integrity by monitoring the activation, propagation, melanocyte migration and pigmentation pathways by modulating activation of T cell, which is seemingly interrelated with melanocyte loss in vitiligo [108]. The immunomodulatory effects of vitamin D3 analogues may also contribute to their action against vitiligo [109]. Vitamin D is also thought to be involved in normal physiology of melanocyte by managing melanogenic cytokines (endothelin-3/ET-3) and the activity of the SCF/c-Kit system, which constitutes one of the most significant controllers of melanocyte bility and maturation [108]. Another mechanism that has been proposed is based on antioxidant properties and regulatory function of Vit D towards the reactive oxygen species, which are produced in large quantities in the vitiligo epidermis [110]. It has been reported that a combination of NB-UVB and topical tacalcitol (vitamin D3 analogue) greatly enhanced the extent of repigmentation and rate of response rate in vitiligo patients in comparison to NBUVB alone [111]. It has also been reported that the repigmentation rate of hands and feet was better with calcipotriol and PUVAsol combination and was quite fast and effective, hence, may be used for shortening the duration of PUVA therapy in vitiligo patients [112].

Cryotherapy

Cryotherapy is mostly used in cases where rapid depigmentation is desirable. It is cost-effective, rapid, causes permanent depigmentation and has shown exceptional beautifying results but over partial areas at a time [113]. Patients with the Koebner phenomenon respond well to cryosurgery, however, tissue damage is irreversible due to intracellular ice formation and melanocytes being more sensitive to cryodamage than any other epidermal cells. The intensity of damage depends on the minimum temperature achieved and the rate of cooling. Development of inflammation occurs within 24 hours of treatment, which further destroys the lesions through immunologically mediated mechanisms. Slight freezing results in the separation of epidermis from the dermis, which is beneficial in treating epidermal lesions [98].

Prior to cryopathy, spot testing is performed by a single freeze-thaw cycle, and once edema and erythema diminish, the patches are subsequently treated with cryotherapy 3-6 weeks later. Both carbon dioxide (CO_2) and liquid nitrogen (N_2) can be used. This technique utilizes a flat-topped and round cryoprobe nearly 40 mm from the skin surface. The intact patch can be frozen with a single freeze-thaw cycle from the periphery and then by forming consecutive rows inward. However, the procedure should be ended when a thin (< 1 mm) frost rim appears around the periphery of the cryoprobe. This rim can develop within 10-20 seconds by a cryogen linked to a container with pressure above 80 kg/cm^2. Cryoprobes with small diameters are mostly required for patchy areas of the nose lesions or for lesions around the orbits. Only one freeze-thaw cycle is recommended [98]. Within a period of a week, depigmented, non-scarred, somewhat atrophic, and erythematous smooth and even area appears. The finest results are obtained within 4 weeks of treatment. It results in permanent depigmentation, however, for partially depigmented lesions, more than one session may be required with an interval of 4-6 weeks intervals, till complete depigmentation occurs. Side effects associated with the therapy are pain, edema, and bulla formation, permanent scarring If cryotherapy is performed aggressively [113].

This method has been proposed to depigment MBEH-resistant skin. It does not require any anesthesia, can be done in an outpatient department, is simple, easy to perform, safe, and does not need any dressing, sedatives or antibiotics. In addition, preparation time is brief, the procedure is cost-effective, infection risk is low and wound care is negligible. It leads to permanent depigmentation, and patients mostly desire a single short-term procedure rather than using a highly expensive compound for a longer duration with erratic effects and a considerable failure rate [98].

Depigmenting Agents

Imatinib

Imatinib mesylate as a depigmenting agent was first used in patients with chronic myeloid leukemia, in whom it resulted in gradual depigmentation. On discontinuation of the drug, the skin turned darker and lightened again once treatment was resumed. It is suggested that this depigmenting agent, being a tyrosine kinase inhibitor, may act by interfering with melanin synthesis, thus, reducing the pigmentation of the skin, and hypopigmentation can usually be observed within 12 weeks [114].

The various side effects associated with the use of imatinib mesylate include periorbital edema, weight gain, musculoskeletal pain, headache, nausea, diarrhoea, and myelosuppression. In addition, a number of other side-effects have been described, such as follicular mucinosis, erythroderma, and lichenoid eruption. It can also induce local or generalized hyperpigmentation. The use of imatinib in children can delay normal growth, though a proportion will experience catch-up growth during puberty [87].

Imiquimod

It is a novel imidazoquinoline immune response modifier that acts by increasing the production of proinflammatory cytokines, mainly necrosis factor (TNF)-α, interferon (IFN)-α, and interleukins. All of these mediators act by enhancing the response of type 1 helper T-cell (TH1), which plays an important role in the pathogenesis of vitiligo [87]. It also stimulates CD8 cells to turn them cytotoxic and enhancentigen presentation [115]. It has also been reported that imiquimod, when applied topically, binds to a toll-like receptor 7 (TLR7) expressed by human melanocytes, and thus, stimulates various cytokines, which results in inducing T lymphocytic response [116]. Direct action on melanocytes is exerted by imiquimod *via* decreased expression of Bcl-2 and/or an increase in the proapoptotic stimulus [117]. Thus, it is likely that it may cause the elimination of melanocytes either directly acting on the cells or indirectly by inducing acquired immunity and vitiligo-like hypopigmented lesions.

Its use may be followed by erythema which gradually changes to depigmented areas over a period of 3 months and after depigmentation, no evidences of repigmentation have been reported till 6 months, and depigmentation is specifically restricted to areas treated with imiquimod [118].

Common side-effects reported with its twice-daily application include pain, erythema, erosions, burning sensation, itching, and scabbing/crusting [87].

Diphencyprone (DPCP)

It has been observed that topical application of DPCP used for treating patients with alopecia areata produced depigmentation as a side effect. Patients with alopecia total, when treated with DPCP, reported erythema and edema on the forearm after 3 days of treatment, but the scalp showed insignificant macular erythema. However, the reaction on the forearm diminished within 2 weeks and eventually, after 6 weeks, turned to a depigmented patch. Similarly, depigmented on the nape of the neck and the midline of the back were observed for any change, but these persisted for 2 years after stopping the therapy. Vitiligo induced by DPCP is infrequent and may symbolize a Koebner phenomenon in susceptible persons. Adverse effects associated with DPCP include localised eczema with blistering, regional lymphadenopathy, hyper or hypopigmentation, and vitiligo [119].

Intradermal Therapy/ Mesotherapy

It is a novel treatment approach used for treating vitiligo. It makes use of intradermal injections of vitamin and mineral complexes as antioxidants into affected areas. The persistent effect on re-pigmentation of vitiligo after the injections of antioxidants and the increasing effect with a repeated course, support the theory of involvement of oxidative stress in the pathogenesis of vitiligo. The incidental monitoring of the response to mesotherapy with bio revitalizant NCTF135 in the vitiligo-affected areas and a subsequent study of its composition, evoked the idea of using it as an antioxidant in the treatment of vitiligo [120]. NCTF135 constitutes a complex of 55 active ingredients (23 amino acids, 6 minerals, 13 vitamins, 6 nucleotides, co-enzymes, glutathione and hyaluronic acid). It includes antioxidants such as glutathione, hyaluronic and ascorbic acid, and tocopherol (vitamin E). All of these antioxidants are important elements in cellular protection from reactive oxygen species (ROS). An increase in the intracellular concentration of glutathione promotes antioxidant cells protection and enhances cellular metabolism. Hyaluronic acid promotes neo-angiogenesis and improves skin microcirculation in the injected areas, improving absorption of vitamins and microelements [120].

The process involves intradermally injecting 3.0ml of NCTF135 in depigmented areas once a week for 5 weeks and it was observed that patients completely retained the pigment in the treated areas, which nearly accounted for 30% of the affected skin, after 6 months of completion of the course of mesotherapy, patients recorded "mosaic" re-pigmentation in all treated areas. In addition, the discrete border between the affected and normal skin disappeared. No cases of an allergic response and other side effects were reported. However, the use of SPF50+ sunscreens is recommended [120]. It has also been observed that intradermal fluorouracil injection is an effective treatment of localized vitiligo [121].

Inhibition of IL-15 Signalling With Anti-CD122 Antibody

The existence of resident memory T cells (TRM) in vitiligo lesional skin of both humans and mice was first confirmed by Richmond *et al.* Since, TRM cells require IL15 for their survival, inhibition of IL15 signalling provides a reasonable target to deplete TRM cells. It has been observed in a mouse model of vitiligo that inhibition of IL-15 signalling by long-term systemic treatment with an anti-CD122 antibody depleted TRM from lesional skin and resulted in durable reversal of disease symptoms. With short-term local intradermal anti-CD122 antibody treatment, inhibition of TRM production of interferon (IFN)γ was observed, resulting in long-term skin repigmentation [122]. Targeting tissue-resident memory T cells may allow for long-lasting therapy as it acts by inhibiting the generation of effector T cells which ultimately attack melanocytes [123]. However, clinical trials to fully elucidate the effectiveness of this therapy are still in progress.

Janus Kinase (JAK) Inhibitors

JAK inhibitors such as ruxolitinib and tofacitinib have been considered good and effective novel therapeutic agents in vitiligo. Several IFN-γ-dependent cytokines produced *via* the JAK-STAT pathway have been implicated in the pathogenesis of vitiligo, thus making JAK- STAT pathway a prominent therapeutic target. With several JAK inhibitors undergoing clinical trials for vitiligo, their approvals will bring new hope and an entirely novel strategy for treating this disease [124]. Use of ruxolitinib cream revealed significant repigmentation of vitiligo lesions up to 52 weeks of treatment, suggesting it is an effective treatment option [125]. It has also been observed that simultaneous UVB phototherapy appears to enhance the efficacy of JAK inhibitors for vitiligo [126]. With monotherapy, the maintenance of repigmentation may be achieved. These conclusions support the fact that JAK inhibitors overpower T cell mediators, and successive irradiation is essential for melanocyte regeneration [127]. The combination of micro-focused phototherapy with tofacitinib citrate provides better clinical results in terms of repigmentation rate [128].

Alpha-Melanocyte Stimulating Hormone Agonistic Analog-Afamelanotide

Afamelanotide is an evolving treatment modality for vitiligo. It is a long-lasting synthetic analog of alpha-melanocyte–stimulating hormone (α-MSH) [129]. It has been observed that patients with vitiligo display defects in the melanocortin system, which manifest as decreased levels of α-MSH in both systemic circulation and skin lesions. Afamelanotide thus acts by binding to the melanocortin-1 receptor and subsequently stimulating melanocyte proliferation and melanogenesis [130]. It has been observed that an implant of 16 mg afamelantotide in combination with NBUVB produced faster repigmentation of facial and upper extremity lesions than NB-UVB alone and also promoted differentiation, proliferation of melanoblasts and eumelanogenesis [131]. Adverse reactions associated with afamelanotide include hyperpigmentation of normal skin, nausea, and abdominal pain [129]. However, Concurrent administration of afamelanotide can reduce the NBUVB dose and potential adverse effects.

Combination of Climatotherapy and Pseudocatalase Cream (PC-KUS)

Short term Climatotherapy (21 days) at the dead sea in combination with pseudocatalase cream (PC-KUS) has revealed significantly faster initiation of repigmentation in vitiligo in comparison to either conventional climatotherapy at the Dead Sea alone or with placebo cream in combination with climatotherapy or narrowband UVB activated pseudocatalase cream (PC-KUS) treatment alone [132].

Antioxidants

Antioxidant supplementation has been observed to be useful in vitiligo patients. Alpha lipoic acid, an organosulfur compound with antioxidant properties, has thus been proposed in treating vitiligo to stop the destruction of melanocytes by free radicals. It is commonly used as an adjuvant therapy in association with other conventional treatment modalities (*e.g.*, corticosteroids, phototherapy). It has been associated with a high safety profile and effectiveness in terms of acceleration of cutaneous repigmentation in vitiligo patients [133, 134]. It has also been observed that oral supplementation with an antioxidant pool containing alpha-lipoic acid before and during NBUVB significantly enhances the effectiveness of NB-UVB and subsequently reduces vitiligo-associated oxidative stress [133]. Another well-known antioxidant Glutathione- is able to protect cellular components from oxidative stress damage and is reported to be lower in vitiligo-affected individuals than in normal individuals, however, its potential use in vitiligo needs further consideration [135]. L-Carnosine (Beta-Alanyl-L-Histidine) is a dipeptide with antioxidant properties, thus, protecting cell membranes from oxidative stress and reducing mitochondrial dysfunction. It has been proposed to be a promising therapeutic agent in vitiligo, as mitochondrial dysfunction causing in cell damage in vitiligo keratinocytes has been reported to be one of the pathophysiological mechanisms in vitiligo. However, its use needs further investigation [136].

Microneedling

Microneedling is a novel technique that is believed to induce pigmentation in vitiliginous areas by physically moving melanocytes from the normally pigmented areas into the depigmented areas with the needle so that they can serve as reservoirs for melanogenesis and hence, be used as a transdermal drug delivery modality. Microneedling in combination with TCI (tacrolimus), 5-fluorouracil (5-FU), betamethasone, topical calcipotriol, NBUVB, and triamcinolone acetonide solution revealed more efficacy than with microneedling alone [137]. This technique involves the insertion of needle into normally pigmented skin on the edge of vitiliginous patch, and is subsequently pushed into the centre of patch, theoretically moving healthy, pigmented skin cells into the patch. During the process of needling, the needle is attached to a syringe filled with a steroid, which is then injected into the patch enabling delivery of the steroid directly to the affected area [138].

It has been observed that the addition of microneedling with triamcinolone acetonide to NB-UVB therapy is quite reasonable, well-tolerated combination treatment for patients with a resistant form of vitiligo and comparison of results of needling plus a topical steroid with NB-UVB, needling yielded a good response in 45% of cases, whereas combining needling with NBUVB increased that percentage to 70%. The incidence of side effects was minimal, except for pain, which can be diminished by using topical anesthetics before sessions [139]. Hence, this technique is safe and effective in treating vitiligo and thus, can be used as an alternative therapy in patients resistant to other conventional therapies.

Prostaglandins

Prostaglandins (PGs) have been shown to play an active role in melanogenesis, proliferation and maturation of melanocytes, immunomodulation and an increased melanocyte density was observed on topical application of PGE2 in animal studies [33]. Application of PGE2 gel twice daily for 6 months has revealed promising therapeutic results in stable localized vitiligo with minimal side effects such as transient burning sensation [140]. Latanoprost (LT), a PGF2α analogue that is generally used in the treatment of glaucoma, was also found to induce skin pigmentation in guinea pigs and in addition, caused periocular and iridal pigmentation as a side effect. Its effect on skin repigmentation could be enhanced by exposure to NBUVB [141].

HERBALS IN VITILIGO

Due to the limited success and significant risks associated with the current therapy herbal therapy could be one of the safe and effective treatment alternatives. Although there are thousands of herbal remedies which have been identified for their skin-lightening effects, very little data on the hyperpigmentation effect of these drugs is available [142]. However, various plants and their constituents, such as psoralen-rich herbs, including *Psoralea corylifolia, Ammi majus*, piperine extracts, khellin extracts, and others, have experimentally demonstrated a major potential in the vitiligo treatment. The more effective and lesser side effects of herbal medicines have made their more promising treatment choices for vitiligo.

Ammi Majus (Common Name: Bishop's Weed; Family: Apiaceae)

The plant extract consisting of ammoidin and ammidin has experimentally shown a specific action in vitiligo. The drug is given topically, orally, and in combination with phototherapy, achieved significant pigmentation rates, especially in combination therapy [143]. However, the therapy of *A.majus* fruit in combination with exposure of skin to the sun has reportedly caused phototoxic dermatitis [144].

Azadirachta Indica (Common Name: Neem; Family: Meliaceae)

It is one of the ingredients of the Herbo-mineral capsule (ALG-06) used in the treatment of vitiligo [145]. Neem oil causes a reversal of discoloration when applied to the affected areas. Oral dosage of leaves four grams three times a day before each meal is also suggested [146].

Cassia Occidentalis (Common Name: Coffee Senna, Kasaunda; Family: Caesalpiniaceae)

C. occidentalis is used in various ayurvedic medicines to treat various diseases. The plant has a well-known anti-inflammatory, antibacterial and anticancer effect. Experimental analysis of pod extract of *C. occidentalis* has demonstrated potential effects in melanoblastactivity, suggesting its use in vitiligo. The extract has induced an effective differentiation and migration of melanoblast experimentally [147].

Cucumis Melo (Common Name: Melon; Family: Cucurbitaceae)

Superoxide dismutase (SOD) and catalase found in *C. Melo* be effective in stopping the melanocyte deconstruction in vitiligo. The topical gel preparation of the drug has been found protective against skin irradiation but with no significant repigmentation. Given along with that, phenylalanine and acetyl-cysteine are more effective [148].

Ginkgo Biloba (Common Name: Maiden Hair Tree; Family: Ginkgoacea)

Ginkgo biloba has well-known antioxidant, anti-inflammatory, and immunomodulatory properties. Extracts of the drug have shown their effectiveness in treating and significantly controlling the progress of depigmentation and inducing a marked repigmentation [149]. Oral tablet formulations are available, which are to be taken daily for more than 3 months. The drug is safe and well-tolerated. GIT disorders and restlessness may be a result of excessive daily doses >240 mg. Intake with anticoagulants is advised only under medical supervision [5].

Lespedeza Bicolor (Common Name: Shrubby Bushclover; Family: Leguminosae)

L. bicolor is used as a traditional medicine used for the treatment of vitiligo & leucoderma. The stem extract of the plant has enhanced melanogenesis and tyrosinase activity experimentally, indicating its use in vitiligo. The extract has also shown an effect on vitiligo-associated hair graying by increasing the concentration of melanin and eumelanin in hair follicles [150].

Malytea Scurfpea (Common Name: Buguzhi; Family: Fabaceae)

The effect of the fruit extract of this drug has been studied on human melanocyte migration and adhesion. The drug has been shown to act by promoting melanocyte adhesion and migration, and thus this regulation of melanocyte function could possibly suggest its use in the vitiligo treatment [151].

Nigella Sativa (Common Name: Black Cumin; Family: Ranunculaceae)

The oil of this plant has been suggested as adjuvant therapy for the treatment of vitiligo. The application of *N. Sativa* seed oil in the cream formulation has achieved significant repigmentation [152]. Also, the active constituent thymoquinone and lyophilized extract of seed have caused skin darkening in wall lizard melanophores [153].

Picrorhiza Kurroa (Common Name: Kutki; Family: Plantaginaceae)

P. kurroa has known hepatoprotective, antioxidant, and immunomodulatory properties [154]. The drug has experimentally been shown to potentiate phytochemotherapy in vitiligo [155]. The drug has provided better results in inducing repigmentation when given in association with other therapies [156].

Piper Nigrum (Common Name: Black Pepper; Family: Piperaceae)

Extract of *P. nigrum* fruit and its main alkaloidal constituent, piperine, has been shown to promote the proliferation of melanocytes in vitiligo [157]. Both the fruit extract and piperine promoted the repigmentation process, and the extract has shown faster and more remarkable results, especially when used in association with travoprost (prostaglandin F2α analogue) [158].

Polypodium Leucotomos (Common Name: Calaguala; Family: Polypodiaceae)

P. leucotomos, due to its antioxidant, photoprotective, and immunomodulatory properties, has been suggested as an alternative therapy along with narrow-band NBUVB for vitiligo. The drug therapy has been shown to increase the repigmentation rates in vitiligo Vulgaris affecting head and neck regions [159].

Psoralea Corylifolia (Common Name: Babchi; Family: Fabaceae)

P. corylifolia seed powder formulated in the hydrophilic ointment preparation has been suggested as effective monotherapy in the treatment of small circular white lesions of vitiligo [160]. A clinical trial of the topical ayurvedic preparation of the drug given along with oral *Gandhaka Rasayana* has shown maximum early improvements [161].

Pyrostegia Venusta (Common Name: Flamevine; Family: Bignoniaceae)

P. venusta is commonly known for its anti-inflammatory, antioxidant, and melanogenic properties [154]. Pre-Clinical evidence of *P. venusta* has shown its evident hyperpigmentation and anti-inflammatory properties, and the leaf extract has revealed significant activity in treating the disease [162].

Rhododendron Schlippenbachii (Common Name: Royal Azalea; Family: Ericaceae)

The effect of *R. schlippenbachii* ethanol extract has been evaluated on melanocyte activity and tyrosinase activity. Enhancement in melanogenesis and increased tyrosinase activity in cultured melanoma cells have proposed its use in vitiligo.

The drug also improved hair graying in vitiligo by increasing the concentration of melanin and eumelanin [163].

Salvia Miltiorrhiza (Common Name: Red Sage; Family: Lamiaceae)

S. miltiorrhiza is a widely used herb in Chinese traditional medicine to treat ischemic stroke, hyperlipidemia, and angina pectoris. The leaf extract has been suggested for use in hypopigmentation disorders and preventing hair graying because the drug has been shown to enhance melanin content and tyrosinase activity experimentally [164].

CONCLUSION

At present, there are no means to avert vitiligo, however, current treatment protocols intend to stop the progression of the disease and have revealed favourable outcomes in most of the patients. The main goals of treatment are to create a uniform tone between the normal skin and vitiliginous patches by either restoring color or removing the remaining color. Appropriate knowledge about the disease and consulting a physician who really knows about the disease, its prognosis and suitable treatment options is key to stopping the progression of the disease. In addition, superlative treatment modality should be adapted for each patient depending on the extent, distribution and rate of progression of the lesions. Phototherapy and Topical corticosteroids are still the mainstays for treating vitiligo however, novel treatment modalities and phytotherapy have presented a new choice for treating vitiligo patients and have offered a number of benefits over conventional treatment modalities. Further, current research is enriching our conceptions regarding various newer pathways involved in the pathogenesis of vitiligo and potential newer ways to treat it. There is also a dire necessity to have public-private partnerships and enduring strategies to descry, develop, and deliver new drugs for treating vitiligo, and reevaluation of treatment options using surrogate theories might find a preemptive therapy.

REFERENCES

[1]   Njoo MD, Westerhof W. Vitiligo. Am J Clin Dermatol 2001; 2(3): 167-81.
        [http://dx.doi.org/10.2165/00128071-200102030-00006] [PMID: 11705094]

[2]   Huang CL, Nordlund JJ, Boissy R. Vitiligo. Am J Clin Dermatol 2002; 3(5): 301-8.
        [http://dx.doi.org/10.2165/00128071-200203050-00001] [PMID: 12069635]

[3]   Mahajan V, Vashist S, Chauhan P, Mehta KS, Sharma V, Sharma A. Clinico-epidemiological profile
        of patients with vitiligo: A retrospective study from a tertiary care center of North India. Indian
        Dermatol Online J 2019; 10(1): 38-44.
        [http://dx.doi.org/10.4103/idoj.IDOJ_124_18] [PMID: 30775297]

[4]   Tamesis MEB, Morelli JG. Vitiligo treatment in childhood: a state of the art review. Pediatr Dermatol
        2010; 27(5): 437-45.
        [http://dx.doi.org/10.1111/j.1525-1470.2010.01159.x] [PMID: 20553403]

[5]   Gianfaldoni S, Wollina U, Tirant M, *et al.* Herbal compounds for the treatment of vitiligo: a review. Open Access Maced J Med Sci 2018; 6(1): 203-7.
[http://dx.doi.org/10.3889/oamjms.2018.048] [PMID: 29484024]

[6]   Bhatia PS, Mohan L, Pandey ON, Singh KK, Arora SK, Mukhija RD. Genetic nature of vitiligo. J Dermatol Sci 1992; 4(3): 180-4.
[http://dx.doi.org/10.1016/0923-1811(92)90017-6] [PMID: 1286069]

[7]   Boldyrev AA. Oxidative stress and the brain. Soros Obraz Zh 2001; 7: 21-7.

[8]   Hazneci E, Karabulut AB, Oztürk C, *et al.* A comparative study of superoxide dismutase, catalase, and glutathione peroxidase activities and nitrate levels in vitiligo patients. Int J Dermatol 2005; 44(8): 636-40.
[http://dx.doi.org/10.1111/j.1365-4632.2004.02027.x] [PMID: 16101862]

[9]   Arican O, Kurutas EB. Oxidative stress in the blood of patients with active localized vitiligo. Acta Dermatovenerol Alp Panonica Adriat 2008; 17(1): 12-6.
[PMID: 18454264]

[10]   Gauthier Y, Andre MC, Taïeb A. A critical appraisal of vitiligo etiologic theories. Is melanocyte loss a melanocytorrhagy? Pigment Cell Res 2003; 16(4): 322-32.
[http://dx.doi.org/10.1034/j.1600-0749.2003.00070.x] [PMID: 12859615]

[11]   Grimes PE. New insights and new therapies in vitiligo. JAMA 2005; 293(6): 730-5.
[http://dx.doi.org/10.1001/jama.293.6.730] [PMID: 15701915]

[12]   Roelandts R. Photo(chemo) therapy for vitiligo. Photodermatol Photoimmunol Photomed 2003; 19(1): 1-4.
[http://dx.doi.org/10.1034/j.1600-0781.2003.00003.x] [PMID: 12713546]

[13]   Kanwar AJ, Dogra S, Parsad D, Kumar B. Narrow-band UVB for the treatment of vitiligo: an emerging effective and well-tolerated therapy. Int J Dermatol 2005; 44(1): 57-60.
[http://dx.doi.org/10.1111/j.1365-4632.2004.02329.x] [PMID: 15663664]

[14]   Ortonne JP. Psoralen therapy in vitiligo. Clin Dermatol 1989; 7(2): 120-35.
[http://dx.doi.org/10.1016/0738-081X(89)90062-X] [PMID: 2667737]

[15]   Grimes PE. Psoralen photochemotherapy for vitiligo. Clin Dermatol 1997; 15(6): 921-6.
[http://dx.doi.org/10.1016/S0738-081X(97)00133-8] [PMID: 9404695]

[16]   Levau M. The treatment of vitiligo with psoralen derivatives. Arch Dermatol 1958; 78: 597.
[http://dx.doi.org/10.1001/archderm.1958.01560110043006]

[17]   Pathak MA, Mosher DB, Fitzpatrick TB. Safety and therapeutic effectiveness of 8-methoxypsoralen, 4,5′,8-trimethylpsoralen, and psoralen in vitiligo. Natl Cancer Inst Monogr 1984; 66: 165-73.
[PMID: 6531024]

[18]   Ling TC, Clayton TH, Crawley J, *et al.* British Association of Dermatologists and British Photodermatology Group guidelines for the safe and effective use of psoralen–ultraviolet A therapy 2015. Br J Dermatol 2016; 174(1): 24-55.
[http://dx.doi.org/10.1111/bjd.14317] [PMID: 26790656]

[19]   Moseley H, Cox NH, Mackie RM. The suitability of sunglasses used by patients following ingestion of psoralen. Br J Dermatol 1988; 118(2): 247-53.
[http://dx.doi.org/10.1111/j.1365-2133.1988.tb01782.x] [PMID: 3348970]

[20]   Bulat V, Situm M, Dediol I, Ljubicić I, Bradić L. The mechanisms of action of phototherapy in the treatment of the most common dermatoses. Coll Antropol 2011; 35 (Suppl. 2): 147-51.
[PMID: 22220423]

[21]   Norris DA, Horikawa T, Morelli JG. Melanocyte destruction and repopulation in vitiligo. Pigment Cell Res 1994; 7(4): 193-203.
[http://dx.doi.org/10.1111/j.1600-0749.1994.tb00049.x]

[22]   Abdel-Naser MB, Hann SK, Bystryn JC. Oral psoralen with UV-A therapy releases circulating growth factor(s) that stimulates cell proliferation. Arch Dermatol 1997; 133(12): 1530-3.
[http://dx.doi.org/10.1001/archderm.1997.03890480050007] [PMID: 9420537]

[23]   Gupta AK, Anderson TF. Psoralen photochemotherapy. J Am Acad Dermatol 1987; 17(5): 703-34.
[http://dx.doi.org/10.1016/S0190-9622(87)70255-2] [PMID: 3316316]

[24]   Morison WL. Phototherapy and photochemotherapy: An update. Semin Cutan Med Surg 1999; 18(4): 297-306.
[http://dx.doi.org/10.1016/S1085-5629(99)80029-7] [PMID: 10604796]

[25]   Wolff K. Side-effects of psoralen photochemotherapy (PUVA). Br J Dermatol 1990; 122(s36): 117-25.
[http://dx.doi.org/10.1111/j.1365-2133.1990.tb02889.x]

[26]   George SA, Ferguson J. Liquid formulations of 8-methoxypsoralen (8-MOP) and 5-MOP: a prospective double-blind crossover assessment of acute non-phototoxic adverse effects. Photodermatol Photoimmunol Photomed 1992; 9(1): 33-5.
[PMID: 1390121]

[27]   Westerhof W, Nieuweboer-Krobotova L. Treatment of vitiligo with UV-B radiation *vs* topical psoralen plus UV-A. Arch Dermatol 1997; 133(12): 1525-8.
[http://dx.doi.org/10.1001/archderm.1997.03890480045006] [PMID: 9420536]

[28]   Njoo M, Bos J, Westerhof W. Treatment of generalized vitiligo in children with narrow-band (TL-01) UVB radiation therapy. J Am Acad Dermatol 2000; 42(2): 245-53.
[http://dx.doi.org/10.1016/S0190-9622(00)90133-6] [PMID: 10642680]

[29]   Anstey A, Asawanonda P, Taylor C. Narrowband (TL-01) UVB phototherapy beyond psoriasis. J Dermatolog Treat 1999; 10(1): 53-7.
[http://dx.doi.org/10.3109/09546639909055911]

[30]   Parsad D, Bhatnagar A, De D. Narrowband ultraviolet B for the treatment of vitiligo. Expert Rev Dermatol 2010; 5(4): 445-59.
[http://dx.doi.org/10.1586/edm.10.34]

[31]   Englaro W, Bahadoran P, Bertolotto C, *et al.* Tumor necrosis factor alpha-mediated inhibition of melanogenesis is dependent on nuclear factor kappa B activation. Oncogene 1999; 18(8): 1553-9.
[http://dx.doi.org/10.1038/sj.onc.1202446] [PMID: 10102625]

[32]   Imokawa G, Miyagishi M, Yada Y. Endothelin-1 as a new melanogen: coordinated expression of its gene and the tyrosinase gene in UVB-exposed human epidermis. J Invest Dermatol 1995; 105(1): 32-7.
[http://dx.doi.org/10.1111/1523-1747.ep12312500] [PMID: 7615973]

[33]   Parsad D, Pandhi R, Dogra S, Kumar B. Topical prostaglandin analog (PGE2) in vitiligo - a preliminary study. Int J Dermatol 2002; 41(12): 942-5.
[http://dx.doi.org/10.1046/j.1365-4362.2002.01612.x] [PMID: 12492997]

[34]   Sapam R, Agrawal S, Dhali TK. Systemic PUVA *vs.* narrowband UVB in the treatment of vitiligo: a randomized controlled study. Int J Dermatol 2012; 51(9): 1107-15.
[http://dx.doi.org/10.1111/j.1365-4632.2011.05454.x] [PMID: 22909369]

[35]   Kunisada M, Kumimoto H, Ishizaki K, Sakumi K, Nakabeppu Y, Nishigori C. Narrow-band UVB induces more carcinogenic skin tumors than broad-band UVB through the formation of cyclobutane pyrimidine dimer. J Invest Dermatol 2007; 127(12): 2865-71.
[http://dx.doi.org/10.1038/sj.jid.5701001] [PMID: 17687389]

[36]   Don P, Iuga A, Dacko A, Hardick K. Treatment of vitiligo with broadband ultraviolet B and vitamins. Int J Dermatol 2006; 45(1): 63-5.
[http://dx.doi.org/10.1111/j.1365-4632.2005.02447.x] [PMID: 16426381]

[37]   Carlie G, Ntusi NBA, Hulley PA, Kidson SH. KUVA (khellin plus ultraviolet A) stimulates proliferation and melanogenesis in normal human melanocytes and melanoma cells *in vitro*. Br J Dermatol 2003; 149(4): 707-17.
[http://dx.doi.org/10.1046/j.1365-2133.2003.05577.x] [PMID: 14616361]

[38]   Hönigsmann H, Ortel B. Khellin photochemotherapy of vitiligo. Photodermatology 1985; 2(4): 193-4.
[PMID: 4059075]

[39]   Hofer A, Kerl H, Wolf P. Long-term results in the treatment of vitiligo with oral khellin plus UVA. Eur J Dermatol 2001; 11(3): 225-9.
[PMID: 11358729]

[40]   Schulpis CH, Antoniou C, Michas T, Strarigos J. Phenylalanine plus ultraviolet light: preliminary report of a promising treatment for childhood vitiligo. Pediatr Dermatol 1989; 6(4): 332-5.
[http://dx.doi.org/10.1111/j.1525-1470.1989.tb00921.x] [PMID: 2616391]

[41]   Cormane RH, Siddiqui AH, Westerhof W, Schutgens RBH. Phenylalanine and UVA light for the treatment of vitiligo. Arch Dermatol Res 1985; 277(2): 126-30.
[http://dx.doi.org/10.1007/BF00414110] [PMID: 3885873]

[42]   Kim SM, Lee HS, Hann SK. The efficacy of low-dose oral corticosteroids in the treatment of vitiligo patients. Int J Dermatol 1999; 38(7): 546-50.
[http://dx.doi.org/10.1046/j.1365-4362.1999.00623.x] [PMID: 10440289]

[43]   Bagherani N. State Art Ther Endocrinol. State Art Ther Endocrinol 2012.
[http://dx.doi.org/10.5772/48384]

[44]   Matin R. Vitiligo in adults and children. BMJ Clin Evid 2011; 2011.

[45]   Coskun B, Saral Y, Turgut D. Topical 0.05% clobetasol propionate *versus* 1% pimecrolimus ointment in vitiligo. Eur J Dermatol 2005; 15(2): 88-91.
[PMID: 15757818]

[46]   Lepe V, Moncada B, Castanedo-Cazares JP, Torres-Alvarez MB, Ortiz CA, Torres-Rubalcava AB. A double-blind randomized trial of 0.1% tacrolimus *vs* 0.05% clobetasol for the treatment of childhood vitiligo. Arch Dermatol 2003; 139(5): 581-5.
[http://dx.doi.org/10.1001/archderm.139.5.581] [PMID: 12756094]

[47]   Gawkrodger DJ, Ormerod AD, Shaw L, *et al.* Vitiligo: concise evidence based guidelines on diagnosis and management. Postgrad Med J 2010; 86(1018): 466-71.
[http://dx.doi.org/10.1136/pgmj.2009.093278] [PMID: 20709768]

[48]   Njoo MD, Spuls PI, Bos JD, Westerhof W, Bossuyt PMM. Nonsurgical repigmentation therapies in vitiligo. Meta-analysis of the literature. Arch Dermatol 1998; 134(12): 1532-40.
[http://dx.doi.org/10.1001/archderm.134.12.1532] [PMID: 9875190]

[49]   Clayton R. A double-blind trial of 0.05% clobetasol proprionate in the treatment of vitiligo. Br J Dermatol 1977; 96(1): 71-3.
[http://dx.doi.org/10.1111/j.1365-2133.1977.tb05188.x] [PMID: 320996]

[50]   Mahmoud BH, Hexsel CL, Hamzavi IH. An update on new and emerging options for the treatment of vitiligo. Skin Therapy Lett 2008; 13(2): 1-6.
[PMID: 18373041]

[51]   Ference JD, Last AR. Choosing topical corticosteroids. Am Fam Physician 2009; 79(2): 135-40.
[PMID: 19178066]

[52]   Seiter S, Ugurel S, Tilgen W, Reinhold U. Use of high-dose methylprednisolone pulse therapy in patients with progressive and stable vitiligo. Int J Dermatol 2000; 39(8): 624-7.
[http://dx.doi.org/10.1046/j.1365-4362.2000.00006.x] [PMID: 10971735]

[53]   Radakovic-Fijan S, Fürnsinn-Friedl AM, Hönigsmann H, Tanew A. Oral dexamethasone pulse treatment for vitiligo. J Am Acad Dermatol 2001; 44(5): 814-7.

[http://dx.doi.org/10.1067/mjd.2001.113475] [PMID: 11312430]

[54]   Oiso N, Suzuki T, Wataya-kaneda M, *et al.* Guidelines for the diagnosis and treatment of vitiligo in Japan. J Dermatol 2013; 40(5): 344-54.
[http://dx.doi.org/10.1111/1346-8138.12099] [PMID: 23441960]

[55]   Berti S, Buggiani G, Lotti T. Use of tacrolimus ointment in vitiligo alone or in combination therapy. Skin Therapy Lett 2009; 14(4): 5-7.
[PMID: 19585060]

[56]   Kostovic K, Pasic A. New treatment modalities for vitiligo: focus on topical immunomodulators. Drugs 2005; 65(4): 447-59.
[http://dx.doi.org/10.2165/00003495-200565040-00002] [PMID: 15733009]

[57]   Phiske M, Patil B, Bharda Z, Jerajani H. Tacrolimus *versus* pimecrolimus in localised stable vitiligo. Pigment Cell Melanoma Res 2011; 24: 833.

[58]   Kang HY, Choi YM. FK506 increases pigmentation and migration of human melanocytes. Br J Dermatol 2006; 155(5): 1037-40.
[http://dx.doi.org/10.1111/j.1365-2133.2006.07467.x] [PMID: 17034537]

[59]   Lee KY, Jeon SY, Hong JW, *et al.* Endothelin-1 enhances the proliferation of normal human melanocytes in a paradoxical manner from the TNF-α-inhibited condition, but tacrolimus promotes exclusively the cellular migration without proliferation: a proposed action mechanism for combination t. J Eur Acad Dermatol Venereol 2013; 27(5): 609-16.
[http://dx.doi.org/10.1111/j.1468-3083.2012.04498.x] [PMID: 22404745]

[60]   Jung H, Oh ES. FK506 positively regulates the migratory potential of melanocyte-derived cells by enhancing syndecan-2 expression. Pigment Cell Melanoma Res 2016; 29(4): 434-43.
[http://dx.doi.org/10.1111/pcmr.12480] [PMID: 27060922]

[61]   Xu P, Chen J, Tan C, Lai RS, Min ZS. Pimecrolimus increases the melanogenesis and migration of melanocytes *in vitro*. Korean J Physiol Pharmacol 2017; 21(3): 287-92.
[http://dx.doi.org/10.4196/kjpp.2017.21.3.287] [PMID: 28461770]

[62]   Lan C-CE, Wu C-S, Chen G-S, Yu H-S. Yu H-S. FK506 (tacrolimus) and endothelin combined treatment induces mobility of melanoblasts: new insights into follicular vitiligo repigmentation induced by topical tacrolimus on sun-exposed skin. Br J Dermatol 2011; 164(3): 490-6.
[http://dx.doi.org/10.1111/j.1365-2133.2010.10113.x]

[63]   Park OJ, Park GH, Choi JR, *et al.* A combination of excimer laser treatment and topical tacrolimus is more effective in treating vitiligo than either therapy alone for the initial 6 months, but not thereafter. Clin Exp Dermatol 2016; 41(3): 236-41.
[http://dx.doi.org/10.1111/ced.12742] [PMID: 26299799]

[64]   Lubaki LJ, Ghanem G, Vereecken P, *et al.* Time-kinetic study of repigmentation in vitiligo patients by tacrolimus or pimecrolimus. Arch Dermatol Res 2010; 302(2): 131-7.
[http://dx.doi.org/10.1007/s00403-009-0973-3] [PMID: 19547993]

[65]   Majid I. Does topical tacrolimus ointment enhance the efficacy of narrowband ultraviolet B therapy in vitiligo? A left-right comparison study. Photodermatol Photoimmunol Photomed 2010; 26(5): 230-4.
[http://dx.doi.org/10.1111/j.1600-0781.2010.00540.x] [PMID: 20831696]

[66]   Kanwar AJ, Parsad D, Vinay K, Satyanarayan HS. Efficacy and tolerability of combined treatment with NB-UVB and topical tacrolimus *versus* NB-UVB alone in patients with vitiligo vulgaris: A randomized intra-individual open comparative trial. Indian J Dermatol Venereol Leprol 2013; 79(4): 525-7.
[http://dx.doi.org/10.4103/0378-6323.113091] [PMID: 23760325]

[67]   Mehrabi D, Pandya AG. A randomized, placebo-controlled, double-blind trial comparing narrowband UV-B Plus 0.1% tacrolimus ointment with narrowband UV-B plus placebo in the treatment of generalized vitiligo. Arch Dermatol 2006; 142(7): 927-9.

[http://dx.doi.org/10.1001/archderm.142.7.927] [PMID: 16847214]

[68] Fai D, Cassano N, Vena GA. Narrow-band UVB phototherapy combined with tacrolimus ointment in vitiligo: a review of 110 patients. J Eur Acad Dermatol Venereol 2007; 21(7): 916-20.
[http://dx.doi.org/10.1111/j.1468-3083.2006.02101.x] [PMID: 17659000]

[69] Kawalek AZ, Spencer JM, Phelps RG. Combined excimer laser and topical tacrolimus for the treatment of vitiligo: a pilot study. Dermatol Surg 2004; 30(2): 130-5.
[http://dx.doi.org/10.1097/00042728-200402000-00002] [PMID: 14756638]

[70] Hu W, Xu Y, Ma Y, Lei J, Lin F, Xu AE. Efficacy of the topical calcineurin inhibitors tacrolimus and pimecrolimus in the treatment of vitiligo in infants under 2 years of age: a randomized, open-label pilot study. Clin Drug Investig 2019; 39(12): 1233-8.
[http://dx.doi.org/10.1007/s40261-019-00845-x] [PMID: 31522334]

[71] Khunger N, Kathuria S, Ramesh V. Tissue grafts in vitiligo surgery - past, present, and future. Indian J Dermatol 2009; 54(2): 150-8.
[http://dx.doi.org/10.4103/0019-5154.53196] [PMID: 20101311]

[72] van Geel N, Ongenae K, Naeyaert JM. Surgical techniques for vitiligo: a review. Dermatology 2001; 202(2): 162-6.
[http://dx.doi.org/10.1159/000051626] [PMID: 11306848]

[73] Thakur P, Sacchidanand S, Nataraj HV, Savitha AS. A study of hair follicular transplantation as a treatment option for vitiligo. J Cutan Aesthet Surg 2015; 8(4): 211-7.
[http://dx.doi.org/10.4103/0974-2077.172192] [PMID: 26865785]

[74] Parsad D, Gupta S. Standard guidelines of care for vitiligo surgery. Indian J Dermatol Venereol Leprol 2008; 74 (Suppl.): S37-45.
[PMID: 18688102]

[75] Boersma BR, Westerhof W, Bos JD. Repigmentation in vitiligo vulgaris by autologous minigrafting: Results in nineteen patients. J Am Acad Dermatol 1995; 33(6): 990-5.
[http://dx.doi.org/10.1016/0190-9622(95)90292-9] [PMID: 7490371]

[76] Ozdemir M, Cetinkale O, Wolf R, *et al.* Comparison of two surgical approaches for treating vitiligo: a preliminary study. Int J Dermatol 2002; 41(3): 135-8.
[http://dx.doi.org/10.1046/j.1365-4362.2002.01391.x] [PMID: 12010337]

[77] Mehra A. Vitiligo Surgery by Aakriti Mehra. Bombay Hosp J 2017; 59.

[78] Falabella R. Surgical approaches for stable vitiligo. Dermatol Surg 2005; 31(10): 1277-84.
[http://dx.doi.org/10.1097/00042728-200510000-00003] [PMID: 16188179]

[79] Brysk MM, Newton RC, Rajaraman S, *et al.* Repigmentation of vitiliginous skin by cultured cells. Pigment Cell Res 1989; 2(3): 202-7.
[http://dx.doi.org/10.1111/j.1600-0749.1989.tb00186.x] [PMID: 2475866]

[80] Njoo MD, Westerhof W, Bos JD, Bossuyt PMM. A systematic review of autologous transplantation methods in vitiligo. Arch Dermatol 1998; 134(12): 1543-9.
[http://dx.doi.org/10.1001/archderm.134.12.1543] [PMID: 9875191]

[81] Mysore V, Salim T. Cellular grafts in management of leucoderma. Indian J Dermatol 2009; 54(2): 142-9.
[http://dx.doi.org/10.4103/0019-5154.53194] [PMID: 20101310]

[82] Savant S. Surgical therapy of vitiligo: Current status. Indian J Dermatol Venereol Leprol 2005; 71(5): 307-10.
[http://dx.doi.org/10.4103/0378-6323.16778] [PMID: 16394452]

[83] Chen YF, Yang PY, Hu DN, Kuo FS, Hung CS, Hung CM. Treatment of vitiligo by transplantation of cultured pure melanocyte suspension: analysis of 120 cases. J Am Acad Dermatol 2004; 51(1): 68-74.
[http://dx.doi.org/10.1016/j.jaad.2003.12.013] [PMID: 15243526]

[84] Redondo P, del Olmo J, García-Guzman M, Guembe L, Prósper F. Repigmentation of vitiligo by transplantation of autologous melanocyte cells cultured on amniotic membrane. Br J Dermatol 2008; 158(5): 1168-71.
[http://dx.doi.org/10.1111/j.1365-2133.2008.08521.x] [PMID: 18363745]

[85] Halaban R, Ghosh S, Baird A. bFGF is the putative natural growth factor for human melanocytes. In Vitro Cell Dev Biol 1987; 23(1): 47-52.
[http://dx.doi.org/10.1007/BF02623492] [PMID: 3027025]

[86] Abu Tahir M, Pramod K, Ansari SH, Ali J. Current remedies for vitiligo. Autoimmun Rev 2010; 9(7): 516-20.
[http://dx.doi.org/10.1016/j.autrev.2010.02.013] [PMID: 20149899]

[87] AlGhamdi KM, Kumar A. Depigmentation therapies for normal skin in vitiligo universalis. J Eur Acad Dermatol Venereol 2011; 25(7): 749-57.
[http://dx.doi.org/10.1111/j.1468-3083.2010.03876.x] [PMID: 21054565]

[88] Bolognia JL, Lapia K, Somma S. Depigmentation therapy. Dermatol Ther 2001; 14(1): 29-34.
[http://dx.doi.org/10.1046/j.1529-8019.2001.014001029.x]

[89] Kasraee B, Fallahi MR, Ardekani GS, *et al.* Retinoic acid synergistically enhances the melanocytotoxic and depigmenting effects of monobenzylether of hydroquinone in black guinea pig skin. Exp Dermatol 2006; 15(7): 509-14.
[http://dx.doi.org/10.1111/j.1600-0625.2006.00441.x] [PMID: 16761959]

[90] van den Boorn JG, Melief CJ, Luiten RM. Monobenzone-induced depigmentation: from enzymatic blockade to autoimmunity. Pigment Cell Melanoma Res 2011; 24(4): 673-9.
[http://dx.doi.org/10.1111/j.1755-148X.2011.00878.x] [PMID: 21689385]

[91] Lyon CC, Beck MH. Contact hypersensitivity to monobenzyl ether of hydroquinone used to treat vitiligo. Contact Dermat 1998; 39(3): 132-3.
[http://dx.doi.org/10.1111/j.1600-0536.1998.tb05863.x] [PMID: 9771988]

[92] Guidelines of care for vitiligo. J Am Acad Dermatol 1996; 35(4): 620-6.
[http://dx.doi.org/10.1016/S0190-9622(96)90691-X]

[93] Njoo MD, Vodegel RM, Westerhof W. Depigmentation therapy in vitiligo universalis with topical 4-methoxyphenol and the Q-switched ruby laser. J Am Acad Dermatol 2000; 42(5): 760-9.
[http://dx.doi.org/10.1067/mjd.2000.103813] [PMID: 10775851]

[94] Nair X, Parab P, Suhr L, Tramposch KM. Combination of 4-hydroxyanisole and all-trans retinoic acid produces synergistic skin depigmentation in swine. J Invest Dermatol 1993; 101(2): 145-9.
[http://dx.doi.org/10.1111/1523-1747.ep12363627] [PMID: 8345215]

[95] Zanini M, Machado Filho CDAS. Terapia despigmentante para vitiligo generalizado com solução tópica de fenol 88%. An Bras Dermatol 2005; 80(4): 415-6.
[http://dx.doi.org/10.1590/S0365-05962005000400013]

[96] Thissen M, Westerhof W. Laser treatment for further depigmentation in vitiligo. Int J Dermatol 1997; 36(5): 386-8.
[http://dx.doi.org/10.1046/j.1365-4362.1997.00144.x] [PMID: 9199992]

[97] Rao J, Fitzpatrick RE. Use of the Q-switched 755-nm alexandrite laser to treat recalcitrant pigment after depigmentation therapy for vitiligo. Dermatol Surg 2004; 30(7): 1043-5.
[http://dx.doi.org/10.1111/j.1524-4725.2004.30313.x] [PMID: 15209798]

[98] Di Nuzzo S, Masotti A. Depigmentation therapy in vitiligo universalis with cryotherapy and 4-hydroxyanisole. Clin Exp Dermatol 2010; 35(2): 215-6.
[http://dx.doi.org/10.1111/j.1365-2230.2009.03412.x] [PMID: 20447090]

[99] Hadi S, Tinio P, Al-Ghaithi K, *et al.* Treatment of vitiligo using the 308-nm excimer laser. Photomed Laser Surg 2006; 24(3): 354-7.

[http://dx.doi.org/10.1089/pho.2006.24.354] [PMID: 16875444]

[100] Passeron T, Ortonne JP. Use of the 308-nm excimer laser for psoriasis and vitiligo. Clin Dermatol 2006; 24(1): 33-42.
[http://dx.doi.org/10.1016/j.clindermatol.2005.10.024] [PMID: 16427504]

[101] Patel NS, Paghdal KV, Cohen GF. Advanced treatment modalities for vitiligo. Dermatol Surg 2012; 38(3): 381-91.
[http://dx.doi.org/10.1111/j.1524-4725.2011.02234.x] [PMID: 22288899]

[102] Nicolaidou E, Antoniou C, Stratigos A, Katsambas AD. Narrowband ultraviolet B phototherapy and 308-nm excimer laser in the treatment of vitiligo: A review. J Am Acad Dermatol 2009; 60(3): 470-7.
[http://dx.doi.org/10.1016/j.jaad.2008.07.053] [PMID: 19157641]

[103] Whitton ME, Pinart M, Batchelor J, *et al.* Interventions for vitiligo. Cochrane Libr 2015; (2): CD003263.
[http://dx.doi.org/10.1002/14651858.CD003263.pub5] [PMID: 25710794]

[104] Hofer A, Hassan AS, Legat FJ, Kerl H, Wolf P. Optimal weekly frequency of 308-nm excimer laser treatment in vitiligo patients. Br J Dermatol 2005; 152(5): 981-5.
[http://dx.doi.org/10.1111/j.1365-2133.2004.06321.x] [PMID: 15888156]

[105] Kakourou T. Vitiligo in children. World J Pediatr 2009; 5(4): 265-8.
[http://dx.doi.org/10.1007/s12519-009-0050-1] [PMID: 19911140]

[106] Milde P, Hauser U, Simon T, *et al.* Expression of 1,25-dihydroxyvitamin D3 receptors in normal and psoriatic skin. J Invest Dermatol 1991; 97(2): 230-9.
[http://dx.doi.org/10.1111/1523-1747.ep12480255] [PMID: 1649228]

[107] Schallreuter-Wood KU, Pittelkow MR, Swanson NN. Defective calcium transport in vitiliginous melanocytes. Arch Dermatol Res 1996; 288(1): 11-3.
[http://dx.doi.org/10.1007/BF02505036] [PMID: 8750928]

[108] Birlea S, Costin GE, Norris D. Cellular and molecular mechanisms involved in the action of vitamin D analogs targeting vitiligo depigmentation. Curr Drug Targets 2008; 9(4): 345-59.
[http://dx.doi.org/10.2174/138945008783954970] [PMID: 18393827]

[109] Zügel U, Asadullah K, Steinmeyer A, Giesen C. A novel immunosuppressive 1α,25-dihydroxyvitamin D3 analog with reduced hypercalcemic activity. J Invest Dermatol 2002; 119(6): 1434-42.
[http://dx.doi.org/10.1046/j.1523-1747.2002.19623.x] [PMID: 12485451]

[110] AlGhamdi K, Kumar A, Moussa N. The role of vitamin D in melanogenesis with an emphasis on vitiligo. Indian J Dermatol Venereol Leprol 2013; 79(6): 750-8.
[http://dx.doi.org/10.4103/0378-6323.120720] [PMID: 24177606]

[111] Leone G, Pacifico A, Iacovelli P, Vidolin AP, Picardo M. Tacalcitol and narrow-band phototherapy in patients with vitiligo. Clin Exp Dermatol 2006; 31(2): 200-5.
[http://dx.doi.org/10.1111/j.1365-2230.2005.02037.x] [PMID: 16487090]

[112] Parsad D, Saini R, Verma N. Combination of PUVAsol and topical calcipotriol in vitiligo. Dermatology 1998; 197(2): 167-70.
[http://dx.doi.org/10.1159/000017991] [PMID: 9732168]

[113] Radmanesh M. Depigmentation of the normally pigmented patches in universal vitiligo patients by cryotherapy. J Eur Acad Dermatol Venereol 2000; 14(3): 149-52.
[http://dx.doi.org/10.1046/j.1468-3083.2000.00038.x] [PMID: 11032055]

[114] Leong KW, Lee TC, Goh AS. Imatinib mesylate causes hypopigmentation in the skin. Cancer 2004; 100(11): 2486-7.
[http://dx.doi.org/10.1002/cncr.20267] [PMID: 15160360]

[115] Brown T, Zirvi M, Cotsarelis G, Gelfand JM. Vitiligo-like hypopigmentation associated with imiquimod treatment of genital warts. J Am Acad Dermatol 2005; 52(4): 715-6.

[http://dx.doi.org/10.1016/j.jaad.2004.10.861] [PMID: 15793538]

[116] Kang HY, Park TJ, Jin SH. Imiquimod, a toll-like receptor 7 agonist, inhibits melanogenesis and proliferation of human melanocytes. J Invest Dermatol 2009; 129(1): 243-6.
[http://dx.doi.org/10.1038/jid.2008.184] [PMID: 18596825]

[117] Kim CH, Ahn JH, Kang SU, *et al.* Imiquimod induces apoptosis of human melanocytes. Arch Dermatol Res 2010; 302(4): 301-6.
[http://dx.doi.org/10.1007/s00403-009-1012-0] [PMID: 20033192]

[118] Senel E, Seckin D. Imiquimod-induced vitiligo-like depigmentation. Indian J Dermatol Venereol Leprol 2007; 73(6): 423.
[http://dx.doi.org/10.4103/0378-6323.37065] [PMID: 18032867]

[119] Duhra P, Foulds IS. Persistent vitiligo induced by diphencyprone. Br J Dermatol 1990; 123(3): 415-6.
[http://dx.doi.org/10.1111/j.1365-2133.1990.tb06306.x] [PMID: 2206982]

[120] Konstantinova V, Olisova O, Gladko V, Burova EP. Vitiligo – New Treatment Approach. Clin Cosmet Investig Dermatol 2019; 12: 911-7.
[http://dx.doi.org/10.2147/CCID.S229175] [PMID: 31908514]

[121] Zohdy HAEW, Hussein MS. Intradermal injection of Fluorouracil *versus* triamcinolone in localized vitiligo treatment. J Cosmet Dermatol 2019; 18(5): 1430-4.
[http://dx.doi.org/10.1111/jocd.12820] [PMID: 30444065]

[122] Crunkhorn S. Reversing vitiligo. Nat Rev Drug Discov 2018; 17(9): 622-2.
[http://dx.doi.org/10.1038/nrd.2018.142] [PMID: 30160255]

[123] Richmond JM, Strassner JP, Zapata L Jr, *et al.* Antibody blockade of IL-15 signaling has the potential to durably reverse vitiligo. Sci Transl Med 2018; 10(450): eaam7710.
[http://dx.doi.org/10.1126/scitranslmed.aam7710] [PMID: 30021889]

[124] Jesitus J. JAK inhibitors offer hope for vitiligo patients.

[125] Rosmarin D, Pandya AG, Lebwohl M, *et al.* Ruxolitinib cream for treatment of vitiligo: a randomised, controlled, phase 2 trial. Lancet 2020; 396(10244): 110-20.
[http://dx.doi.org/10.1016/S0140-6736(20)30609-7] [PMID: 32653055]

[126] Phan K, Phan S, Shumack S, Gupta M. Repigmentation in vitiligo using janus kinase (JAK) inhibitors with phototherapy: systematic review and Meta-analysis. J Dermatolog Treat 2022; 33(1): 173-7.
[http://dx.doi.org/10.1080/09546634.2020.1735615] [PMID: 32096671]

[127] Liu LY, Strassner JP, Refat MA, Harris JE, King BA. Repigmentation in vitiligo using the Janus kinase inhibitor tofacitinib may require concomitant light exposure. J Am Acad Dermatol 2017; 77(4): 675-682.e1.
[http://dx.doi.org/10.1016/j.jaad.2017.05.043] [PMID: 28823882]

[128] Gianfaldoni S, Tchernev G, Wollina U, *et al.* Micro - focused phototherapy associated to Janus kinase inhibitor: a promising valid therapeutic option for patients with localized vitiligo. Open Access Maced J Med Sci 2018; 6(1): 46-8.
[http://dx.doi.org/10.3889/oamjms.2018.042] [PMID: 29483979]

[129] Lim HW, Grimes PE, Agbai O, *et al.* Afamelanotide and narrowband UV-B phototherapy for the treatment of vitiligo: a randomized multicenter trial. JAMA Dermatol 2015; 151(1): 42-50.
[http://dx.doi.org/10.1001/jamadermatol.2014.1875] [PMID: 25230094]

[130] Graham A, Westerhof W, Thody AJ. The expression of α-msh by melanocytes is reduced in vitiligo. Ann N Y Acad Sci 1999; 885(1): 470-3.
[http://dx.doi.org/10.1111/j.1749-6632.1999.tb08715.x]

[131] Grimes PE, Hamzavi I, Lebwohl M, Ortonne JP, Lim HW. The efficacy of afamelanotide and narrowband UV-B phototherapy for repigmentation of vitiligo. JAMA Dermatol 2013; 149(1): 68-73.
[http://dx.doi.org/10.1001/2013.jamadermatol.386] [PMID: 23407924]

[132] Schallreuter KU, Moore J, Behrens-Williams S, Panske A, Harari M. Rapid initiation of repigmentation in vitiligo with Dead Sea climatotherapy in combination with pseudocatalase (PC-KUS). Int J Dermatol 2002; 41(8): 482-7.
[http://dx.doi.org/10.1046/j.1365-4362.2002.01463.x] [PMID: 12207762]

[133] Dell'Anna ML, Mastrofrancesco A, Sala R, *et al.* Antioxidants and narrow band-UVB in the treatment of vitiligo: a double-blind placebo controlled trial. Clin Exp Dermatol 2007; 32(6): 631-6.
[http://dx.doi.org/10.1111/j.1365-2230.2007.02514.x] [PMID: 17953631]

[134] Li L, Li L, Wu Y, Gao XH, Chen HD. Triple-combination treatment with oral α-lipoic acid, betamethasone injection, and NB-UVB for non-segmental progressive vitiligo. J Cosmet Laser Ther 2016; 18(3): 182-5.
[http://dx.doi.org/10.3109/14764172.2015.1114646] [PMID: 26735264]

[135] Schäfer M, Dütsch S, auf dem Keller U, *et al.* Nrf2 establishes a glutathione-mediated gradient of UVB cytoprotection in the epidermis. Genes Dev 2010; 24(10): 1045-58.
[http://dx.doi.org/10.1101/gad.568810] [PMID: 20478997]

[136] Lotti TM, Hercogová J, Schwartz RA, *et al.* Treatments of vitiligo: what's new at the horizon. Dermatol Ther 2012; 25 (Suppl. 1): S32-40.
[http://dx.doi.org/10.1111/dth.12011] [PMID: 23237036]

[137] Salloum A, Bazzi N, Maalouf D, Habre M. Microneedling in vitiligo: a systematic review. Dermatol Ther 2020; 33(6): e14297.
[http://dx.doi.org/10.1111/dth.14297] [PMID: 32940387]

[138] Trials C. Assessing the efficacy of needling with or without corticosteroids in the repigmentation of vitiligo, 2021. Available from: https://classic.clinicaltrials.gov/ct2/show/NCT02191748

[139] Elshafy Khashaba SA, Elkot RA, Ibrahim AM. Efficacy of NB-UVB, microneedling with triamcinolone acetonide, and a combination of both modalities in the treatment of vitiligo: A comparative study. J Am Acad Dermatol 2018; 79(2): 365-7.
[http://dx.doi.org/10.1016/j.jaad.2017.12.054] [PMID: 29291952]

[140] Kapoor R, Phiske MM, Jerajani HR. Evaluation of safety and efficacy of topical prostaglandin E$_2$ in treatment of vitiligo. Br J Dermatol 2009; 160(4): 861-3.
[http://dx.doi.org/10.1111/j.1365-2133.2008.08923.x] [PMID: 19014395]

[141] Anbar TS, El-Ammawi TS, Abdel-Rahman AT, Hanna MR. The effect of latanoprost on vitiligo: a preliminary comparative study. Int J Dermatol 2015; 54(5): 587-93.
[http://dx.doi.org/10.1111/ijd.12631] [PMID: 25545321]

[142] Moreira CG, Carrenho LZB, Pawloski PL, Soley BS, Cabrini DA, Otuki MF. Pre-clinical evidences of Pyrostegia venusta in the treatment of vitiligo. J Ethnopharmacol 2015; 168: 315-25.
[http://dx.doi.org/10.1016/j.jep.2015.03.080] [PMID: 25862965]

[143] Sidi E, Bourgeois-Gavardin J. The treatment of vitiligo with Ammi Majus Linn; a preliminary note. J Invest Dermatol 1952; 18(5): 391-5.
[http://dx.doi.org/10.1038/jid.1952.46] [PMID: 14927989]

[144] Ossenkoppele PM, van der Sluis WG, van Vloten WA. Phototoxic dermatitis following the use of Ammi majus fruit for vitiligo. Ned Tijdschr Geneeskd 1991; 135(11): 478-80.
[PMID: 2023655]

[145] Narayanaswamy R, Ismail IS. Role of herbal medicines in vitiligo treatment-current status and future perspectives. Asian J Pharm Clin Res 2018; 11(9): 19.
[http://dx.doi.org/10.22159/ajpcr.2018.v11i9.26830]

[146] Bhowmik D, Chiranjib YJ, Tripathi KK, Kumar KS. Herbal remedies of Azadirachta indica and its medicinal application. J Chem Pharm Res 2010; 2: 62-72.

[147] Babitha S, Shin JH, Nguyen DH, *et al.* A stimulatory effect of Cassia occidentalis on melanoblast

differentiation and migration. Arch Dermatol Res 2011; 303(3): 211-6.
[http://dx.doi.org/10.1007/s00403-011-1127-y] [PMID: 21328088]

[148]   Buggiani G, Tsampau D, Hercogovà J, Rossi R, Brazzini B, Lotti T. Clinical efficacy of a novel topical formulation for vitiligo: compared evaluation of different treatment modalities in 149 patients. Dermatol Ther 2012; 25(5): 472-6.
[http://dx.doi.org/10.1111/j.1529-8019.2012.01484.x] [PMID: 23046028]

[149]   Parsad D, Pandhi R, Juneja A. Effectiveness of oral *Ginkgo biloba* in treating limited, slowly spreading vitiligo. Clin Exp Dermatol 2003; 28(3): 285-7.
[http://dx.doi.org/10.1046/j.1365-2230.2003.01207.x] [PMID: 12780716]

[150]   Ha SY, Jung JY, Kang HY, Kim TH, Yang JK. Tyrosinase activity and melanogenic effects of Lespedeza bicolor extract *in vitro* and *in vivo*. BioResources 2020; 15(3): 6244-61.
[http://dx.doi.org/10.15376/biores.15.3.6244-6261]

[151]   Mou KH, Zhang XQ, Yu B, Zhang ZL, Feng J. Promoting of melanocyte adhesion and migration by Malytea Scurfpea fruit *in vitro*. Methods Find Exp Clin Pharmacol 2004; 26(3): 167-70.
[http://dx.doi.org/10.1358/mf.2004.26.3.809721] [PMID: 15148520]

[152]   Sarac G, Kapicioglu Y, Sener S, *et al.* Effectiveness of topical *Nigella sativa* for vitiligo treatment. Dermatol Ther 2019; 32(4): e12949.
[http://dx.doi.org/10.1111/dth.12949] [PMID: 31025474]

[153]   Ali SA, Meitei KV. *Nigella sativa* seed extract and its bioactive compound thymoquinone: the new melanogens causing hyperpigmentation in the wall lizard melanophores. J Pharm Pharmacol 2011; 63(5): 741-6.
[http://dx.doi.org/10.1111/j.2042-7158.2011.01271.x] [PMID: 21492177]

[154]   Gianfaldoni S, Wollina U, Tirant M, *et al.* Herbal compounds for the treatment of vitiligo: a review. Open Access Maced J Med Sci 2018; 6(1): 203-7.
[http://dx.doi.org/10.3889/oamjms.2018.048] [PMID: 29484024]

[155]   Bedi KL, Zutshi U, Chopra CL, Amla V. Picrorhiza kurroa, an ayurvedic herb, may potentiate photochemotherapy in vitiligo. J Ethnopharmacol 1989; 27(3): 347-52.
[http://dx.doi.org/10.1016/0378-8741(89)90009-3] [PMID: 2615440]

[156]   Gianfaldoni S, Wollina U, Tirant M, *et al.* Herbal Compounds for the Treatment of Vitiligo: A Review. Open Access Maced J Med Sci 2018; 6(1): 203-7.
[http://dx.doi.org/10.3889/oamjms.2018.048] [PMID: 29484024]

[157]   Lin Z, Hoult JRS, Bennett DC, Raman A. Stimulation of mouse melanocyte proliferation by Piper nigrum fruit extract and its main alkaloid, piperine. Planta Med 1999; 65(7): 600-3.
[http://dx.doi.org/10.1055/s-1999-14031] [PMID: 10575373]

[158]   Mihăilă B, Dinică R, Tatu A, Buzia O. New insights in vitiligo treatments using bioactive compounds from *Piper nigrum*. Exp Ther Med 2018; 1039-44.
[http://dx.doi.org/10.3892/etm.2018.6977] [PMID: 30679971]

[159]   Middelkamp-Hup MA, Bos JD, Rius-Diaz F, Gonzalez S, Westerhof W. Treatment of vitiligo vulgaris with narrow-band UVB and oral *Polypodium leucotomos* extract: a randomized double-blind placebo-controlled study. J Eur Acad Dermatol Venereol 2007; 21(7): 942-50.
[http://dx.doi.org/10.1111/j.1468-3083.2006.02132.x] [PMID: 17659004]

[160]   Hussain I, Hussain N, Manan A, Rashid A, Khan B, Bukhsh S. Fabrication of anti-vitiligo ointment containing *Psoralea corylifolia*: *in vitro* and *in vivo* characterization. Drug Des Devel Ther 2016; 10: 3805-16.
[http://dx.doi.org/10.2147/DDDT.S114328] [PMID: 27920496]

[161]   Khushboo PS, Jadhav VM, Kadam VJ, Sathe NS. Psoralea corylifolia Linn.-"Kushtanashini". Pharmacogn Rev 2010; 4(7): 69-76.
[http://dx.doi.org/10.4103/0973-7847.65331] [PMID: 22228944]

[162] Moreira CG, Carrenho LZB, Pawloski PL, Soley BS, Cabrini DA, Otuki MF. Pre-clinical evidences of Pyrostegia venusta in the treatment of vitiligo. J Ethnopharmacol 2015; 168: 315-25.
[http://dx.doi.org/10.1016/j.jep.2015.03.080] [PMID: 25862965]

[163] Ha SY, Jung JY, Kang HY, Kim T-H, Yang J-K. Tyrosinase activity and melanogenic effects of *Rhododendron schlippenbachii* Extract *in vivo* and *in vitro*. Mogjae Gonghag 2020; 48(2): 166-80.
[http://dx.doi.org/10.5658/WOOD.2020.48.2.166]

[164] Shu-Hua Chiang . The enhancement effect of Salvia miltiorrhiza on melanin production of B16F10 melanoma cells. J Med Plants Res 2012; 6(26)
[http://dx.doi.org/10.5897/JMPR12.544]

CHAPTER 5

Atopic Dermatitis Prevalence and How to Manage It

Edith Filaire[1,*], **Jacques Peyrot**[2] and **Jean-Yves Berthon**[3]

[1] *University Clermont Auvergne, UMR 1019 INRA-UcA, UNH (Human Nutrition Unity), ECREIN Team, 63000 Clermont-Ferrand, France*

[2] *Cabinet de Dermatologie, 43 Rue Blatin, 63000 Clermont-Ferrand, France*

[3] *GREENTECH, Biopôle Clermont-Limagne, 63360 Saint Beauzire, France*

Abstract: Atopic dermatitis (AD) is a common inflammatory skin disorder characterized by recurrent eczematous lesions and intense itch. More precisely, the earliest lesion is a small erythematous papule or papulovesicle. These papules may then later become erythematous plaques with clinical features of weeping, crusting, or scaling, depending on the severity of the lesions. The most problematic symptom of AD is itch. The "itch-scratch" cycle involves the act of scratching affected areas of the skin to relieve AD-associated itch, which can further worsen the disease.

This skin disorder affects people of all ages and ethnicities, has a substantial psychosocial impact on patients and relatives, and is the leading cause of the global burden of skin disease. Moreover, AD persistence has been reported in 60% of adults who had the disease as children.

AD is associated with an increased risk of multiple comorbidities, including food allergy, asthma, allergic rhinitis, and mental health disorders. The pathophysiology is complex and involves a strong genetic predisposition, epidermal dysfunction, and T-cell-driven inflammation. There is increasing evidence that AD involves multiple immune pathways. Currently, there is no cure, but increasing numbers of innovative targeted therapies hold promise for achieving disease control. As effective medical treatments for this condition are limited in number, many patients have turned to alternative therapies, including so-called natural products, such as herbs and algae. In this chapter, we summarized and discussed advances in the understanding of the disease and its implications for prevention, management, and future research, with a focus on natural solutions.

Keywords: Atopic dermatitis, Filaggrin, Genetic, IgE, Microbiota, Natural solutions, Skin barrier, Treatment, Th2.

---

[*] **Corresponding author Edith Filaire:** University Clermont Auvergne, UMR 1019 INRA-UcA, UNH (Human Nutrition Unity), ECREIN Team, 63000 Clermont-Ferrand, France; Tel: 0033648035198; E-mail: edith.filaire@univ-orleans.fr

Heba Abd El-Sattar El-Nashar, Mohamed El-Shazly & Nouran Mohammed Fahmy (Eds.)

INTRODUCTION

Prevalence and Economic Impact

Atopic dermatitis (AD) is one of the most common inflammatory skin diseases, often of early-life onset, for which the prevalence continues to increase in industrialized countries [1]. The prevalence of AD in adults ranges from 2% to 10% (reported by the World Allergy Organization), and from 15% to 20% in children [2, 3]. Both sexes are affected, and the prevalence varies among races and ethnic groups. While the majority of patients (>85%) develop AD within the first 5 years of life, only half achieve significant improvement by 7 years of age [4]. It is important to note that the risk of atopic eczema is 40% for children with one atopic parent. When both parents are affected by the same manifestation of atopy (*i.e.*, father and mother with atopic eczema), the risk is between 70% and 80%. This prevalence has increased by 2 to 3-fold during the past decade in Western countries [5]. Although the cause of this increase remains unknown, the role of the microbiome in the pathogenesis of AD has been suggested [6].

It is well established that AD has large cost implications, as the disease clearly causes a major financial burden to both individual families and national healthcare systems. Aside from its economic cost, this skin disease bears a significant burden on society. However, assessing the economic burden of AD is complex as it consists of costs for medical care and non-medical care as well as indirect costs (*i.e.*, loss of education and workdays), given that the degree to which medical costs are an individual (out-of-pocket) burden or a collective burden largely depends on each country's respective healthcare system. More precisely, direct costs include prescription medicines, visits to health care providers, hospitalizations, and transportation. Indirect costs include missed days or lost productivity at work or school, career modification, and reduced quality of life [7].

The diversity of the healthcare system of each country is reflected in several studies. Two studies from the USA reported direct and indirect costs of approximately USD 3300 per person per year (PPPY) for children [8] and adults [9]. Three European studies reported out-of-pocket costs for medical care as €351 PPPY for French adults and €927 for adults with moderate-to-severe AD in nine European countries [10, 11]. The burden of AD can also be evaluated using the disability-adjusted life-years (DALYs), a measure of the difference between living a life in perfect health *versus* living with the disease. This measure is the sum of the years of life lost due to premature death and the years lived with a disability within a given population [12]. These authors noted that AD has the highest DALY burden of all skin diseases and ranks 15th among all nonfatal diseases globally. A total of five European countries rank top in age-standardized DALYs: Sweden, the UK, Iceland, Finland and Denmark. However, it appears that the global burden of AD expressed in DALYs remained stable during the data collection period from 1990 to 2017 [12].

Generally, healthcare costs continue to rise around the world. Finding ways to reduce costs by more efficiently managing AD will continue to be important for physicians, patients and society. By reducing the incidence of AD, it is possible that fewer patients will require more expensive interventions, which is of particular concern as emerging biologics become available for this disorder.

ETIOLOGY AND PATHOGENESIS

AD is an inflammatory, chronically relapsing, intensely pruritic skin disease characterized by dry skin [13]. Furthermore, it is the highest-ranked skin disease with respect to DALYs and years lived with a disease. This pathology is characterized by eczematous, pruritic skin patches and plaques as well as itching that can severely affect quality of life [14]. Furthermore, the itch has been associated with mental distress and increased risk for suicidal ideation in those with AD [15]. Of note, emotional stress has also been shown to increase itching, implying a bidirectional relationship between these features [16].

Nevertheless, AD is a "diffuse" skin condition. The definition of the whole disease seems as imprecise as the limits of the affected skin areas. Sometimes the term "involved" skin is questionable, especially when dermato-histopathological investigations show signs of inflammation in also clinically "uninvolved" skin areas. The susceptibility to environmental influences, especially on the psychosocial level, underlines the strong variability of this dermatosis. In addition, this disease manifests itself differently in different age groups and different body regions.

AD is often accompanied by other atopic disorders, such as allergic rhinoconjunctivitis, asthma, food allergies, and less often, eosinophilic esophagitis. These conditions may appear simultaneously or develop in succession.

AD is also associated with sleep disruption (mainly due to pruritus), with worse sleep disruption observed in more severe diseases. In addition, AD is associated with decreased work productivity, depression, and anxiety, all of which carry additional health and economic burdens for patients and their families.

It is also important to note that there is a link between AD and obesity [17]. Indeed, the few investigations addressing AD and obesity in infancy or early childhood (age < 2 years) noted that there is a positive association between overweight/ adiposity in infancy and the development of AD in early life. Even if the underlying mechanisms between obesity and AD are incompletely understood, it seems that obesity has been shown to alter the skin's epidermal barrier, leading to increased transepidermal water loss (TEWL) and dry skin, which may aggravate underlying barrier defects in AD [18]. Moreover, it is well known that obesity is associated with persistent low-grade systemic inflammation [19]. Adipose tissue produces adipokines, the two important adipokines being leptin and adiponectin. It is well known that leptin stimulates the production of inflammatory mediators. Low adiponectin concentrations have also been associated with an increased prevalence of AD.

Although the pathophysiology of AD is not completely understood, several models have been proposed, including skin barrier dysfunction, dysfunctional cell-mediated immunity, alteration of the microbiome, and environmental and lifestyle factors [20, 21].

Initial studies focused on the role of altered immune responses, particularly T helper (Th) type 2 and immunoglobulin E (IgE) responses, as major drivers of the disease [22]. The so-called inside-out hypothesis postulated that immune dysregulation induces skin barrier alteration, emitting allergens and pathogens to penetrate the skin [23]. However, the discovery of inherited defects in factors that contribute to the skin barrier posited the alternative outside-in hypothesis, wherein an underlying barrier dysfunction allows antigen penetration to induce altered immune responses. Models then incorporated aspects of both, including an outside- inside-outside model wherein the skin microbiome and environmental factors penetrate the body from the outside through epidermal barrier defects and subsequently trigger immune dysregulation, which further exacerbates skin barrier defects [24].

Role of the Epidermal Barrier

Epidermal barrier defects, including filaggrin (FLG) gene mutation, lipid defects, proteases, irritants, pH changes, and influx of bacteria and other pathogens, are implicated in the development of AD [25]. The epidermis plays a crucial role as a physical and functional barrier, prevents TEWL, and excludes invading pathogens and environmental antigens. FLG, transglutaminases, keratins, and intercellular proteins are key proteins responsible for the epidermal function. Defects in these proteins facilitate allergen and microbial penetration into the skin [26]. Proteins defects also lead to dysregulated immune responses to external antigens and drive skin and systemic inflammatory responses [27].

Lesional AD skin demonstrates elevated levels of endogenous serine proteases (*i.e.*, kallikrein 5 and 7 (KLK5/7)), due to an imbalance in the activities of these proteolytic enzymes and protease inhibitors such as the lymphoepithelial Kazal-type trypsin inhibitor (LEKTI) encoded by *SPINK5*. Other factors that enhance proteolysis include increased skin surface pH and exogenous proteases from allergens (*i.e.*, house dust mites, pollens), *Staphylococcus aureus*, and *Malassezia.*

Abnormalities in the epidermal lipid layer are also involved in AD onset. The epidermal layer plays an important role in barrier formation by maintaining lubrication and preventing dehydration as well as having antimicrobial activity [28]. Lipids, such as ceramides, long-chain free fatty acids (FFAs), and cholesterol, constitute the lipid matrix that is organized in lamellar bodies and located between corneocytes. During epidermal differentiation, precursor lipids are stored in lamellar bodies within the upper cell layers of the epidermis and extruded into the extracellular domain. Subsequent enzymic processing produces the major lipid classes, which are necessary to maintain the integrity of the epidermal barrier. Altered lipid composition is observed in lesional and nonlesional AD skin [29]. In particular, long-chain EO ceramides are essential because they are covalently bound to cornified-envelope proteins and cover the surface of each corneocyte. It seems that Th2 cytokines reduce levels of long-chain FFAs and EO ceramides in a STAT6-dependent manner. Li *et al.* [30] noted that the concentrations of long-chain ceramides were decreased in patients with AD and as well as in skin colonized with *S. aureus* compared with skin that was not colonized. TEWL was also negatively correlated with levels of these ceramides. It has been suggested that the topical application of lipids could be a promising alternative treatment strategy in mild and moderate AD. Topical application of lipids could involve either non-physiological lipids such as petrolatum or, beeswax, or lipids similar to the intrinsic pool of lipids present in the lamellar bodies: however, the mechanism of action of the later remains unknown [28].

Environmental Factors

Any environmental factor that adversely impacts skin barrier integrity increases both AD risk onset and severity [31]. The most important local environmental factor is mechanical damage, including repetitive scratching, use of detergents and release of exogenous proteases. Washing the skin may also contribute to mechanical damage, and controversy surrounds the optimal bathing frequency for children with AD. Properties of the water used for washing may also play an important role. Finally, climatic effects on the skin barrier are also thought to be relevant, and previous observations have suggested a positive linear association between country-level AD prevalence and certain metrics of ultraviolet radiation exposure [32].

Genetic and Epigenetic Factors

Genetic and epigenetic factors also seem to play a role in the occurrence of AD, in particular *FLG* gene, which encodes FLG, a major structural protein in the *stratum corneum* (SC). Three primary reviews about the genetics of AD have been performed in the last decade. The first review was published in 2010 and compiled all the existing genetic studies related to AD [33]. Barnes [33] reported variants in 81 genes, 46 of which had shown a positive association with the disease. Bin and Leung [34] published an update that included a review of genetic and epigenetic studies from 2009 to June 2016. Recently, Martin *et al.* [35] conducted a systematic literature review using three scientific publication databases (PubMed, Cochrane Library, and Scopus). The search was restricted to publications indexed from July 2016 to December 2019, and keywords related to atopic dermatitis genetics and epigenetics were used. A total of 62 genes and 5 intergenic regions were described as associated with AD.

FLG loss-of-function mutations were the genetic variants for AD most significantly associated with AD. FLG is a key protein in the differentiation of the epidermis and the formation of the skin barrier, which is necessary to prevent water loss through the epidermis and to inhibit the penetration of allergens, toxins, and pathogens [36]. Its precursor profilaggrin is encoded by the *FLG* gene, which is located on chromosome 1q21.3 within a region known as the epidermal differentiation complex (EDC) comprising over 50 genes encoding proteins involved in terminal differentiation and cornification of keratinocytes. *FLG* mutations lead to functional epidermal barrier defects, increase skin permeability and subsequent allergic sensitization, promote the Th2 inflammatory response, and eventually lead to asthma [37]. The "outside–inside" theory of AD pathogenesis proposes that epidermal Antigen Presenting Cells (APC) in patients with AD are overexposed to danger signals because of their impaired skin barrier, leading to APC maturation and T-cell-mediated inflammatory skin disease. Some genes associated with AD have been related to innate immune system pathways, providing solid evidence of the relationship between the innate immune system with the disease and its progression. Genes associated with innate immune pathways (*ADAM33, MIF, MMP9, ORM2, RETN,* and *TLR2*) are related to neutrophil degranulation that contributes to inflammation of the tissue in AD. Prior evidence has also linked an association between AD and genes such as *ADAM33, CARD11,* and *DEFB1*. *CARD11* is required for B- and T-cell receptor signal transduction and activation of the NF-κB transcription factor. *DEFB1* is an antimicrobial peptide implicated in the resistance of epithelial surfaces to microbial colonization, and it has been proposed as a link between the innate and adaptive immune systems. Studies by Heine *et al.* [38] and Suzuki *et al.* [39] also support the idea that AD is linked to vitamin D receptor polymorphisms and cytochrome P450 family 27 subfamily A member 1 (*CYP27A1*), *CYP27A1* being involved in the metabolism of vitamin D3 which plays an essential role in immune modulation.

Most of the research on AD epigenetic regulation has focused on the posttranscriptional regulation mediated by microRNAs (miRNAs) [35]. miRNAs constitute a class of small, non-coding RNAs, with a size ranging from 17 to 25 nucleotides, and a sequence that allows them to bind to specific messengers RNAs (mRNAs). This key feature permits the posttranscriptional modulation of targeted genes by triggering mRNA degradation and/or inhibition of translation [40]. According to several functional studies, miRNAs are involved in virtually every cellular process and are also related to immune system regulation. The most extensively studied miRNAS include miR-21, miR-146a, and mIR-155. A role in the regulation of the immune response and tissue inflammation in allergic diseases is well known. Even though the data remain under debate, developments in genetics and epigenetics technology offer opportunities to improve the diagnosis of AD. These advancements allow ascribing patients to specific genetic groups and enable the tailoring of therapy with the most optimal response to ensure the most convenient patient care.

Immune Dysregulation

AD is an inflammatory skin disease in which immune dysregulation results in subsequent systemic immune complications. Acute AD lesions have a predominance of Th2 cytokines. More precisely, activated T cells release cytokines into the skin, mainly interleukin (IL)-4, interleukin-13, and interleukin-31, which activate downstream Janus kinase (JAK) pathways. The cytokines promote inflammation, pruritus, and the production of antigen-specific IgE by activating B cells and plasma cells.

Recent studies have expanded on this Th2 paradigm to include the roles of other immune subsets, such as Th17, Th22, T regulatory cells (Tregs), and Th9 cells in part associated with race or ethnic group [24].

The innate immune system also significantly contributes to the development of AD skin inflammation, including IL-5 and IL-13 from group 2 innate lymphoid cells, IL-4 from basophils, and IL-25, IL-33, and TSLP from epithelial cells [20]. This immune milieu is dependent on a patient's age, sex, and ethnic background, thereby adding to the complexity of this disease [41].

Recent studies demonstrated that skin-resident group 2 innate lymphoid cells (ILC2) play a role in the pathogenesis of AD. ILC2s were found to produce IL-5 and IL-13, which include the development of an AD-like skin lesion [42]. Similarly, human skin ILC2s are highly enriched in the lesional skin of patients with AD and activated by epithelial cell–derived cytokines such as IL-25, IL-33, and/or TSLP [43]. This leads to the production of type 2 cytokines and skin allergic inflammation. Mohapatra *et al.* [44] also suggested that human primary keratinocytes secrete several inflammatory cytokines, such as IL-32, contributing to allergic inflammation.

Antimicrobial peptides (AMPs), including cathelicidin (LL-37) and human β-defensins, are produced by keratinocytes and play a pivotal role in host defense as well as control of host physiologic functions, such as inflammation and wound healing. AMP expressions are inhibited by Th2 cytokines, which are highly produced in AD skin [42]. The decreased expression of AMPs is associated with a higher predisposition to *Staphylococcus aureus* colonization, which can aggravate AD.

Impact of the Microbiome

The human microbiome refers to the collective genetic information of microorganisms that inhabit the human body. It is considered a counterpart of the human genome, which is the collection of all genetic information in an individual. With the discovery that microorganisms have a substantial impact on human health, the microbiome has been termed the 'second genome' and is being widely studied [45]. The microbiome takes part in a number of human biological processes, such as metabolism, epithelial development, and immunity. Long-standing diseases such as obesity, inflammatory bowel diseases, allergic rhinitis, and AD are reportedly linked to the human microbiome in a non-causal manner.

The skin is a shelter to a countless number of microbial communities which live on the tissue surface, in addition to the appendages such as the sweat glands and the hair follicles. About 1 million bacteria are found per square centimeter across the skin surface, totaling over 10^{10} bacterial cells in total. The human skin flora, possibly the most diverse within the body, is recognized as a crucial component in host defense. Commensal skin flora protects humans from pathogens and helps to maintain the delicate balance of the immune system in regard to effective protection and damaging inflammation [42]. Evidence accumulated in the past decade has also shown that specific strains within the community of resident skin bacteria suppress inflammation, stimulate the adaptive and innate immune system, and produce diverse molecules with antimicrobial activity [5].

The composition of microbial communities is linked to the skin site. Changes in the relative abundance of bacterial taxa are associated with moist, dry and sebaceous microenvironments. Sebaceous sites were dominated by lipophilic *Propionibacterium* species, whereas bacteria that thrive in humid environments, such as *Staphylococcus* and *Corynebacterium* species, were preferentially abundant in moist areas. Fungi of the genus *Malassezia* predominated at the core body and arm sites [46].

Besides skin microbiota, the gut is naturally home to an array of phyla. The exact composition of microbes varies even between healthy individuals, and it can be influenced by sex, age, or diet. Phyla making up a healthy adult gut microbiome are considered to be actinobacteria, bacteroidetes, firmicutes, and proteobacteria [47]. Differences in diversity and reoccurring strains of bacteria have been reported in several diseases, including obesity [48]. It is also the case in AD, a disease in which the *Bifidobacterium* counts were significantly lower than in young healthy subjects [49]. At the same time, a higher frequency of *Staphylococcus* was noted in patients with AD compared with healthy controls. Moreover, significant dysbiosis of *F. prausnitzii* species was reported in the fecal sample patients with AD [50]. Concurrent decrease of short-chain fatty acids, which takes part in keeping the integrity of the epithelial barrier and exhibit an anti-inflammatory effect, was also noted. It seems that these modifications propel skin inflammation by enabling the penetration of toxins into the systemic circulation, thereby inducing a severe Th2 response in skin and causing significant tissue damage [51].

Changes in the skin microbiota are often investigated in cutaneous disease, with "dysbiosis," or an imbalance of microbial inhabitants on the skin, often highlighted. However, Flowers and Grice [52] reported that the causal links between dysbiotic states and skin pathologies are questionable, with the relevance of "who is there?" being less relevant than "what are they doing?". This being said, a species that repeatedly appears and dominates the microbiota in association with skin disorders is *S. aureus*, which is often found where there is a breach in the skin barrier (*i.e.*, AD). Byrd *et al.* [53] noted in a murine model of cutaneous colonization that *S. aureus* isolates from more severe AD flares elicited increased epidermal thickening and promoted T cell infiltration in the skin, compared with strains from less severe disease and/or healthy individuals. Higaki *et al.* [54] noted that AD skin lesions have an estimated 90% *S. aureus* colonization rate that correlates with increased disease burden. Clonotypic analysis of *S. aureus* clinical isolates shows that highly pathogenic, antimicrobial-resistant, toxigenic strains predominantly found in AD skin also correlate with disease severity [55].

In addition to microbiota, it appears that mycobiota also plays a role in the incidence of AD [56]. More precisely, *Malassezia* has been implicated in AD pathogenesis, as patients are more often hypersensitive with specific IgE antibodies against *Malassezia* in comparison with healthy individuals, a subtype of AD called 'head and neck dermatitis' [57]. *Candida* is another commensal yeast that has been suggested to contribute to the onset and exacerbation of AD [58]; however, the data are still in debate [59]. Furthermore, a wide range of environmental molds, such as *Aspergillus* and *Cladosporium* species, can induce type I allergic responses, where greater incidence rates have been reported among atopic patients compared to the general population [60]. Viruses including *Herpes simplex virus* (HSV) may also lead to an exacerbation of the condition [48]. Recently, Edslev *et al.* [56] noted an increase prevalence of the skin mite *Demodex folliculorum* on AD skin, and reports suggest colonization with *Demodex spp.* may be associated with folliculitis and rosacea [60]. Thus, it would thus be clinically relevant to examine if *D. folliculorum* can contribute to skin inflammation in AD.

The interactions between barrier dysfunction, dysbiosis, and immune dysregulation are crucial factors in the pathogenesis of AD [24]. Indeed, disruptions to barrier function can result in deleterious changes to the microbiome, changes of which are referred to as dysbiosis. Overall, dysbiosis can also have consequences for skin barrier function. Defective barrier function also plays a role in the immune dysregulation seen in AD, and immune dysregulation can also have profound effects on skin barrier function. These interactions are summarized in Fig. (**1**).

DIAGNOSIS OF ATOPIC DERMATITIS

The diagnosis of AD is established clinically through an extensive history and physical examination that relies strongly on clinical presentation. The clinical picture of AD varies substantially depending on the age of the patient [61], and the presence of at least four different kinds of clinical features have been defined as follows: infantile, childhood, adolescent/adult, and elderly [62]. Several international groups have proposed formal sets of criteria to aid in the diagnosis of AD, and there is now a guideline for the management of this disease [63]. Based on the American Academy of Dermatology recommendations, Table **1** presents these criteria [63].

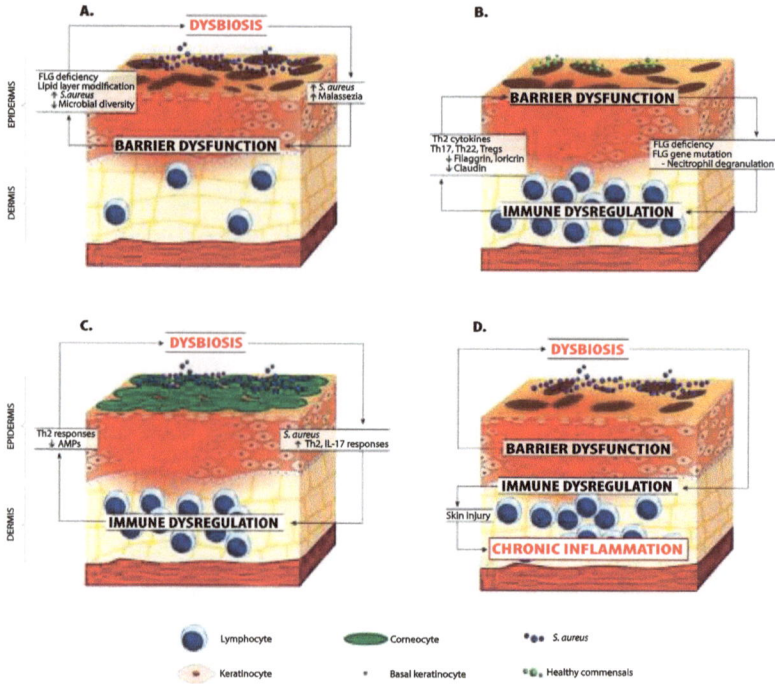

Fig. (1). Systemic relations between inflammation, skin barrier and microbiota.

Table 1. Features to be considered in the diagnosis of patients with AD.

Essential and sufficient features for the diagnosis
• Pruritus
• Eczema (acute, subacute, chronic)
- Typical morphology and age-specific distribution patterns, including facial, neck, and extensor involvement in infants and children, flexural lesions in any age, sparing of the groin, and axillary regions
- Chronic or relapsing history
Important features, seen in most cases, to support the diagnosis
• Early age of onset
• Atopy
- Personal and/or family history (IgE reactivity)
- Xerosis
Associated features to support the diagnosis of AD
Not be used for defining or detecting AD for research and epidemiologic studies
• Atypical vascular responses (*i.e.*, facial pallor, white dermographism, delayed blanch response)
• Filaggrin deficiency-associated conditions:
- Keratosis pilaris, hyperlinear palms, ichthyosis
- Ocular changes: recurrent conjunctivitis
- Other regional findings: perioral or periauricular lesions
- Follicular accentuation: lichenification, prurigo lesions
Exclusionary conditions
• Seborrheic dermatitis
• Contact dermatitis (irritant or allergic)
• Cutaneous T-cell lymphoma
• Psoriasis
• Photosensitivity dermatoses
• Immune deficiency diseases
• Erythroderma of other causes

Patients with presumed atopic dermatitis should have their diagnosis based on the criteria summarized in Table **1**. A punch skin biopsy may be necessary for patients with atypical presentations to rule out other skin conditions that may resemble AD. These conditions include other inflammatory dermatoses (seborrheic dermatitis, psoriasis, allergic or irritant contact dermatitis, and pityriasis lichenoides), primary ichthyosis, infestations (scabies), infections (fungal, human immunodeficiency virus), malignancies (most commonly cutaneous T-cell lymphoma), and metabolic disorders [64]. Other tests such as serum immunoglobulin E, potassium hydroxide preparation, patch testing, and/or genetic testing) may be helpful to rule out other or associated skin conditions.

Even if the diagnosis remains clinical, it is important to note that biomarkers may also assist in diagnosis. The discovery of new T-lymphocyte subsets and novel cytokines and chemokines have created opportunities for the development of new biomarkers, including serum levels of CD30, macrophage-derived chemoattractant (MDC), interleukins (IL-12, IL-16, IL-18, IL-31), and thymus and activation-regulated chemokine (TARC). However, even if some of these biomarkers have correlated with AD severity, none have shown reliable sensitivity to support regular clinical use for diagnosis and monitoring.

TREATMENT

Management of AD includes education of patients and parents, gentle skin care, moisturizer use, and anti-inflammatory therapy to control subclinical inflammation as well as overt flares. Therapy is selected according to the clinical stage of disease (mild, moderate, or severe), the extent of body-surface area involved, age, coexisting conditions and medications being taken by the patient, the severity of pruritus, the degree to which quality of life is impaired, and the goals of the patient [65].

Topical agents represent the mainstay of treatment. Nevertheless, physicians who take care of patients with AD are well aware of the high degree of heterogeneity of the clinical phenotype and the debated role of IgE-mediated sensitization. Despite the obvious complexity of the clinical phenotype, the treatment of AD is often based on a "one-size-fits-all" approach that neglects a more differentiated method based on stratification of AD [62]. This being said, the guidelines of care for the management of AD from the Journal of the American Academy of Dermatology comprise recommendations for the use of topical therapies such as emollients, antihistamines, calcineurin inhibitors, glucocorticoids, phototherapy, antimicrobials and antiseptics [66]. Table **2** summarizes some therapeutic proposals mainly available on a daily-basis.

Table 2. Therapeutic proposals.

Nonpharmacologic interventions
Moisturizers ; bathing practices ; emollient devices
Topical pharmacotherapies
Corticosteroids; Wet wrap therapy
Calcineurin inhibitors
Systemic immunosuppressants
IL-32 gamma
JAK inhibition
Spleen tyrosine kinase (SYK)
Nonpharmacologic recommendations
Ultraviolet light therapy
Prebiotic and probiotic treatments

Corticosteroids

Most reviews and guidelines do not encourage the use of systemic corticosteroids due to their adverse effect profile. Systemic corticosteroids should be limited to use for no more than two weeks for the management of acute flares, or as a bridging treatment to another systemic agent [67]. Topical corticosteroids are available in a wide range of potencies, from the class VII corticosteroids (*i.e.*, hydrocortisone acetate) to the class I. Adverse effects can be induced using topical corticosteroids for long periods (Table **3**). The face and intertriginous areas are the most susceptible sites and may show local effects, even when weaker steroids are used for prolonged periods. Due to their increased body surface area-to-weight ratio, small children have the greatest risk of systemic absorption of topically applied steroids. Group I corticosteroids are not recommended for patients younger than the age of 12 years. Moreover, a rest period is required after 14 days of use.

Table 3. Potential side effects of topical corticosteroids.

Local Cutaneous Side Effects
1. Atrophy
2. Striae
3. Periorificial granulomatous dermatitis
4. Acne
5. Telangiectasia
6. Erythema
7. Hypopigmentation
8. Ocular effects
9. Cataracts
10. HPA axis suppression*

*: HPA: Hypothalamo-Pituitary-Axis.

Considering the widespread use of topical corticosteroids, few local adverse reactions occur when topical steroids are carefully chosen and used appropriately based on the site of application and severity of the dermatitis. As such, even potent topical corticosteroids may safely be used in small areas for short periods.

In order to treat severe recalcitrant AD or during an acute flare period, it may be interesting to resort to Wet wrap therapy (WWT), which consists of a topical corticosteroid application (sometimes diluted), followed by an inner wet layer and outer dry layer of cotton gauze or garments; they are left in place eight to 24 hours per day. The treatment duration of WWT should not exceed two weeks. The penetration of topical corticosteroids can be enhanced through the use of dressings, which can increase skin hydration, and act as a barrier to scratching. Nevertheless, evidence that WWT is more effective than conventional treatment with topical steroids for AD is in debate, and further clinical trials should be done to prove the efficacy of WWT in AD [68].

Calcineurin Inhibitors

To decrease the topical application of steroids, non-steroidal anti-inflammatory agents have been offered to patients, such as topical calcineurin inhibitors (TCI) (Tacrolimus ointment 0.03% and Pimecrolimus-cream 1%), which have been approved as an alternative therapy for AD in children older than 2 years of age. TCI is a distinct class of steroid-sparing, anti-inflammatory agents. Evidence of their efficacy against acute flares and maintenance therapy of AD in both adults and children over 2 years of age have been noted [69]. They inhibit calcineurin-dependent T-cell activation inducing a decrease of proinflammatory cytokines and mediators. More precisely, Tacrolimus and Pimecrolimus prevent the formation of a complex that includes calcineurin, a phosphatase. Without this complex, the phosphate group from the nuclear factor of activated T cells (NF-AT) cannot be cleaved, the NF-AT transcription factor cannot be transported to the nucleus, and the production of cytokines associated with T-cell activation is inhibited. Tacrolimus and Pimecrolimus also inhibit mediator release from mast cells and basophils and decrease IgE receptor expression on cutaneous Langerhans cells.

Burning or pruritus after application of calcineurin inhibitors have been noted in children, stimulation of TRPV1 receptors being the cause of this sensation.

Calcineurin inhibitors do not show the atrophogenic potential of the corticosteroids and can be safely used on the head, neck, and intertriginous areas. Furthermore, no adverse effects on the eyes have been found, allowing safe application in periorbital areas.

Like psoriasis, AD is now considered a primarily T cell–driven disease [70]. Inhibition of the calcineurin phosphatase induces an impaired release of IL-2 and a suppression of T-cell proliferation. Safety and efficacy of cyclosporine (CyA) in AD have been noted, the treatment being effective after 6 to 8 weeks [71]. Sometimes, CyA is used for patients with severe AD but as short-term rescue therapy (<1-2 years) because of nephrotoxicity [72]. Finding the minimal dose of efficacy is, therefore, key in that setting.

Phosphodiesterase 4 Topical Inhibitor

Crisaborole ointment 2% (Eucrisa™) is an anti-inflammatory inhibitor of phosphodiesterase 4 (PDE4) that is available in the US for the topical treatment of mild-to-moderate AD in patients aged $\geq$ 2 years [73]. PDE-4 induces an increase in cytokines production, including IL-10 and IL-4.

Systemic Immunosuppressants

Systemic anti-inflammatory medications can be used for children and adults with moderate-to-severe AD when these patients had no good results with other topical treatments. The risk–benefit profile should be considered before starting an immunosuppressive agent, and side effects must be detected. Association of systemic treatment with topical corticosteroid therapy is frequently required to optimize the benefit [70].

It seems that methotrexate therapy can be an effective therapeutic alternative for late-onset AD as an immunosuppressant in adult AD because of its anti-inflammatory properties and allergen-specific T-cell activity reduction [74].

Monoclonal Antibodies Directed Against IL-13

Correlations between high IL-13 concentrations and disease severity have been noted, suggesting that IL-13 may be a therapeutic target in the treatment of AD [75]. Three monoclonal antibody treatments for refractory AD have been proposed: Dupilumab, Tralokinumab, and Lebrikizumab. Even if this treatment is yet in the debate because of ophthalmic complications such as conjunctival redness, hyperaemia, blepharitis, dryness, and discharge, Th2 cytokines can be blocked by Dupilumab [76, 77].

Tralokinumab is a humanized monoclonal IgG_4 antibody (MAB) that neutralizes IL-13, while Lebrikizumab is a MAB that binds IL-13 and inhibits the dimerization of IL-13Rα1 and IL-4Rα [78]. These novel agents have previously demonstrated efficacy [72].

Monoclonal Antibodies Targeting the Th 17 Way

These molecules are indicated in psoriasis, but they could be interesting in the DA, given the participation of a Th17 response in the DA as well.

Therapeutic Perspectives

IL-32, secreted by keratinocytes, contributes to allergic inflammation. Lee *et al.* [79] noted that a novel role of an isoform of IL-32, IL-32 gamma, inhibits NF-kB activation, leading to altered miR-205 expression, which leads to decreased in the development of T-cell–mediated severe AD pathology. These observations open the door to new therapeutic development.

The Janus kinase (JAK)-signal transducer and activator of transcription (STAT) signaling, as well as the spleen tyrosine kinase (SYK) pathways, have been implicated in AD, psoriasis, alopecia areata (AA), and other autoimmune and inflammatory diseases [80]. Modulation of several immune pathways involved in AD, including Th2 (IL-4, IL-5, IL-6, IL-10, IL-13, IL-31), Th1 (IL-2, IFN-γ, and *TNF-β*), and Th17 (IL-17A, IL-17F, IL-21, IL-22, IL-23R) are under the control of these two pathways [81]. JAK inhibition may be linked to more rapid anti-pruritic effects than other drug classes.

Guttman-Yassky *et al.* [81] showed that Upadacitinib monotherapy has good efficacy and noted a favorable benefit/risk profile as compared to placebo in adults with moderate-to-severe AD. Baracitinib, Abrocitinib, and Upadacitinib also show promising for decreasing AD severity and disease-related symptoms. However, it remains to compare in terms of the safety and efficacy of narrow-acting agents, like single interleukin inhibitors, with acting agents, such as JAK inhibitors [82].

SYK, which regulates IL-17 to stimulate CCL20 production in keratinocytes and recruit Th17 cells to the skin, is a non-receptor tyrosine kinase involved in several cytokine signaling pathways. The SYK pathway is also involved in B cell survival, proliferation, and activation, along with dendritic cell differentiation [83]. JAK and SYK inhibitors are small molecules that block the JAK-STAT and SYK pathways, respectively, thereby antagonizing cytokine activity across [81] Thus, this could have synergistic effects that provide added therapeutic benefit to AD. In this line, ASN002 is an oral dual inhibitor of the JAK and SYK pathways. A 12-week study is ongoing that will shed light on the safety and efficacy of ASN002 in AD (NCT03531957).

Cerdulatinib (RVT-502), which is currently evaluated as a topical therapy in phase 1 clinical trials for dermatologic conditions (AD, AA, and vitiligo), is a dual JAK and SYK inhibitor. Efficacy of this drug has been noted in lymphoma when administered as oral therapy (NCT01994382). Improvement in Topical Cerdulatinib was recently assessed in a mouse model of AD and showed significantly improved epidermal hyperplasia, hyperkeratosis, and inflammatory cell infiltration with 0.2% and 0.4% Cerdulatinib gel daily [84].

Even if promising AD treatments begin to be available, larger-scale, longer-term clinical trials are still required to assess the use of JAK and SYK inhibitors in AD treatment. Moreover, future research will determine if specific immunomodulators work better for certain subtypes of patients with AD.

Treatment of Secondary Cutaneous Infections

Secondary infections, also called superinfections, can occur in patients with AD, who are predisposed to the development of secondary staphylococcal infections (including *S. aureus*), or/and who may also be subject to a defective immune response.

Topical antibiotic therapy such as Mupirocin or Fusidic acid or general antibiotic treatment may be offered depending on the severity of the staphylococcal infection. It should be noted that resistance to Fusidic acid is increasingly reported in studies, hence the interest in limiting its use.

To reduce flare-ups in moderate to severe AD, dilute sodium hypochlorite (bleach) baths are suggested as a maintenance measure. The addition of ½ cup of 5% to 6% sodium hydroxide per full tub of water (1 mL.L^{-1} or 4 mL per gallon) markedly reduces the severity and extent of dermatitis in children with a history of staphylococcal infections.

Nakatsuji *et al.* [85] evaluated the safety and mechanisms of action of *Staphylococcus hominis* A9 (*Sh*A9), a bacterium isolated from healthy human skin, as a topical therapy for AD. They noted that *Sh*A9 killed *S. aureus* on the skin of mice and inhibited the expression of an inflammatory toxin from *S. aureus* (*psmα*). This new therapeutic approach appears to be safe over a seven-day period. Further investigation is needed to evaluate the benefits of this method for bacteriotherapy.

Nonpharmacologic Recommendations

Besides pharmacological interventions, some nonpharmacologic recommenda-tions often include topical therapies. When used in conjunction with other interventions, topical therapies can target different components of AD pathog-enesis [69]. It is the case for Moisturizers, which can be used as primary therapy, especially for mild AD and adjunctive therapy for moderate-to-severe AD. Indeed, they improve skin barrier function and reduce transepidermal water loss and decrease signs and symptoms of AD such as erythema, pruritus, thus impeding the "itch-scratch" cycle.

Specific skin barrier alteration can be reversed using emollient, a topical nonsteroidal agent, even though the data have been largely controversial [69].

Severe atopic dermatitis can be treated using phototherapy with UV light by preventing bacterial infections, one of the important problems in this skin disease [86]. The Association of UVA and UVB seems to have a more efficacy effect as compared to UVA or UVB light alone.

Recent years have brought about additional data on the benefits of prebiotics and probiotics treatment in patients with AD. Several studies have evaluated the probiotics such as lactobacilli (*L. rhamnosus* GG, *L. rhamnosus* LC705, *L. salivarius*), bifidobacteria (*B. longum reuter*, *B. longer infantis*, *B. breve*) or combinations [87] in patients with AD. However, data do not yet offer yet answers on the issues involving optimal dosing, duration of treatment needed to experience benefit, or the optimal time to start therapy, knowing that most studies suggest that administration of probiotics for at least 8 weeks is needed to obtain efficacy in improving severity scoring of AD.

INTERESTS IN NATURAL SOLUTIONS (ALGAE AND HERBAL MEDICINE)

Topical glucocorticosteroids, calcineurin inhibitors, ultraviolet irradiation, lifestyle modification, systemic anti-inflammatory treatment, and immunotherapy are recommended for the treatment of AD [88]. Individualized treatment that includes complementary and integrative medicine also has much interest in managing AD [89].

Natural products derived from sea, such as algae, may also be suitable candidates [90]. Algae are broadly classified as Rhodophyta (red algae), Phaeophyta (brown algae), and Chlorophyta (green algae) and classified by size as macroalgae or microalgae [90]. Macroalgae (seaweed) are multicellular, large-size algae, while microalgae are microscopic single cells and may be prokaryotic, like cyanobacteria (Chloroxybacteria), or eukaryotic, like green algae (Chlorophyta) [91]. Due to their ability to live in extreme environments, microalgae produce bioactive compounds with interesting properties for medical, pharmaceutical, cosmetic, and biofuel industries [92]. Indeed, some of these bioactive compounds have anticancer, antidiabetic, and anti-oxidative activities (*i.e.*, fatty acids, phycobiliproteins, chlorophylls, carotenoids, and vitamins) [93]. Anti-inflammatory components are also one of the important biological features that have been exhibited by different metabolites from microalgae and cyanobacteria like *Chlorella, Dunaliella, and Phaeodactylum*. The chemical structures of these metabolites are classified as polysaccharides, polyunsaturated fatty acids, and carotenoids.

These metabolites target enzymatic activities, inducing a regulation of cellular activities, in particular the NF-ƙβ and MAPKs pathways, thus inhibiting skin inflammation.

Peptides extracted from Chlorella have been proposed to inhibit synthesis of intercellular cell adhesion molecule-1 (ICAM-1), endothelial cell selectin (E-selectin), and vascular cell adhesion molecule-1 (VCAM-1). In addition, they limit pro-inflammatory cytokine monocyte chemoattractant protein-1 (MCP-1) concentrations [94]. It also seems that mast cell degranulation and histamine release can be reduced after Chlorella treatment [95].

Astaxanthin, a lipid-soluble pigment synthesized by microalgae, is known to have anti-inflammatory properties [96]. This molecule also decreases the expression levels of inducible nitric oxide synthase (iNOS), cycloosygenase-2 (COX-2) and the synthesis of PGE_2 [97]. Nevertheless, even if microalgae, through their bioactive compounds, have several health properties, further investigations are needed to understand how they are involved in skin diseases.

Other alternative treatments in association with conventional treatments for AD have been proposed, such as herbal medicine [98]. Indeed, due to their low toxicity, polysaccharides and polyphenol such as Schizandrin, derived from *Schizandra chinensis*, have beneficial effects. Through the limitation of mast cell degranulation and proinflammatory cytokine, this molecule may decrease the urge to scratch [99]. Other compounds, such as linoleic acid and linoleic acid, could have antioxidant and anti-inflammatory effects, which are interesting for skin pathologies [100, 101]. Chinese herbal medicine has anti-proliferative and anti-differential effects on CD4 + T cells, which can further lead to the inhibition of Th1-, Th2-, and Th17-mediated cell differentiation [66]. In addition, the constituents in Traditional Chinese Medicine (TCM) can decrease the concentrations of cytokines such as TNF-α, INF-γ, IL-4, IL-5, IL-6, IL-13, IL-33 and IL-1α, as well as chemokines such as CCL2, CCL7, and CCL8.

Nevertheless, the safety profiles of herbal medicine as adjuvant therapy, particularly in terms of herb-drug, require further elucidation. Generally, interactions between herbs and conventional AD medications have been largely understudied.

Besides herbal and microalgal solutions, nutritional supplementation can also have beneficial effects in moderate AD. It is the case for vitamin D, which stimulates the expression of antimicrobial peptides, decreases pro-inflammatory cytokine expression, and increases regulatory cytokine expression leading to reduced T-cell activation. Huang *et al.* [4] noted a negative correlation between vitamin D levels and the severity of AD, but most of the data remain controversial [102]. Serum IgE in atopic patients also seems to decrease after Vitamin E supplementation [103]; however, like for Vitamin D, data are also in debate [104].

CONCLUDING REMARKS

While several studies have found promising benefits with novel isolated pharmacological and natural compounds, further studies are needed before drug discovery can be achieved to better understand the different genetic and immunological mechanisms underlying the broad spectrum of disease phenotypes that will help change the landscape of AD care.

REFERENCES

[1]   Boothby IC, Gonzalez JR, Scharschmidt TC. Atlas of atopic dermatitis. J Allergy Clin Immunol 2020; 145(6): 1558-9.
[http://dx.doi.org/10.1016/j.jaci.2020.03.040] [PMID: 32344054]

[2]   Avena-Woods C. Overview of atopic dermatitis. Am J Manag Care 2017; 23(8) (Suppl.): S115-23.
[PMID: 28978208]

[3]   Weidinger S, Novak N. Atopic dermatitis. Lancet 2016; 387(10023): 1109-22.
[http://dx.doi.org/10.1016/S0140-6736(15)00149-X] [PMID: 26377142]

[4]   Huang E, Ong PY. Severe atopic dermatitis in children. Curr Allergy Asthma Rep 2018; 18(6): 35.
[http://dx.doi.org/10.1007/s11882-018-0788-4] [PMID: 29748919]

[5]   Nakatsuji T, Hata TR, Tong Y, *et al.* Development of a human skin commensal microbe for bacteriotherapy of atopic dermatitis and use in a phase 1 randomized clinical trial. Nat Med 2021; 27(4): 700-9.
[http://dx.doi.org/10.1038/s41591-021-01256-2] [PMID: 33619370]

[6]   Kim J, Kim BE, Leung DYM. Pathophysiology of atopic dermatitis: clinical implications. Allergy Asthma Proc 2019; 40(2): 84-92.
[http://dx.doi.org/10.2500/aap.2019.40.4202] [PMID: 30819278]

[7]   Adamson AS. The economics burden of atopic dermatitis. Adv Exp Med Biol 2017; 1027: 79-92.
[http://dx.doi.org/10.1007/978-3-319-64804-0_8] [PMID: 29063433]

[8]   Filanovsky MG, Pootongkam S, Tamburro JE, Smith MC, Ganocy SJ, Nedorost ST. The financial and emotional impact of atopic dermatitis on children and their families. J Pediatr 2016; 169: 284-290.e5.
[http://dx.doi.org/10.1016/j.jpeds.2015.10.077] [PMID: 26616249]

[9]   Drucker AM, Qureshi AA, Amand C, *et al.* Health care resource utilization and costs among adults with atopic dermatitis in the United States: a claims-based analysis. J Allergy Clin Immunol Pract 2018; 6(4): 1342-8.
[http://dx.doi.org/10.1016/j.jaip.2017.10.024] [PMID: 29174063]

[10]   Launois R, Ezzedine K, Cabout E, *et al.* Importance of out-of-pocket costs for adult patients with atopic dermatitis in France. J Eur Acad Dermatol Venereol 2019; 33(10): 1921-7.

[http://dx.doi.org/10.1111/jdv.15581] [PMID: 30887577]

[11]   Zink A, Arents B, Fink-Wagner A, *et al.* Out-of-pocket costs for individuals with atopic eczema: a cross-sectional study in nine European countries. Acta Derm Venereol 2019; 99(3): 263-7.
[http://dx.doi.org/10.2340/00015555-3102] [PMID: 30521060]

[12]   Laughter MR, Maymone MBC, Mashayekhi S, *et al.* The global burden of atopic dermatitis: lessons from the Global Burden of Disease Study 1990–2017. Br J Dermatol 2021; 184(2): 304-9.
[http://dx.doi.org/10.1111/bjd.19580] [PMID: 33006135]

[13]   Nahm DH. Personalized immunomodulatory therapy for atopic dermatitis: an allergist's view. Ann Dermatol 2015; 27(4): 355-63.
[http://dx.doi.org/10.5021/ad.2015.27.4.355] [PMID: 26273148]

[14]   Chung J, Simpson EL. The socioeconomics of atopic dermatitis. Ann Allergy Asthma Immunol 2019; 122(4): 360-6.
[http://dx.doi.org/10.1016/j.anai.2018.12.017]

[15]   Halvorsen JA, Lien L, Dalgard F, Bjertness E, Stern RS. Suicidal ideation, mental health problems, and social function in adolescents with eczema: a population-based study. J Invest Dermatol 2014; 134(7): 1847-54.
[http://dx.doi.org/10.1038/jid.2014.70] [PMID: 24496238]

[16]   Langenbruch A, Radtke M, Franzke N, Ring J, Foelster-Holst R, Augustin M. Quality of health care of atopic eczema in Germany: results of the national health care study atopic health. J Eur Acad Dermatol Venereol 2014; 28(6): 719-26.
[http://dx.doi.org/10.1111/jdv.12154] [PMID: 23560545]

[17]   Ali Z, Ulrik CS. Obesity and asthma: A coincidence or a causal relationship? A systematic review. Respir Med 2013; 107(9): 1287-300.
[http://dx.doi.org/10.1016/j.rmed.2013.03.019] [PMID: 23642708]

[18]   Löffler H, Aramaki JUN, Effendy I. The influence of body mass index on skin susceptibility to sodium lauryl sulphate. Skin Res Technol 2002; 8(1): 19-22.
[http://dx.doi.org/10.1046/j.0909-752x] [PMID: 12005116]

[19]   Ali Z, Suppli Ulrik C, Agner T, Thomsen SF. Is atopic dermatitis associated with obesity? A systematic review of observational studies. J Eur Acad Dermatol Venereol 2018; 32(8): 1246-55.
[http://dx.doi.org/10.1111/jdv.14879] [PMID: 29444366]

[20]   Brunner PM, Leung DYM, Guttman-Yassky E. Immunologic, microbial, and epithelial interactions in atopic dermatitis. Ann Allergy Asthma Immunol 2018; 120(1): 34-41.
[http://dx.doi.org/10.1016/j.anai.2017.09.055] [PMID: 29126710]

[21]   Kim BE, Leung DYM. Significance of skin barrier dysfunction in atopic dermatitis. Allergy Asthma Immunol Res 2018; 10(3): 207-15.
[http://dx.doi.org/10.4168/aair.2018.10.3.207] [PMID: 29676067]

[22]   Vestergaard C, Yoneyama H, Murai M, *et al.* Overproduction of Th2-specific chemokines in NC/Nga mice exhibiting atopic dermatitis-like lesions. J Clin Invest 1999; 104 1097e105

[23]   Leung DY, Harbeck R, Bina P, *et al.* Presence of IgE antibodies to staphylococcal exotoxins on the skin of patients with atopic dermatitis evidence for a new group of allergens. J Clin Invest 1993; 92 1374e80.

[24]   Garret JP, Archer NK, Miller LS. Which way do we go? Complex unteractions in atopic dermatitis pathogenesis. J Investig Dermatol 2021; 141 274e284.

[25]   Criton S, Gangadharan G. Nonpharmacological management of atopic dermatitis. Indian J Paediatr Dermatol 2017; 18(3): 166-73.
[http://dx.doi.org/10.4103/2319-7250.207605]

[26]   Kim J, Kim BE, Leung DYM. Pathophysiology of atopic dermatitis: clinical implications. Allergy

Asthma Proc 2019; 40(2): 84-92.
[http://dx.doi.org/10.2500/aap.2019.40.4202] [PMID: 30819278]

[27]   Schleimer RP, Berdnikovs S. Etiology of epithelial barrier dysfunction in patients with type 2 inflammatory diseases. J Allergy Clin Immunol 2017; 139(6): 1752-61.
[http://dx.doi.org/10.1016/j.jaci.2017.04.010] [PMID: 28583447]

[28]   Bhattacharya N, Sato WJ, Kelly A, *et al.* Epidermal lipids: key mediators of atopic dermatitis pathogenesis. Trends Mol Med 2019; 25 551e62.

[29]   Berdyshev E, Goleva E, Bronova I, *et al.* Lipid abnormalities in atopic skin are driven by type 2 cytokines. JCI Insight 2018; 3(4): e98006.
[http://dx.doi.org/10.1172/jci.insight.98006] [PMID: 29467325]

[30]   Li S, Villarreal M, Stewart S, *et al.* Altered composition of epidermal lipids correlates with *Staphylococcus aureus* colonization status in atopic dermatitis. Br J Dermatol 2017; 177(4): e125-7.
[http://dx.doi.org/10.1111/bjd.15409] [PMID: 28244066]

[31]   Chan G, Ong PY. Pathophysiology, diagnosis, and management of infections in atopic dermatitis. Curr Dermatol Rep 2019; 8(2): 73-9.
[http://dx.doi.org/10.1007/s13671-019-0256-y]

[32]   Tsakok T, Woolf R, Smith CH, Weidinger S, Flohr C. Atopic dermatitis: the skin barrier and beyond. Br J Dermatol 2019; 180(3): 464-74.
[http://dx.doi.org/10.1111/bjd.16934] [PMID: 29969827]

[33]   Barnes KC. An update on the genetics of atopic dermatitis: Scratching the surface in 2009. J Allergy Clin Immunol 2010; 125(1): 16-29.e11.
[http://dx.doi.org/10.1016/j.jaci.2009.11.008] [PMID: 20109730]

[34]   Bin L, Leung DYM. Genetic and epigenetic studies of atopic dermatitis. Allergy Asthma Clin Immunol 2016; 12(1): 52.
[http://dx.doi.org/10.1186/s13223-016-0158-5] [PMID: 27777593]

[35]   Martin MJ, Estravís M, García-Sánchez A, Dávila I, Isidoro-García M, Sanz C. Genetics and epigenetics of atopic dermatitis: an updated systematic review. Genes (Basel) 2020; 11(4): 442.
[http://dx.doi.org/10.3390/genes11040442] [PMID: 32325630]

[36]   Kaufman BP, Guttman-Yassky E, Alexis AF. Atopic dermatitis in diverse racial and ethnic groups-Variations in epidemiology, genetics, clinical presentation and treatment. Exp Dermatol 2018; 27(4): 340-57.
[http://dx.doi.org/10.1111/exd.13514] [PMID: 29457272]

[37]   Marenholz I, Nickel R, Rüschendorf F, *et al.* Filaggrin loss-of-function mutations predispose to phenotypes involved in the atopic march. J Allergy Clin Immunol 2006; 118(4): 866-71.
[http://dx.doi.org/10.1016/j.jaci.2006.07.026] [PMID: 17030239]

[38]   Heine G, Hoefer N, Franke A, *et al.* Association of vitamin D receptor gene polymorphisms with severe atopic dermatitis in adults. Br J Dermatol 2013; 168(4): 855-8.
[http://dx.doi.org/10.1111/bjd.12077] [PMID: 23034014]

[39]   Suzuki H, Makino Y, Nagata M, *et al.* A rare variant in CYP27A1 and its association with atopic dermatitis with high serum total IgE. Allergy 2016; 71(10): 1486-9.
[http://dx.doi.org/10.1111/all.12950] [PMID: 27259383]

[40]   Makeyev EV, Maniatis T. Multilevel regulation of gene expression by microRNAs. Science 2008; 319(5871): 1789-90.
[http://dx.doi.org/10.1126/science.1152326] [PMID: 18369137]

[41]   Brunner PM, Guttman-Yassky E. Racial differences in atopic dermatitis. Ann Allergy Asthma Immunol 2019; 122 449e55

[42]   Kim J, Kim H. Microbiome of the skin and gut in atopic dermatitis (AD) Understanding the

pathophysiology and finding novel management strategies. J Clin Med 2019; 8(4): 444.
[http://dx.doi.org/10.3390/jcm8040444] [PMID: 30987008]

[43]   Salimi M, Barlow JL, Saunders SP, *et al.* A role for IL-25 and IL-33–driven type-2 innate lymphoid cells in atopic dermatitis. J Exp Med 2013; 210(13): 2939-50.
[http://dx.doi.org/10.1084/jem.20130351] [PMID: 24323357]

[44]   Mohapatra SS, Mohapatra S, McGill AR, Green R. Molecular mechanism–driven new biomarkers and therapies for atopic dermatitis. J Allergy Clin Immunol 2020; 146(1): 72-3.
[http://dx.doi.org/10.1016/j.jaci.2020.04.039] [PMID: 32416110]

[45]   Grice EA, Segre JA. The human microbiome: our second genome. Annu Rev Genomics Hum Genet 2012; 13(1): 151-70.
[http://dx.doi.org/10.1146/annurev-genom-090711-163814] [PMID: 22703178]

[46]   Oh J, Byrd AL, Deming C, Conlan S, Kong HH, Segre JA. Biogeography and individuality shape function in the human skin metagenome. Nature 2014; 514(7520): 59-64.
[http://dx.doi.org/10.1038/nature13786] [PMID: 25279917]

[47]   Gensollen T, Blumberg RS. Correlation between early-life regulation of the immune system by microbiota and allergy development. J Allergy Clin Immunol 2017; 139(4): 1084-91.
[http://dx.doi.org/10.1016/j.jaci.2017.02.011] [PMID: 28390575]

[48]   Pothmann A, Illing T, Wiegand C, Hartmann AA, Elsner P. The microbiome and atopic dermatitis: a review. Am J Clin Dermatol 2019; 20(6): 749-61.
[http://dx.doi.org/10.1007/s40257-019-00467-1] [PMID: 31444782]

[49]   Watanabe S, Narisawa Y, Arase S, *et al.* Differences in fecal microflora between patients with atopic dermatitis and healthy control subjects. J Allergy Clin Immunol 2003; 111(3): 587-91.
[http://dx.doi.org/10.1067/mai.2003.105] [PMID: 12642841]

[50]   Song H, Yoo Y, Hwang J, Na YC, Kim HS. Faecalibacterium prausnitzii subspecies–level dysbiosis in the human gut microbiome underlying atopic dermatitis. J Allergy Clin Immunol 2016; 137(3): 852-60.
[http://dx.doi.org/10.1016/j.jaci.2015.08.021] [PMID: 26431583]

[51]   Johnson CC, Ownby DR. The infant gut bacterial microbiota and risk of pediatric asthma and allergic diseases. Transl Res 2017; 179: 60-70.
[http://dx.doi.org/10.1016/j.trsl.2016.06.010] [PMID: 27469270]

[52]   Flowers L, Grice EA. The skin microbiota: balancing risk and reward. Cell Host Microbe 2020, 28(2). 190-200.
[http://dx.doi.org/10.1016/j.chom.2020.06.017] [PMID: 32791112]

[53]   Byrd AL, Deming C, Cassidy SKB, *et al.* *Staphylococcus aureus* and *Staphylococcus epidermidis* strain diversity underlying pediatric atopic dermatitis. Sci Transl Med 2017; 9(397): eaal4651.
[http://dx.doi.org/10.1126/scitranslmed.aal4651] [PMID: 28679656]

[54]   Higaki S, Morohashi M, Yamagishi T, *et al.* Comparative study of Staphylococci from the skin of atopic dermatitis patients and from healthy subjects. Int J Dermatol 1999; 38 265e9

[55]   Pascolini C, Sinagra J, Pecetta S, *et al.* Molecular and immunological characterization of *Staphylococcus aureus* in pediatric atopic dermatitis: implications for prophylaxis and clinical management. Clin Dev Immunol 2011; 2011: 1-7.
[http://dx.doi.org/10.1155/2011/718708] [PMID: 22110527]

[56]   Edslev SM, Andersen PS, Agner T, *et al.* Identification of cutaneous fungi and mites in adult atopic dermatitis: analysis by targeted 18S rRNA amplicon sequencing. BMC Microbiol 2021; 21(1): 72.
[http://dx.doi.org/10.1186/s12866-021-02139-9] [PMID: 33663381]

[57]   Prohic A, Jovovic Sadikovic T, Krupalija-Fazlic M, Kuskunovic-Vlahovljak S. *Malassezia* species in healthy skin and in dermatological conditions. Int J Dermatol 2016; 55(5): 494-504.
[http://dx.doi.org/10.1111/ijd.13116] [PMID: 26710919]

[58] Javad G, Taheri SM, Hedayati MT, Hajheydari Z, Yazdani J, Shokohi T. Evaluation of Candida colonization and specific Humoral responses against *Candida albicans* in patients with atopic dermatitis. BioMed Res Int 2015; 2015: 1-5.
[http://dx.doi.org/10.1155/2015/849206] [PMID: 25945349]

[59] Simon-Nobbe B, Denk U, Pöll V, Rid R, Breitenbach M. The spectrum of fungal allergy. Int Arch Allergy Immunol 2008; 145(1): 58-86.
[http://dx.doi.org/10.1159/000107578] [PMID: 17709917]

[60] Elston CA, Elston DM. Demodex mites. Clin Dermatol 2014; 32(6): 739-43.
[http://dx.doi.org/10.1016/j.clindermatol.2014.02.012] [PMID: 25441466]

[61] Avena-Woods C. Overview of atopic dermatitis. Am J Manag Care 2017; 23(8) (Suppl.): S115-23.
[PMID: 28978208]

[62] Bieber T, Bussmann C. Atopic dermatitis. In: Bolognia JL, Lorizzo JL, Schaffer JV, Eds. Dermatology. St Louis: Mosby 2012; pp. 203-16.

[63] Eichenfield LF, Tom WL, Chamlin SL, *et al.* Guidelines of care for the management of atopic dermatitis. J Am Acad Dermatol 2014; 70(2): 338-51.
[http://dx.doi.org/10.1016/j.jaad.2013.10.010] [PMID: 24290431]

[64] Maliyar K, Sibbald C, Pope E, Gary Sibbald R. Diagnosis and management of atopic dermatitis: a review. Adv Skin Wound Care 2018; 31(12): 538-50.
[http://dx.doi.org/10.1097/01.ASW.0000547414.38888.8d] [PMID: 30475283]

[65] Ständer S. Atopic dermatitis. N Engl J Med 2021; 384(12): 1136-43.
[http://dx.doi.org/10.1056/NEJMra2023911] [PMID: 33761208]

[66] Yan F, Li F, Liu J, *et al.* The formulae and biologically active ingredients of Chinese herbal medicines for the treatment of atopic dermatitis. Biomed Pharmacother 2020; 127: 110142.
[http://dx.doi.org/10.1016/j.biopha.2020.110142] [PMID: 32330795]

[67] Drucker AM, Eyerich K, de Bruin-Weller MS, *et al.* Use of systemic corticosteroids for atopic dermatitis: International Eczema Council consensus statement. Br J Dermatol 2018; 178(3): 768-75.
[http://dx.doi.org/10.1111/bjd.15928] [PMID: 28865094]

[68] González-López G, Ceballos-Rodríguez RM, González-López JJ, Feito Rodríguez M, Herranz-Pinto P. Efficacy and safety of wet wrap therapy for patients with atopic dermatitis: a systematic review and meta-analysis. Br J Dermatol 2017; 177(3): 688-95.
[http://dx.doi.org/10.1111/bjd.15165] [PMID: 27861727]

[69] Eichenfield LF, Ahluwalia J, Waldman A, Borok J, Udkoff J, Boguniewicz M. Current guidelines for the evaluation and management of atopic dermatitis: A comparison of the joint task force practice parameter and American academy of dermatology guidelines. J Allergy Clin Immunol 2017; 139(4): S49-57.
[http://dx.doi.org/10.1016/j.jaci.2017.01.009] [PMID: 28390477]

[70] Bußmann C, Novak N. Systemic therapy of atopic dermatitis. Allergol Select 2017; 1(1): 1-8.
[http://dx.doi.org/10.5414/ALX01285E] [PMID: 30402595]

[71] Arakawa A, Siewert K, Stöhr J, *et al.* Melanocyte antigen triggers autoimmunity in human psoriasis. J Exp Med 2015; 212(13): 2203-12.
[http://dx.doi.org/10.1084/jem.20151093] [PMID: 26621454]

[72] Berth-Jones J, Graham-Brown RAC, Marks R, *et al.* Long-term efficacy and safety of cyclosporin in severe adult atopic dermatitis. Br J Dermatol 1997; 136(1): 76-81.
[http://dx.doi.org/10.1046/j.1365-2133.1997.d01-1146.x] [PMID: 9039299]

[73] Guttman-Yassky E, Thaçi D, Pangan AL, *et al.* Upadacitinib in adults with moderate to severe atopic dermatitis: 16-week results from a randomized, placebo-controlled trial. J Allergy Clin Immunol 2020; 145(3): 877-84.

[http://dx.doi.org/10.1016/j.jaci.2019.11.025] [PMID: 31786154]

[74]   Zoller L, Ramon M, Bergman R. Low dose methotrexate therapy is effective in late-onset atopic dermatitis and idiopathic eczema. Isr Med Assoc J 2008; 10(6): 413-4.
[PMID: 18669134]

[75]   Hoy SM. Crisaborole ointment 2%: a review in mild to moderate atopic dermatitis. Am J Clin Dermatol 2017; 18(6): 837-43.
[http://dx.doi.org/10.1007/s40257-017-0327-4] [PMID: 29076116]

[76]   Wollenberg A, Howell MD, Guttman-Yassky E, *et al.* Treatment of atopic dermatitis with tralokinumab, an anti–IL-13 mAb. J Allergy Clin Immunol 2019; 143(1): 135-41.
[http://dx.doi.org/10.1016/j.jaci.2018.05.029] [PMID: 29906525]

[77]   Akinlade B, Guttman-Yassky E, Bruin-Weller M, *et al.* Conjunctivitis in dupilumab clinical trials. Br J Dermatol 2019; 181(3): 459-73.
[http://dx.doi.org/10.1111/bjd.17869] [PMID: 30851191]

[78]   Simpson EL, Flohr C, Eichenfield LF, *et al.* Efficacy and safety of lebrikizumab (an anti-IL-13 monoclonal antibody) in adults with moderate-to-severe atopic dermatitis inadequately controlled by topical corticosteroids: A randomized, placebo-controlled phase II trial (TREBLE). J Am Acad Dermatol 2018; 78(5): 863-871.e11.
[http://dx.doi.org/10.1016/j.jaad.2018.01.017] [PMID: 29353026]

[79]   Lee YS, Han SB, Ham HJ, *et al.* IL-32γ suppressed atopic dermatitis through inhibition of miR-205 expression *via* inactivation of nuclear factor-kappa B. J Allergy Clin Immunol 2020; 146(1): 156-68.
[http://dx.doi.org/10.1016/j.jaci.2019.12.905] [PMID: 31931018]

[80]   Cotter DG, Schairer D, Eichenfield L. Emerging therapies for atopic dermatitis: JAK inhibitors. J Am Acad Dermatol 2018; 78(3) (Suppl. 1): S53-62.
[http://dx.doi.org/10.1016/j.jaad.2017.12.019] [PMID: 29248518]

[81]   He H, Guttman-Yassky E. JAK inhibitors for atopic dermatitis: an update. Am J Clin Dermatol 2019; 20(2): 181-92.
[http://dx.doi.org/10.1007/s40257-018-0413-2] [PMID: 30536048]

[82]   Newsom M, Bashyam AM, Balogh EA, Feldman SR, Strowd LC. New and emerging systemic treatments for atopic dermatitis. Drugs 2020; 80(11): 1041-52.
[http://dx.doi.org/10.1007/s40265-020-01335-7] [PMID: 32519223]

[83]   Ackermann JA, Nys J, Schweighoffer E, McCleary S, Smithers N, Tybulewicz VLJ. Syk tyrosine kinase is critical for B cell antibody responses and memory B cell survival. J Immunol 2015; 194(10): 4650-6.
[http://dx.doi.org/10.4049/jimmunol.1500461] [PMID: 25862820]

[84]   McHale K, Harrington W, Roeloffs R, Lee J. 1083 Effect of RVT-502 therapy in the NC/Nga mouse model of atopic dermatitis. J Invest Dermatol 2018; 138(5): S184.
[http://dx.doi.org/10.1016/j.jid.2018.03.1096]

[85]   Nakatsuji T, Hata TR, Tong Y, *et al.* Development of a human skin commensal microbe for bacteriotherapy of atopic dermatitis and use in a phase 1 randomized clinical trial. Nat Med 2021; 27(4): 700-9.
[http://dx.doi.org/10.1038/s41591-021-01256-2] [PMID: 33619370]

[86]   Katayama I, Aihara M, Ohya Y, *et al.* The Japanese society of allergolog: Japanese guidelines for atopic dermatitis. Allerg Int 2017; 66 230e247.

[87]   Rusu E, Enache G, Cursaru R, *et al.* Prebiotics and probiotics in atopic dermatitis. Exp Ther Med 2019; 18(2): 926-31.
[PMID: 31384325]

[88]   LePoidevin LM, Lee DE, Shi VY. A comparison of international management guidelines for atopic dermatitis. Pediatr Dermatol 2019; 36(1): 36-65.

[http://dx.doi.org/10.1111/pde.13678] [PMID: 30303557]

[89] Hon KL, Leung AKC, Leung TNH, Lee VWY. Complementary, alternative and integrative medicine for childhood atopic dermatitis. Recent Pat Inflamm Allergy Drug Discov 2017; 11(2): 114-24.
[http://dx.doi.org/10.2174/1872213X11666171128142333] [PMID: 29189188]

[90] Patras D, Moraru CV, Socaciu C. Bioactive ingredients from microalgae: food and feed applications. Bull Univ Agric Sci Vet Med Cluj-Napoca Food Sci Technol 2019; 76(1): 1-9.
[http://dx.doi.org/10.15835/buasvmcn-fst:2018.0018]

[91] García JL, de Vicente M, Galán B. Microalgae, old sustainable food and fashion nutraceuticals. Microb Biotechnol 2017; 10(5): 1017-24.
[http://dx.doi.org/10.1111/1751-7915.12800] [PMID: 28809450]

[92] Remize M, Brunel Y, Silva JL. Microalgae n-3 PUFAs production and use in food and feed industries. Marine Drugs 2021; 18(1): 113.

[93] Barkia I, Saari N, Manning SR. Microalgae for high-value products towards human health and nutrition. Marine Drugs 2019; 17(5): 304.
[http://dx.doi.org/10.3390/md17050304] [PMID: 31137657]

[94] Shih M, Chen L, Cherng J. Chlorella 11-peptide inhibits the production of macrophage-induced adhesion molecules and reduces endothelin-1 expression and endothelial permeability. Marine Drugs 2013; 11(10): 3861-74.
[http://dx.doi.org/10.3390/md11103861] [PMID: 24129228]

[95] Bae MJ, Shin HS, Chai OH, Han JG, Shon DH. Inhibitory effect of unicellular green algae (*Chlorella vulgaris*) water extract on allergic immune response. J Sci Food Agric 2013; 93(12): 3133-6.
[http://dx.doi.org/10.1002/jsfa.6114] [PMID: 23426977]

[96] Spiller GA, Dewell A. Safety of an astaxanthin-rich Haematococcus pluvialis algal extract: a randomized clinical trial. J Med Food 2003; 6: 51-6.
[http://dx.doi.org/10.1089/109662003765184741] [PMID: 12804020]

[97] Yoshihisa Y, Rehman M, Shimizu T. Astaxanthin, a xanthophyll carotenoid, inhibits ultraviolet-induced apoptosis in keratinocytes. Exp Dermatol 2014; 23(3): 178-83.
[http://dx.doi.org/10.1111/exd.12347] [PMID: 24521161]

[98] Kwon CY, Lee B, Kim S, Lee J, Park M, Kim N. Effectiveness and safety of herbal medicine for atopic dermatitis: an overview of systematic reviews. Evid Based Complement Alternat Med 2020; 2020: 1-15.
[http://dx.doi.org/10.1155/2020/4140692] [PMID: 32724323]

[99] Lee B, Bae EA, Trinh HT, *et al.* Inhibitory effect of schizandrin on passive cutaneous anaphylaxis reaction and scratching behaviors in mice. Biol Pharm Bull 2007; 30(6): 1153-6.
[http://dx.doi.org/10.1248/bpb.30.1153] [PMID: 17541172]

[100] Park G, Kim HG, Lim S, Lee W, Sim Y, Oh MS. Coriander alleviates 2,4-dinitrochlorobenzen--induced contact dermatitis-like skin lesions in mice. J Med Food 2014; 17(8): 862-8.
[http://dx.doi.org/10.1089/jmf.2013.2910] [PMID: 24963872]

[101] Man M, Hu L, Elias PM. Herbal medicines prevent the development of atopic dermatitis by multiple mechanisms. Chin J Integr Med 2019; 25(2): 151-60.
[http://dx.doi.org/10.1007/s11655-015-2438-1] [PMID: 26740223]

[102] HYPPöNEN ELINA, Sovio U, Wjst M, *et al.* Infant vitamin d supplementation and allergic conditions in adulthood: northern Finland birth cohort 1966. Ann N Y Acad Sci 2004; 1037(1): 84-95.
[http://dx.doi.org/10.1196/annals.1337.013] [PMID: 15699498]

[103] Faghihi G, Jaffary F, Mokhtarian A, Hosseini S. Effects of oral vitamin E on treatment of atopic dermatitis: A randomized controlled trial. J Res Med Sci 2015; 20(11): 1053-7.
[http://dx.doi.org/10.4103/1735-1995.172815] [PMID: 26941808]

[104] Bath-Hextall FJ, Jenkinson C, Humphreys R, Williams HC. Dietary supplements for established atopic eczema. Cochrane Database Syst Rev 2012; (2): CD005205.
[PMID: 22336810]

CHAPTER 6

Epidemiology, Diagnosis, Prevention, Policy and Treatment Schemes of Skin Infections in Developing Countries

Taha Hussein Musa[1,2]**, Tosin Yinka Akintunde**[3,4]**, Idriss Hussein Musa**[5]**, Haroon Elrasheid Tahir**[6] **and Hassan Hussein Musa**[7,*]

[1] *Biomedical Research Institute, Darfur University College, Nyala, Sudan*

[2] *Department of Epidemiology and Health Statistics, School of Public Health, Southeast University, Nanjing, 210009, Jiangsu Province, China*

[3] *Department of Sociology, School of Public Administration, Hohai University, Nanjing, China*

[4] *Department of Social Work, Chinese University of Hong Kong, Hong Kong*

[5] *School of Medicine and Surgery, Darfur University College, Nyala, Sudan*

[6] *School of Food and Biological Engineering, Jiangsu University, 301 Xuefu Rd., 212013 Zhenjiang, Jiangsu, China*

[7] *Faculty of Medical Laboratory Sciences, University of Khartoum, Khartoum, Sudan*

Abstract: Skin diseases are common public health problems in developing countries. The prevalence is universal and can cause a significant economic burden. Additionally, it is a common cause of morbidity among vulnerable groups, such as children, and affects people of all ages and ethnicities. However, the impact of skin disease on the national public healthcare system is complex and poorly studied, particularly in developing countries. A number of factors, including population aging, genetics, and environment, have contributed to the change in skin disease trends. The combined effects of these factors have severe health implications for people, and their dynamics are not fully understood. It is thus necessary to improve diagnostic techniques in order to provide new therapeutic resources in dermatology in the wake of the scientific revolution and technological innovations. To understand the changes in the prevalence of skin disease age-specific distributions and associated mortality, this study provides comprehensive information on vulnerable populations, epidemiological characteristics, and geographic distributions. Furthermore, the study provides a baseline for the management of skin disorders using medicinal plants. Surveillance, burden, diagnostics, and treatments of skin disease are essential components of developing measurable, influential, and sustainable intervention programs to reduce disease infections. Furthermore, these approaches assist in understanding the pathogenesis and disease process and assist with the development of new therapeutic strategies and prev-

*****Corresponding author Hassan Hussein Musa:** Faculty of Medical Laboratory Sciences, University of Khartoum, Khartoum, Sudan; Tel: 00249-906-547-116; E-mail: hassantahir70@hotmail.com

entive measures against morbidity in underdeveloped and developing countries, as well as establishing a baseline for medicinal plants that contribute significantly to the treatment.

Keywords: Skin diseases, epidemiology, diagnosis, treatment, quality of life, prevention, herbal plants, developing countries.

INTRODUCTION

The skin is a vital organ in human anatomy and performs essential functions crucial for optimal health. Skin functions are critical for human survival: organ protection, regulating the optimal performance of organs, excretion, and electrolyte balance, among other indispensable roles it plays [1]. The skin composition consists of three layers, such as the Epidermis, Dermis, and Fat layer. While the epidermis is a thin keratinocytes cell composite, the dermis is relatively thick and consists of nerve endings, sweat and oil glands (sebaceous glands), hair follicles, and blood vessels. The fat layer, however, has other peculiar functions equally vital for overall health. The impairment or damage to the skin has general implications for health in the human body. Thus, varying conditions may expose the skin to a degenerative state that subsequently results in skin diseases.

Skin disease is a health problem that has triggered severe public health concerns in developing countries [2] and has been plaguing the region for more than a century. The prevalence has consistently affected livelihood, mental health, and overall quality of life in the region [3 - 5]. It is also considered the most common dermatological problem aggravated by migration due to overexposure to the sun and insect bites. Consequently, there are shreds of evidence of considerable morbidity and mortality globally [6]. They are by far the leading cause of an increase in the death rate in developing countries compared with developed countries. Advancements in technology and medical discovery have made it possible to put numerous infectious diseases under control, coupled with improvements in hand and personal hygiene and nutrition and the availability of anti-infective chemotherapy and preventive measures, such as the discovery of vaccines for different skin diseases [7]. There is various evidence of skin diseases affecting all genders, and ages from different countries and ethnic groups; approximately 70% of people in developing countries suffer from skin diseases at some time in their lives [8]. The majority seek medical consultation because of the self-limiting nature of disease or self-treatment options for many people. The prevalence of skin diseases significantly impacts individuals, families, and patients' social lives, and the heavy economic burden on the health community and public health. The prevalence of skin diseases is associated with people's socioeconomic status globally [9], and there is a need to craft a road map and improve on early detection, treatment, and control, especially in the resource-poor region [10, 11].

This chapter explored the epidemiology of skin diseases and the various forms of manifestation evidenced in developing countries. The epidemiology expanded on the most common skin diseases and among whom they are most prevalent. The part consolidated on the risk factors of skin diseases, beginning from bacteria-associated skin diseases and down to autoimmune and environmental-triggered skin diseases. Other parts explored various options available for diagnosing and treating skin diseases and the implementation modality in practice. The later part of the chapter focuses on skin disease patients' quality of Life (QoL), telemedicine, and other technology applications in skin diseases. Policy implications for skin diseases to improve approaches to skin disease were included to facilitate the improvement of health delivery for skin diseases in developing countries.

EPIDEMIOLOGY OF SKIN DISEASES

The most common manifestations of skin diseases in developing countries are pyoderma, anthrax, cutaneous diphtheria, cutaneous tuberculosis, Buruli ulcer, leprosy, scabies, and pediculosis capitis, leishmaniasis, and cutaneous larva migrans [12]. These skin diseases are further categorized as infectious and noninfectious [13, 14]. Similarly, skin disease prevalence in developing countries is rampant among infants, young and old, males and females alike, depending on their circumstances and experiences.

There are reports of skin diseases such as staphylococcal scalded skin Syndrome in neonates [15, 16]. Of 340 pediatric patients in Tanzania recruited for a study, at least 16.5% reported having at least one skin condition affecting boys and girls. The majority of the skin diseases were due to infections, while 28.5% reported eczematous dermatitis and pigmentary disorders (7.4%) [17]. In the same study, 50.7 were fungal infections, bacterial (29.6%), and viral (19.7%) among those with infectious skin diseases. Other evidence shows an increased prevalence of skin diseases like scabies, impetigo, warts, and tinea capitis among male children than among female school children [18]. Similarly, among outpatients in a Bangladesh health complex, among about 2000 patients enrolled for investigation for skin diseases, approximately 33.02% had a parasitic infection, 28.3% suffered from fungal infection, 20.1% bacterial infection and 43% from some noninfectious skin diseases among them 37.79% had eczema, 17.87% had a papulosquamous disease, 14.25% had acne, 14.01% had urticaria, and 8.7% had vitiligo [19].

Skin diseases like crusted scabies are usually immunocompromised patients problems, more in people with immunodeficiency virus, human and T-lymphocytic virus 1 infection, or medical immunosuppression leprosy and developmental disability, including Down syndrome [20]. The region with the most manifestation of scabies is the east and southeast Asia regions, highest in children aged one to four years, and a relatively high but gradually abating prevalence from age 5 to 24 years [21].

Skin cancer is another skin condition that has plagued developing countries and represents a public health burden in the region. Cancer-related skin disease manifests in melanoma, an aggressive malignant neoplasm derived from melanocytes [22] and non-melanoma skin cancer [23]. Melanoma skin cancer has been argued to cause an epidemic if left treated potentially. For instance, almost 50,000 cases of skin cancer were aggregated for a study in Iran, of which 37.45% were women and 62.55% were men [24]. There was evidence of malignant melanoma, squamous cell carcinoma, dermatofibrosarcoma and basal cell carcinoma in Nigeria [25]. Accounts from South Africa show skin cancer has led to mortality with an increasing age-adjusted mortality prevalence in men between 2000 and 2005, which rose to 3 from 2 per 100,000, and in women between 1997 and 2014 to 1.2 per 100,00 from 0.9 per 100,000 [26].

RISK FACTORS OF SKIN DISEASES

Bacterial Diseases

There are many common bacterial skin diseases that are needed to cause a variety of bacterial infections. Most skin infections are required frequent visiting dermatology. The clinic forms of presentations vary regarding deep and location, facts that were in the part condition the topical or systemic treatment or not [27]. Common skin infections include cellulite, erysipelas, impetigo, folliculitis, and furuncles and carbuncles. Cellulitis is an infection of the dermis and subcutaneous tissue with poorly demarcated borders and is usually caused by Streptococcus or Staphylococcus species [28].

Obesity and its metabolic comorbidities are associated with various skin manifestations, such as increased incidence of bacterial and Candida skin infections and onychomycosis, inflammatory skin diseases, and chronic dermatoses like hidradenitis suppurativa, psoriasis, and rosacea [29]. Obesity also increased incidence or aggravation of the symptoms of rare skin disorders, such as keratosis follicularis squamosa, adiposis dolorosa/Dercum disease, granular parakeratosis, lipedema and lymphedematous mucinosis, further leading to the increased risk of skin cancer among obese patients is debatable. Therefore, a better understanding of these clinical signs and the underlying systemic disorders will facilitate better treatment and avoidance of sequelae. Therefore, Obesity requires a multidisciplinary approach by the primary care physician, dermatologist, and others to reduce harmful effects and complications [29].

With the fast-emerging antimicrobial resistance leading to gram-positive infections, one of the significant public health threats globally leading to multidrug resistance, there is difficulty in treating infections with increased morbidity and mortality and hospitalization [30]. Many serious infections and skin diseases can cause by Gram-positive bacteria, which are challenging to treat because many pathogens are now resistant to standard antimicrobial agents [31]. As a result of the emergence and spread of multidrug-resistant such as (Daptomycin, Tigecycline, Linezolid Quinupristin/dalfopristin, and Dalbavancin) have been reported with many adverse effects and complications, including diarrhoea, rash, dizziness, dyspnoea and hypotension [32], has been a significant healthcare concern [33]. However, some antibiotics are still helpful in treating skin diseases caused by bacterial infections.

In some developing countries like Italy, herbal drugs have been recommended in popular Italian medicine to treat bacterial skin diseases between the latter half of the nineteenth century and the early to a mid-twentieth century [34]. Those medicines treat many skin diseases such as Anthrax, Erysipelas, Pustules, Erysipelas, Boils, Whitlow, and Impetigo.

Besides, many plants have also been used to treat dermatological diseases between the latter half of the nineteenth century and the early to mid-twentieth century, showing many antibacterial properties in many patients [34]. These reported antibacterial activities have been determined by measuring the inhibition of bacterial growth n experimental models such as agar diffusion and dilution methods [34].

Viral Diseases

The skin is an active immune organ that functions as the first and largest defense site against the outside environment. Serving as the primary interface between host and pathogen, the skin's early immune responses to viral invaders often determine the course and severity of infection [35]. Cutaneous viral infection presents a unique challenge to the skin's immune system, as viruses can hijack host machinery to advance viral replication. As such, early abrogation of viral pathogenicity by the innate immune response establishes a protective antiviral state and limits the potential for systemic spread [35]. Viral infections are responsible for some of the most common dermatologic presentations in adults, such as oral and genital herpes, warts, and a wide variety of exanthemas [36]. In addition, viral skin infections are common and can be challenging to diagnose, especially in children [36].

Parasitic Diseases

Parasitic cutaneous diseases are caused by insects, worms, protozoa, or coelenterates that may not have a parasitic life [37]. Cutaneous parasitic infections often result in discomfort, debilitation, and even stigmatization [38].

Cutaneous parasitic infections differ in their biological and epidemiological manifestations and life cycles. The cutaneous manifestations of ectoparasitic infections, such as scabies and pediculosis, and endoparasitic infections (cysticercosis and amoebiasis), result in considerable discomfort [38]. Other endoparasitic infections, such as hookworm infection, strongyloidiasis, schistosomiasis, and enterobiasis, are less severe [38].

Fungal Diseases

Fungal infections of the skin are among the most common diseases in our daily practice, and they may cause dermatological conditions that do not involve tissue invasion. It is estimated that 20-25% of the world population may suffer from fungal infections [39]. Fungal infections include superficial and subcutaneous infections. The main groups of fungi causing superficial fungal infections are dermatophytes, yeasts and moulds [39].

Dermatophytes grow on keratin and cause diseases in body sites wherein keratin is present. The presence of hyperkeratosis, such as palmoplantar keratoderma, predisposes to dermatophyte infections. Trichophyton rubrum is the most common cause worldwide for superficial dermatophytosis [39]. Yeasts are not inherently pathogenic, but colonization, infection, and disease can occur when the host's cellular defences, skin function, or normal flora are altered. *Candida albicans* and Malassezia furfur are the best examples that lead to superficial skin infections [39]. Moulds, also called non-dermatophyte filamentous fungi, are ubiquitous but not commonly pathogenic in regular hosts. They are, however, not uncommonly isolated from clinical specimens for fungal culture [39].

Various tropical organisms cause subcutaneous mycoses, usually implanted into the dermis or subcutaneous tissue. The causative agents are commonly found in the soil, leaves, and organic material and are introduced by traumatic injury of the skin. Sporotrichosis, mycetoma, and chromoblastomycosis are more common subcutaneous mycoses than rhinosporidiosis, zygomycosis, pheohyphomycosis, and lobomycosis [40].

In developed, high-income settings, health institutions and residential home outbreaks challenge health and social care services. In resource-poor settings, it is the downstream sequelae of staphylococcal and streptococcal bacteraemia, induced by scratching, that significantly impact communities' long-term health [41]. Scabies is a parasitic infestation of the skin caused by the mite Sarcoptes scabiei. In developed countries, scabies outbreaks are common in residential and nursing care homes, where they cause significant morbidity and distress [42 - 44].

Diagnosis is challenging and often delayed, and management of outbreaks is costly. More than 200 million people are affected globally, with an exceptionally high prevalence in resource-poor tropical regions [44]. The clinical picture varies among the different diseases, but the appearance of a localized nodule, verrucous plaques, ulcerations, granulomatous tissue, subcutaneous tumours with abscesses, and fistulae should alert the clinician to the diagnosis of a subcutaneous mycosis [40]. The isolation of the etiologic agent by either culture or molecular techniques confirms the diagnosis and allows the clinician to select the best [40].

Drug-Related Skin Diseases

In recent years, multiple disorders treated with many drugs, either monotherapy or fixed-dose therapy, have led to increased drug-induced disorders. Morbidity and mortality have increased due to drug-induced disorders [45]. Drug-induced skin disease affects 2-3% of hospitalized patients, and it is estimated that 1 in 1000 hospitalized patients have a severe cutaneous drug reaction [46]. Drug reactions cause changes in skin function or alter the ability of the skin and associated structures (hair and nails) to perform their function normally [45, 46]. Therefore, drugs can cause light-induced eruptions, skin pigmentation, hair disorders such as (Alopecia, Hirsutism/hypertrichosis), acne, lichenoid eruptions, urticarial/ angioedema, exacerbated psoriasis, erythema multiforme, and Stevens-Johnson syndrome and toxic epidermal necrolysis [46].

The skin may be involved in drug hypersensitivity reactions alone or as part of multi-organ involvement. Hypersensitivities can cause by immunological effector mechanisms such as antibodies of different classes or T lymphocytes or by direct chemical effects of the drug. In susceptible intolerant individuals, the drug may directly induce mast cell degranulation or release inflammatory mediators such as leukotrienes that produce clinical syndromes such as urticaria, asthma, or anaphylaxis indistinguishable from true immunological hypersensitivities [47, 48]. It is recommended to understand the fundamental mechanisms underlying cutaneous drug hypersensitivities. These include the drug disposition and how drugs become immunogenic in specific individuals, the nature of the immune response and the immune effector mechanisms generated, and why the skin is involved in some reactions [47]. Farshchian *et al.* (2015) indicated that drug reactions are more common in women and increase with age and the number of medications used [48].

It is essential to understand that the pathogenesis of drug-induced various skin disorders helps achieve a greater appreciation of the disease process, but it is also helpful in guiding treatment methodologies. Resistance can be avoided and can improve treatment adherence [47].

Autoimmune Diseases

Besides regulating internal body temperature, the critical functions of the skin include forming the barrier between the organism and the external environment, which protect against pathogen invasion, chemical and physical assaults, and unregulated loss of water and solutes [49]. Disruption of this protective event causes blisters and erosions of the skin that form in blistering autoimmune diseases where the body produces autoantibodies against structural proteins of the epidermis or the epidermal-dermal junction [49].

Auto-inflammation is a newly expanding concept in medicine with substantial relevance in dermatology, as many auto-inflammatory disorders present with cutaneous findings [50]. The immune system was divided into an effector arm responsible for fighting infections and cancer and a regulatory component that reduces auto-reactivity and maintains immune homeostasis [51]. Cutaneous autoimmunity develops when the equilibrium between these arms is disrupted [51]. Although there is no cure for autoimmune skin blistering diseases, immune-suppressive therapies currently offer disease management opportunities [49 - 51]. Genetic factors play an essential role, as the prevalence of specific skin diseases is different between populations and inherited human leukocyte antigen (HLA) types are associated with auto-reactivity to specific auto-antigens [52]. Multiple HLA alleles have been identified, associated with pemphigus vulgaris [52, 53].

Environmental Factors in Skin Diseases

The skin is the first defensive barrier to our body being in contact with the environment. All the skin cells and layers of the skin play essential roles in the defence and protection of the skin against environmental air pollutants, health, and illness, including physical contacts such as (fingerprints, face, voice and hand geometry), chemical and biological [54] are becoming more important in terms of human health effects [55, 56] besides reducing the high risk of developing dermatitis [57].

Nevertheless, most environmental pollution exposure to harmful substances will occur at work or during exposure to sunlight, producing oxidative stress and making healthy skin more vulnerable [54, 58]. Those factors influence skin, presenting in many categories ranging from sun radiation (ultraviolet radiation, visible light, and infra-red radiation) to air pollution, tobacco smoke, and cosmetic products [54]. In addition to various other environmental factors such as absolute humidity rather than relative humidity, the most significant effect on certain skin diseases [56, 59], like stress, irritation, chemicals, diet, climate, UV-radiation, environment and sun exposure, are factors affecting skin disease. The interaction between the skin and the environment presents attractive and challenging research in the world. Such factors are needed to understand the pathogenesis and the disease process better and develop new therapeutic strategies and preventive measures of skin disease towards non-allergic skin diseases with environmental exposures with the factors regarding increasing incidence of skin cancer [58, 60].

Therefore, better understanding and identification of those harmful environmental factors and treatment are required strategies towards environmental prevention and behavioural prevention, as well as global action is needed to be addressed [58] expressly understand the mechanisms of ageing and development toward keeping the skin healthy and preventing damage happen due to Ultraviolet radiation and others environmental pollution [61]. Besides, identify current gaps in knowledge and guide further research in the field [62].

DIAGNOSIS OF SKIN DISEASES

Skin diseases may cause rashes, inflammation, itchiness, or other skin changes based on clinical signs. In a further critical situation, some skin conditions may be due to genetic or lifestyle factors that may cause others. At the level of the hospital, dermatologists perform a range of tests to diagnose your skin. These tests include a blood test, skin biopsy, X-rays, MRI/CT scans, Allergy testing, swab or culture, dermoscopy, and Tzanck test, examining the fluid from a blister. Therefore, several noninvasive approaches have been developed over the years. The golden rule in skin disease diagnosis remains a skin biopsy histologic examination, a somewhat invasive method [63].

With the advance of molecular biology and the explosion of sciences, there is used for molecular pathology techniques in skin disease diagnosis for better understanding and provides insight into the clinical features in affected individuals and also allows for accurate diagnosis outcome and also provide a platform to develop new drugs to treat genetic skin diseases [64, 65]. From a clinical perspective, the advances in molecular biology provide insight into the clinical features of better genetic counselling and allow for accurate diagnosis and treatment [64].

Skin is the most sensitive part of the humans' body that needs special attention and diagnosis approaches. Skin diseases are the most common form of human disease. Recently, many researchers have advocated and developed many methods to diagnose skin diseases through imaging human vision or the loop approach to visual object recognition. The implementation ranges from the classical, modern method through molecular diagnostic techniques and advanced applications [8, 66 - 70].

With fast development, smartphone-based skin disease diagnosis [71], deep learning, artificial intelligence, a neural network have led numerous researchers to use them for skin lesion classification [72], besides interesting use of application convolutional neural networks in the area of dermatoscopic lesion image processing [73]. In health care and disease diagnosis over the last ten years, were highly contributed to increasing the efficiency of the diagnostic and have provided objectivity and high support for accurate, cost-effective and timely treatment of many skin diseases without the need to touch patients.

In addition, the importance of mobile applications in dermatology. Nowadays, a few mobile applications have been developed to diagnose skin diseases from coloured photographs using lightweight networks application [8]. Although recent advancements in mobile phone technologies and improvements in pattern recognition [8], mobile applications in skin disease diagnosis the technology application are still very limited in the literature [74]. Therefore, using traditional diagnosis methods, molecular data, or smartphone-based skin disease deep learning, artificial intelligent neural network techniques provide a platform to develop new drugs and drug repositioning to treat skin diseases.

Treatment of Skin Diseases

There are different options for treating skin diseases depending on the underlying cause, stage of the disease and health-seeking practice of the infected. The available treatment for skin disease varies depending on region and availability among developing countries. At the hospital level, skin diseases were treated using medications, creams, ointments, or lifestyle changes. However, evidence shows that treatment options for skin disease abound, like surgical, destructive, topical and systemic treatments [75]. Other therapies focus on phototherapy [76] and alternative and traditional treatments [77, 78].

Clinical Treatments

Clinical treatment of skin diseases abounds and has proved efficacious based on the different adoptions and applications. In treating basal cell carcinoma, flap surgery may be conducted or use chemotherapy [75]. The treatment options are not limited to these two methods as other methods are adaptable based on clinical treatments. Clinical treatments focus on the microbiome to investigate the different pathogens and their manifestation in the skin and profer treatment solutions [79].

The use of dermoscopy in diagnosis and treatment monitoring has proved very effective for skin cancer and tumours [80]. Other studies have also found the use of Aryl hydrocarbon receptor as a viable approach in treating skin conditions capable of inhibiting non-melanoma skin cancer, melanoma, and psoriasis [81]. Mycophenolate and methotrexate are also evidenced to support treating sclerosis skin diseases in clinical practices [82]. In a hydroxychloroquine trial among Japanese patients, the application of the drug after 16 weeks of usage produced a remarkable improvement in lupus-related skin disease [83]. The extent of the availability and application of these treatment options in developing countries is yet to be ascertained based on limited empirical evidence to support the practice.

Alternative Treatment

Alternative and herbal medicine has been widely accepted and used globally for centuries by physicians to treat different diseases due to its therapeutic effect on the human body. Studies have stretched the need to integrate the use of traditional herbal medicine in the treatment of diseases. For example, evidence has shown that about 116 plant species belonging to 49 families can treat 73 ailments, including skin disorders [84]. The herbal medicine called "neem" has gained attention globally due to its medicinal properties. Evidence has it that the extract from need contains Nimbinin, nimbandiol as active constituents, alcoholic extract, and has significant blood sugar lowering effect, and the treatment of Dermatitis Eczema, Acne, Bacterial, Fungal infections and various skin conditions [85].

Innovations have encouraged the effective use of nanotized herbal medicine to treat skin cancer [86]. Similarly, Chinese herbal medicine has significantly effectively treated various skin allergies. In a national study, Chinese herbal medicine atopic dermatitis and urticaria skin diseases were among the top prescribed alternative medications, giving credence to their acceptability and usability among the population [77]. Adopting traditional medicine in developing countries promises to improve the quality of life of skin disease patients with adequate management.

The history of herbal medicines proves that many herbal products originated from plants and have been used to preserve or recover human health over several years [87]. While in the past two decades, the use of herbal medicines has grown considerably globally as alternative medicines, especially in developing regions with diverse and multifaceted knowledge on the use of traditional medicine, which is transferred from generation to generation through verbal and communal teaching [88].

Many developing countries, including Africans, have used medicinal plants for various ailments. Most regions are dependent on surrounding plant resources for purposes, including food, shelter, fodder, health care, and other cultural purposes [89]. Additional evidence has shown that traditional western medicine remains valid as an alternative treatment of diseases, and the literature on the most popular herbs is explicitly used for dermatologic disease [90]. These traditional medicines have remained the most credible source of treatment for several diseases and are also sources of medication used in primary health care in many countries (Table. 1) [89, 91 - 97]. There are many antimicrobial potential herbal remedies in other developing countries like Italy to treat and control bacterial skin diseases [34].

Table 1. Example of some Medicinal Plants reported in developing countries used for the treatment of skin disease and other diseases.

Country	Species	Family	Medicinal Uses	Plant Part Use	References
Mauritius	*Annonaceae*	*Centella asiatica (Linn.) Urban*	Skin diseases, dyspeptic complaints, worms, wound healing, fever, and insomnia	Leaves	[89]
Tanzania	*Apocynaceae*	*Mondia whitei (Hook.f.) Skeels*	Skin diseases, nausea, fever, bilharzia, sexual dysfunction, induce labor, abdominal pains anthelmintic, and asthma	Leaves	[98, 99]
Nigeria	*Balanitaceae*	*B. aegyptiaca (L.) Delile*	Skin diseases, whooping cough, wound healing, and leucoderma	Leaves	[100]
South Africa & Sudan	*Bignoniaceae*	*K. africana (Lam.) Benth*	Dysentery, sores, stomach ailments, wounds, rheumatism, skin care, cosmetic	Bark	[92 - 94]

(Table 1) cont.....

Country	Species	Family	Medicinal Uses	Plant Part Use	References
Sudan	*A. sinkatana Rey*	*A. sinkatana Rey*	Skin diseases, fever, diabetic, hemorrhoids against constipation, anthelmintic, colon and inflammation	Leaves	[91, 101, 102]
Sudan	*Meliaceae*	*A. indica A. Juss.*	Skin diseases, antimalarial, fever, jaundice, and helminthiasis	Leaves, roots	[91, 102]
Sudan	*Meliaceae*	*K. senegalensis (Desr.) A. Juss*	Skin diseases, Antimalarial, diabetes, hepatic inflammation, sinusitis, trachoma, and stomach complaints	Stem bark	[91, 101]
Sudan	*Malvaceae*	*G . bicolor Juss.*	Against pustular skin lesions and to facilitate labor	Roots	[91, 103]
Sudan	*Tiliaceae*	*G. tenax (Forssk.) Fiori.*	Antimalarial, skin diseases, and for anemia	Fruits	[91, 104, 105]
Southern Africa	*Burseraceae*	*B. sacra Flueck*	Wound healing, skin diseases, urinary tract infections, gynecological disorders, anti-inflammatory agent	Seeds	[106]
Cameroon	*Clusiaceae*	*H. madagascariensis Lam. ex Poir*	Parasitic skin diseases, antiseptic for treating anemia, asthma, tuberculosis, diarrhea, dysentery, STDs, malaria, wounds, fever, and angina	Leaves	[107, 108]
Mauritians	*Flacourtiaceae*	*A. theiformis Benn.*	Skin infections, dysentery, fever, gastrointenstinal infections, ulcers, jaundice, and stomach pains	Leaves	[109]

Country	Species	Family	Medicinal Uses	Plant Part Use	References
Africa	*Meliaceae*	*H. procumbens (Burch.) DC. ex Meisn.*	Skin injuries, allergies, analgesia, arteriosclerosis, boils, ulcers, sores, childbirth, dysmenorrhea, edema, fever, gastrointestinal disorders, headache, migraine, malaria, myalgia, neuralgia, tendonitis, and urinary tract infections	Tubers	[110]
South Africa & Eastern Cape	*Xanthorrhoeaceae*	*A. ferox Mill*	Skin and wound healing, relief of arthritis, sinusitis, conjunctivitis, and opthalmia, and treatment of infection-related ailments including sexually transmitted infections	Leaves	[95 - 97]
South-western Nigeria & Ghana	*Zingiberaceae*	*Aframomum melegueta (Roscoe) K. Schum.*	Skin wounds, wound healing, skin rushes, mouth sores, boils, fractures, stomachache, cough remedy, measles, yellow fever	Seeds	[111, 112]
German	*Marigold*	*Calendula officionalis*	Heal wounds	Pot	[113]
Asia	*Tea (green tea)*	*Skin cancer*	Skin tumor promotion & protects against psoalen–UV-A- induced photochemical damage to the skin	Leaves	[114, 115]
Lagos, Nigeria, Zambia	*Aloe plants*	*Aloe barbadensis Mill.*	Skin hydration and moisture, and prevents skin ulcers, healing and softening the skin, Skin abrasions, and skin injured by radiation & scabies treatment	leaves	[116 - 119]
Madagascar	*Odiota*	*Asparagus simulans Baker (Asparagaceae), Liana, E*	Skin diseases, treatment of Boil and Pityriasis	Leaves	[120]

(Table 1) cont.....

Country	Species	Family	Medicinal Uses	Plant Part Use	References
Sychelles	*Fandamane*	*Aphloia theiformis*	The root is used to wash different skin infections	Root	[121]
Egypt	*Cruciferae*	*Sinapis alba L.*	Treat skin infections such as scabies, wart, varicose veins and inflammations	Seeds	[122]
Egypt	*Acacia*	*Acacia nilotica*	Skin diseases, vermifuge eases diarrhea, and internal bleeding	-	[123]
	Balsam Apple	*Malus sylvestris*	Skin allergies, soothe headaches, gums and teeth, for asthma, liver stimulant, and weak digestion	-	[123]
Egypt	*Tumeric*	*Curcumae longa*	Dye skin and cloth	-	[123]
Liberia	*Butter tree*	*Pentadesma butyracea, Clusiaceae*	Treatment of skin infection, moisturizer, food oil and soap	Seeds	[124]
India	*Artocarpus lakoocha Roxb.*	*Moraceae*	Diabetes, bacterial and worm infection, skin rash	Bark, fruit	[125]
India	*Azadirachta indica*	*Meliaceae*	Skin disease	Neem. Leaf	[126]
India	*Auguste ferrier*	*Cannaceae*	Skin disease	Akon . Extract	[126]
India	*Curcuma longa*	*Zingiberaceae*	Skin disease	Whole Tumeric	[126]
India	*Cassia fistula*	*Zabaceae*	Skin disease	Cassia Leaf	[126]
India	*Aloe (Aloe vera)*	*Liliaceae*	Juice of *A. vera* used in skin care and tooth and gum protective products, HIV infection, wound healing, antidiabetic, antiulcer, immunomodulatory, antitumor, hepatoprotective	leaves	[127]
Namibia	*Ziziplus mucronata*	*Rharmnaceae*	Skin allergy, skin rash, sore fingers, and Gonorrhoea	Bark, leaves, and rooots	[128]

Country	Species	Family	Medicinal Uses	Plant Part Use	References
Namibia	*Berchemia discolor*	*Omuye*	Skin itching, cold, and bleeding	Bark, leaves,	[128]

Topical Treatment

The topical treatment approach involves the body surface, which means when a skin ailment is involved, the focus is given to the skin's surface for immediate treatment. One of the most used topical treatments that have produced outstanding results is the JAK inhibitor which shows effective results in the oral and topical formulation in treating psoriasis, lichen planus (LP), cutaneous lupus erythematosus (CLE), atopic dermatitis (AD), pyoderma gangrenosum (PG) and alopecia areata (AA) [129]. Other efficacious treatments are an elastic liposomal formulation for RNAi-based treatment for skin disorders like psoriasis [130]. The use of ointment such as crissaborole topical cream was used in phases to establish its efficacy in treating moderate to mild atopic dermatitis [131], while nanostructured supramolecular hydrogel was efficacious in psoriasis and other skin diseases [132]. A guideline issued in Korea on the treatment of Atopic Dermatitis focuses on bathing and skincare, avoiding exacerbation and moisturizers [133]. The approach also focused on the short-term and long-term use of topical corticosteroids and calcineurin to relieve the symptoms of atopic dermatitis. As promising and widely used, topical treatment has shown adverse effects on the body, as some studies have shown that increased topical steroids were a risk factor for lymphoma [134].

QUALITY OF LIFE AND SKIN DISEASE

Quality of life (QoL) is a domain that explores how much an individual enjoys life and can feel comfortable and participate in daily functions. The stress, pain, and psychological impact of skin conditions are primarily responsible for a severe reduction in QoL of skin disease patients [135]. The manifestation of skin diseases in humans may cause severe damage to these functions and life satisfaction. Among patients with vitiligo, evidence has shown that it affects more women than men and thus significantly impairs the affected person's QoL [136]. Similarly, health-related QoL among persons dealing with venous leg ulcers is greatly affected [3]. Also, most common in patients suffering from comorbidity of psoriasis and psoriatic arthritis is the reduced quality of life they experience due to progressive damage [137]. Skin diseases such as acne that can cause permanent damage to the skin can significantly impair QoL [138]. Overall, delay and inadequacy in treating skin disease can harm QoL through psychological distress and affect cognition and daily functions.

SKIN DISEASE AND TELEMEDICINE APPLICATION

Technological advancement has paved the way for telemedicine in treating various diseases, and there are still substantial opportunities yet to be explored in use. Notable is the use of teledermatology in the treatment of skin disorders and cancer [139]. While there have been advancements in integrative medicine in developing countries, telemedicine and mobile health have supported managing patients with skin diseases [140]. In Botswana, the application of telemedicine has enhanced the health of patients with skin disorders [141]. Recent advancement in machine learning has paved the way for the early detection of skin disease [142]. However, adequate financing is necessary to improve teledermatology to enhance the quality of care for skin disease patients in developing countries.

POLICY INTERVENTION FOR THE PREVENTION OF SKIN DISEASE

Addressing the public health problem of skin diseases in developing countries requires global and national stakeholder funding and intervention. A significant amount of studies have attributed the burden of skin diseases as a consequence of poverty [143] and costly medical expenditure in treating skin diseases, even in resource-rich regions [144], ampers progress for developing countries. Thus skin disease problem in resource-poor environments requires particular focus and attention. Stakeholder intervention can facilitate immediate intervention for skin disease in developing regions. The World Health Organization (WHO) role is indispensable, and the national governments' cooperation in promoting intervention is paramount. While funding should be made available to support resource-poor populations prone to or battling skin diseases, an improved approach to diagnosis and treatment should also be considered.

Therefore, more organized actions such as the improved financial capacity for countries' health sectors, the provision and availability of effective hospitals can help relieve the burden of skin diseases in the developing region. Similarly, drug availability should also be intensified for drug-treatable skin diseases. Technological advancement has also birthed a new approach to the treatment of skin diseases. Financing should also target the scaling up of telemedicine, teledermatology and other technologies that may improve the quality of care, diagnosis and treatment of skin diseases. There is also the need to enhance research on skin diseases in developing countries. Funding should be made available for clinical and social research on skin disease to facilitate informative intervention. Clinical research funding supports discovering new approaches to treating infectious and noninfectious skin diseases and may help discover emerging skin diseases. Extensive research on the risk factor and psychosocial impact of skin diseases on the general resource-poor population promises to enhance global intervention.

CONCLUSION

Besides regulating internal body temperature, the critical functions of the skin include forming the barrier between the organism and the external environment, which protects against pathogen invasion. In this study, we presented the epidemiological characteristics and geographic distribution and understood the changes in the prevalence of SD and the associated mortality in developing countries. Bacterial, viral, parasitic, and fungal diseases were significant risk factors for skin diseases. The multiple disorders treated with many drugs lead to increased drug-induced skin disorders. In addition, autoimmunity and environmental factors trigger skin diseases.

Generally, skin diseases are diagnosed based on clinical signs; however, from a clinical perspective, the advances in molecular biology provide insight into the clinical features to better understand genetic counselling and allow for accurate diagnosis and treatment. The standard treatment of skin diseases depends on the underlying cause, stage of the conditions and health-seeking practice of the infected. The treatment options usually are clinical treatment or using alternative herbal medicine. Technological advancement has paved the way for telemedicine in treating various diseases. Notable is the use of teledermatology in treating skin disorders and cancer and using machine learning for the early detection of skin disease. It is necessary to improve teledermatology to enhance the quality of care for skin disease patients in developing countries.

ACKNOWLEDGEMENTS

The authors wish to acknowledge the support of the Biomedical Research Institute, Darfur College, Nyala, Sudan, and the research innovation of the Organization of African Academic Doctors (OAAD) for enhancing collaborations and innovative research in Africa.

REFERENCES

[1]   Tortora GJ, Grabowski SR. Principles of anatomy and physiology. 16th ed. John Wiley & Sons, Inc: Academic Press 2020; p. 1296.

[2]   Ryan TJ. Public health dermatology: regeneration and repair of the skin in the developed transitional and developing world. Int J Dermatol 2006; 45(10): 1233-7.
[http://dx.doi.org/10.1111/j.1365-4632.2006.02671.x] [PMID: 17040450]

[3]   González-Consuegra RV, Verdú J. Quality of life in people with venous leg ulcers: an integrative review. J Adv Nurs 2011; 67(5): 926-44.
[http://dx.doi.org/10.1111/j.1365-2648.2010.05568.x] [PMID: 21241355]

[4]   Alemayehu G, Zewde G, Admassu B. Risk assessments of lumpy skin diseases in Borena bull market chain and its implication for livelihoods and international trade. Trop Anim Health Prod 2013; 45(5): 1153-9.
[http://dx.doi.org/10.1007/s11250-012-0340-9] [PMID: 23274626]

[5]   Mphande FA. Infectious diseases and rural livelihood in developing countries. Infect Dis Rural Livelihood Dev Ctries. Singapore: Springer 2016; p. 187.
[http://dx.doi.org/10.1007/978-981-10-0428-5]

[6]   Boyers LN, Karimkhani C, Naghavi M, *et al.* Global mortality from conditions with skin manifestations. J Am Acad Dermatol 2014; 71(6): 1137-1143.e17.
[http://dx.doi.org/10.1016/j.jaad.2014.08.022] [PMID: 25282129]

[7]   Nothdurft HD, Caumes E, Eds. Epidemiology of health risks and travel. Principles and Practice of Travel Medicine, 2nd ed. Wiley Online Library 2013; pp. 588-600.

[8]   Goceri E. Diagnosis of skin diseases in the era of deep learning and mobile technology. Comput Biol Med 2021; 134: 104458.
[http://dx.doi.org/10.1016/j.compbiomed.2021.104458] [PMID: 34000524]

[9]   Khatami A, San Sebastian M. Skin disease: a neglected public health problem. Dermatol Clin 2009; 27(2): 99-101.
[http://dx.doi.org/10.1016/j.det.2008.11.011] [PMID: 19254651]

[10]   Giesey RL, Mehrmal S, Uppal P, Delost ME, Delost GR. Dermatoses of the world: Burden of skin disease and associated socioeconomic status in the world. J Am Acad Dermatol 2021; 84(2): 556-9.
[http://dx.doi.org/10.1016/j.jaad.2020.05.157] [PMID: 32593635]

[11]   Seth D, Cheldize K, Brown D, Freeman EE. Global burden of skin disease: inequities and innovations. Curr Dermatol Rep 2017; 6(3): 204-10.
[http://dx.doi.org/10.1007/s13671-017-0192-7] [PMID: 29226027]

[12]   Afsar FS. Skin infections in developing countries. Curr Opin Pediatr 2010; 22(4): 459-66.
[http://dx.doi.org/10.1097/MOP.0b013e32833bc468] [PMID: 20601882]

[13]   Dlova NC, Mosam A. Inflammatory noninfectious dermatoses of HIV. Dermatol Clin 2006; 24(4): 439-448, vi.
[http://dx.doi.org/10.1016/j.det.2006.06.002] [PMID: 17010774]

[14]   Piccolo V. Update on dermoscopy and infectious skin diseases. Dermatol Pract Concept 2019; 10(1): e2020003.
[http://dx.doi.org/10.5826/dpc.1001a03] [PMID: 31921490]

[15]   Li MY, Hua Y, Wei GH, Qiu L. Staphylococcal scalded skin syndrome in neonates: an 8-year retrospective study in a single institution. Pediatr Dermatol 2014; 31(1): 43-7.
[http://dx.doi.org/10.1111/pde.12114] [PMID: 23557104]

[16]   Gianfaldoni S, Tchernev G, Tirant M, *et al.* 2020.

[17]   Kiprono SK, Muchunu JW, Masenga JE. Skin diseases in pediatric patients attending a tertiary dermatology hospital in Northern Tanzania: a cross-sectional study. BMC Dermatol 2015; 15(1): 16.
[http://dx.doi.org/10.1186/s12895-015-0035-9] [PMID: 26359248]

[18]   Abd El Aal NH, Mostafa LA, Farag AS, Hassan SH. Epidemiological study of infectious skin diseases among Egyptian school children in urban and rural areas. J Egypt Women's Dermatologic Soc 2013; 10(1): 42-6.
[http://dx.doi.org/10.1097/01.EWX.0000422131.75701.17]

[19]   Biswas C, Das SR. Pattern of skin diseases in patients attending OPD of selected upazilla health complex, Bangladesh. J Taibah Univ Med Sci 2017; 12(5): 3-6.

[20]   Hay RJ, Steer AC, Engelman D, Walton S. Scabies in the developing world-its prevalence, complications, and management. Clin Microbiol Infect 2012; 18(4): 313-23.

[http://dx.doi.org/10.1111/j.1469-0691.2012.03798.x] [PMID: 22429456]

[21]   Karimkhani C, Colombara DV, Drucker AM, *et al.* The global burden of scabies: a cross-sectional analysis from the global burden of disease study 2015. Lancet Infect Dis 2017; 17(12): 1247-54.
[http://dx.doi.org/10.1016/S1473-3099(17)30483-8] [PMID: 28941561]

[22]   Linares MA, Zakaria A, Nizran P. Skin cancer. Prim Care - Clin Off Pract 2015; 42(4): 645-59.
[http://dx.doi.org/10.1016/j.pop.2015.07.006]

[23]   Apalla Z, Nashan D, Weller RB, Castellsagué X. Skin cancer: epidemiology, disease burden, pathophysiology, diagnosis, and therapeutic approaches. Dermatol Ther (Heidelb) 2017; 7(S1) (Suppl. 1): 5-19.
[http://dx.doi.org/10.1007/s13555-016-0165-y] [PMID: 28150105]

[24]   Razi S, Rafiemanesh H, Ghoncheh M, Khani Y, Salehiniya H. Changing trends of types of skin cancer in Iran. Asian Pac J Cancer Prev 2015; 16(12): 4955-8.
[http://dx.doi.org/10.7314/APJCP.2015.16.12.4955] [PMID: 26163621]

[25]   Oseni GO, Olaitan PB, Oluwole A, Olaofe OO, Morakinyo HA, Suleiman OA. Malignant skin lesions in Oshogbo, Nigeria. Pan Afr Med J 2015; 20: 253.
[http://dx.doi.org/10.11604/pamj.2015.20.253.2441] [PMID: 26161176]

[26]   Wright CY, du Preez DJ, Millar DA, Norval M. The epidemiology of skin cancer and public health strategies for its prevention in southern Africa. Int J Environ Res Public Health 2020; 17(3): 1017.
[http://dx.doi.org/10.3390/ijerph17031017] [PMID: 32041101]

[27]   Edlich RF, Winters KL, Britt LD, Long WB III. Bacterial diseases of the skin. J Long Term Eff Med Implants 2005; 15(5): 499-510.
[http://dx.doi.org/10.1615/JLongTermEffMedImplants.v15.i5.40] [PMID: 16218899]

[28]   Stulberg DL, Penrod MA, Blatny RA. Common bacterial skin infections. Am Fam Physician 2002; 66(1): 119-24.
[PMID: 12126026]

[29]   Hirt PA, Castillo DE, Yosipovitch G, Keri JE. Skin changes in the obese patient. J Am Acad Dermatol 2019; 81(5): 1037-57.
[http://dx.doi.org/10.1016/j.jaad.2018.12.070] [PMID: 31610857]

[30]   Kulkarni AP, Nagvekar VC, Veeraraghavan B, *et al.* Current perspectives on treatment of gram-positive infections in india: what is the way forward? Interdiscip Perspect Infect Dis 2019; 2019: 1-8.
[http://dx.doi.org/10.1155/2019/7601847] [PMID: 31080476]

[31]   Banwan K, Senok AC, Rotimi VO. Antibiotic therapeutic options for infections caused by drug-resistant Gram-positive cocci 2009; 2(2009): 62-73.

[32]   Dvorchik BH, Brazier D, DeBruin MF, Arbeit RD. Daptomycin pharmacokinetics and safety following administration of escalating doses once daily to healthy subjects. Antimicrob Agents Chemother 2003; 47(4): 1318-23.
[http://dx.doi.org/10.1128/AAC.47.4.1318-1323.2003] [PMID: 12654665]

[33]   Cornaglia G. Fighting infections due to multidrug-resistant Gram-positive pathogens. Clin Microbiol Infect 2009; 15(3): 209-11.
[http://dx.doi.org/10.1111/j.1469-0691.2009.02737.x] [PMID: 19335367]

[34]   Mazzei R, Leonti M, Spadafora S, Patitucci A, Tagarelli G. A review of the antimicrobial potential of herbal drugs used in popular Italian medicine (1850s–1950s) to treat bacterial skin diseases. J Ethnopharmacol 2020; 250: 112443.
[http://dx.doi.org/10.1016/j.jep.2019.112443] [PMID: 31790819]

[35]   Lei V, Petty AJ, Atwater AR, Wolfe SA, MacLeod AS. Skin viral infections: host antiviral innate immunity and viral immune evasion. Front Immunol 2020; 11: 593901.
[http://dx.doi.org/10.3389/fimmu.2020.593901] [PMID: 33240281]

[36]   Yeroushalmi S, Shirazi JY, Friedman A. New developments in bacterial, viral, and fungal cutaneous
        infections. Curr Dermatol Rep 2020; 9(2): 152-65.
        [http://dx.doi.org/10.1007/s13671-020-00295-1] [PMID: 32435525]

[37]   Cardoso AEC, Cardoso AEO, Talhari C, Santos M. Update on parasitic dermatoses. An Bras Dermatol
        2020; 95(1): 1-14.
        [http://dx.doi.org/10.1016/j.abd.2019.12.001] [PMID: 32001061]

[38]   Belizario V. delos Trinos JPC, Garcia NB, Reyes M. Cutaneous manifestations of selected parasitic
        infections in western pacific and southeast asian regions. Curr Infect Dis Rep 2016; 18(30): 18-30.

[39]   Ho K, Cheng T. Common superficial fungal infections, a short review. Med Bull 2010; 15(11): 23-7.

[40]   Tyring SK, Lupi O, Hengge UR, Eds. Tropical Dermatology. 2nd ed., 2017; p. 463.

[41]   Chandler DJ, Fuller LC. A review of scabies: an infestation more than skin deep. Dermatology 2019;
        235(2): 79-90.
        [http://dx.doi.org/10.1159/000495290] [PMID: 30544123]

[42]   Lassa S, Campbell MJ, Bennett CE. Epidemiology of scabies prevalence in the U.K. from general
        practice records. Br J Dermatol 2011; 164(6): 1329-34.
        [http://dx.doi.org/10.1111/j.1365-2133.2011.10264.x] [PMID: 21574970]

[43]   Hewitt KA, Nalabanda A, Cassell JA. Scabies outbreaks in residential care homes: factors associated
        with late recognition, burden and impact. A mixed methods study in England. Epidemiol Infect 2015;
        143(7): 1542-51.
        [http://dx.doi.org/10.1017/S0950268814002143] [PMID: 25195595]

[44]   Cassell JA, Middleton J, Nalabanda A, *et al.* Scabies outbreaks in ten care homes for elderly people: a
        prospective study of clinical features, epidemiology, and treatment outcomes. Lancet Infect Dis 2018;
        18(8): 894-902.
        [http://dx.doi.org/10.1016/S1473-3099(18)30347-5] [PMID: 30068499]

[45]   Siskin SB, Pharm D. Clinical Pharmacy and Therapeutics. Am J Health Syst Pharm 1975; 32(12):
        1266.
        [http://dx.doi.org/10.1093/ajhp/32.12.1266]

[46]   N P, Srinivasan R. A review on drug induced skin disorders: pathophysiology and therapeutics.
        International Journal of Research in Dermatology 2020; 6(5): 715.
        [http://dx.doi.org/10.18203/issn.2455-4529.IntJResDermatol20203761]

[47]   Ardern-Jones MR, Friedmann PS. Skin manifestations of drug allergy. Br J Clin Pharmacol 2011;
        71(5): 672-83.
        [http://dx.doi.org/10.1111/j.1365-2125.2010.03703.x] [PMID: 21480947]

[48]   Farshchian M, Ansar A, Zamanian A, *et al.* Drug-induced skin reactions: A 2-year study. Clin Cosmet
        Investig Dermatol 2015; 8(default): 53.

[49]   Vorobyev A, Ludwig RJ, Schmidt E. Clinical features and diagnosis of epidermolysis bullosa
        acquisita. Expert Rev Clin Immunol 2017; 13(2): 157-69.
        [http://dx.doi.org/10.1080/1744666X.2016.1221343] [PMID: 27580464]

[50]   Murthy AS, Leslie K. Autoinflammatory skin disease: a review of concepts and applications to general
        dermatology. Dermatology 2016; 232(5): 534-40.
        [http://dx.doi.org/10.1159/000449526] [PMID: 27871068]

[51]   Vesely MD. Getting under the skin: Targeting cutaneous autoimmune disease. Yale J Biol Med 2020;
        93(1): 197-206.
        [PMID: 32226348]

[52]   Vodo D, Sarig O, Sprecher E. The genetics of *Pemphigus vulgaris*. Front Med (Lausanne) 2018; 5:
        226.
        [http://dx.doi.org/10.3389/fmed.2018.00226] [PMID: 30155467]

[53]   Li S, Zhang Q, Wang P, *et al.* Association between HLA-DQB1 polymorphisms and pemphigus vulgaris: A meta-analysis. Immunol Invest 2018; 47(1): 101-12.
[http://dx.doi.org/10.1080/08820139.2017.1385622] [PMID: 29182409]

[54]   Parrado C, Mercado-Saenz S, Perez-Davo A, Gilaberte Y, Gonzalez S, Juarranz A. Environmental stressors on skin aging. Mechanistic insights. Front Pharmacol 2019; 10: 759.
[http://dx.doi.org/10.3389/fphar.2019.00759] [PMID: 31354480]

[55]   Narayanan DL, Saladi RN, Fox JL. Review: Ultraviolet radiation and skin cancer. Int J Dermatol 2010; 49(9): 978-86.
[http://dx.doi.org/10.1111/j.1365-4632.2010.04474.x] [PMID: 20883261]

[56]   Drahanský M, Kanich O, Březinová E. Challenges for Fingerprint Recognition Spoofing, Skin Diseases, and Environmental Effects. In: Tistarelli M, Champod C, Eds. Handbook of Biometrics for Forensic Science Advances in Computer Vision and Pattern Recognition. Cham: Springer 2017; pp. 63-83.
[http://dx.doi.org/10.1007/978-3-319-50673-9_4]

[57]   English JSC, Dawe RS, Ferguson J. Environmental effects and skin disease. Br Med Bull 2003; 68(1): 129-42.
[http://dx.doi.org/10.1093/bmb/ldg026] [PMID: 14757713]

[58]   Mahler V. Skin diseases associated with environmental factors. Bundesgesundheitsblatt Gesundheitsforschung Gesundheitsschutz 2017; 60(6): 605-17.
[http://dx.doi.org/10.1007/s00103-017-2543-8] [PMID: 28516256]

[59]   Dardick K. Imported skin diseases. Emerg Infect Dis 2008; 14(6): 1008.
[http://dx.doi.org/10.3201/eid1406.080223]

[60]   Jones HE, Lewis CW, Aton JK, Sorensen GW, Akers WA. Environmental factors and skin diseases. Mil Med 1976; 141(4): 237-43.
[http://dx.doi.org/10.1093/milmed/141.4.237] [PMID: 817227]

[61]   Burke KE. Mechanisms of aging and development—A new understanding of environmental damage to the skin and prevention with topical antioxidants. Mech Ageing Dev 2018; 172: 123-30.
[http://dx.doi.org/10.1016/j.mad.2017.12.003] [PMID: 29287765]

[62]   Siiskonen H, Smorodchenko A, Krause K, Maurer M, Maurer M. Ultraviolet radiation and skin mast cells: Effects, mechanisms and relevance for skin diseases. Exp Dermatol 2018; 27(1): 3-8.
[http://dx.doi.org/10.1111/exd.13402] [PMID: 28677275]

[63]   Kollias N, Stamatas GN. Optical non-invasive approaches to diagnosis of skin diseases. J Investig Dermatol Symp Proc 2002; 7(1): 64-75.
[http://dx.doi.org/10.1046/j.1523-1747.2002.19635.x] [PMID: 12518795]

[64]   Wessagowit V, McGrath JA. Molecular basis of skin disease. Mol Pathol 2009; 519-50.

[65]   Wessagowit V, Ed. Molecular basis of skin disease. 2nd ed., Essent Concepts Mol Pathol 2020; pp. 463-94.

[66]   Kumar M, Kumar R. An intelligent system to diagnosis the skin disease. ARPN J Eng Appl Sci 2016; 11(19): 11368-73.

[67]   Chiorean R, Mahler M, Sitaru C. Molecular diagnosis of autoimmune skin diseases. Rom J Morphol Embryol 2014; 55(3) (Suppl.): 1019-33.
[PMID: 25607381]

[68]   Yeo DC, Xu C. Simplifying Skin Disease Diagnosis with Topical Nanotechnology. Society for Laboratory Automation and Screening Post, 18th May 2018.

[69]   Liu Y, Jain A, Eng C, *et al.* A deep learning system for differential diagnosis of skin diseases. Nat Med 2020; 26(6): 900-8.
[http://dx.doi.org/10.1038/s41591-020-0842-3] [PMID: 32424212]

[70] Bajwa MN, Muta K, Malik MI, *et al.* Computer-aided diagnosis of skin diseases using deep neural networks. Appl Sci (Basel) 2020; 10(7): 2488.
[http://dx.doi.org/10.3390/app10072488]

[71] Velasco J, Pascion C, Alberio JW, *et al.* A smartphone-based skin disease classification using mobilenet CNN. Int J Adv Trends Comput Sci Eng 2019; 8(5): 2632-7.
[http://dx.doi.org/10.30534/ijatcse/2019/116852019]

[72] Ech-Cherif A, Misbhauddin M, Ech-Cherif M. Deep Neural Network Based Mobile Dermoscopy Application for Triaging Skin Cancer Detection. 2nd Int Conf Comput Appl Inf Secur ICCAIS 2019. 2019; pp. 1-6.
[http://dx.doi.org/10.1109/CAIS.2019.8769517]

[73] Sae-Lim W, Wettayaprasit W, Aiyarak P. Convolutional Neural Networks Using MobileNet for Skin Lesion Classification. JCSSE 2019-16th Int Jt Conf Comput Sci Softw Eng Knowl Evol Towar Singul Man-Machine Intell. 2019; pp. 242-7.
[http://dx.doi.org/10.1109/JCSSE.2019.8864155]

[74] Goceri E. Impact of Deep Learning and Smartphone Technologies in Dermatology: Automated Diagnosis. 2020 10th Int Conf Image Process Theory, Tools and Applications (IPTA 2020), Paris, France, 2020. 2020; pp. 1-6.

[75] Garcovich S, Colloca G, Sollena P, *et al.* Skin cancer epidemics in the elderly as an emerging issue in geriatric oncology. Aging Dis 2017; 8(5): 643-61.
[http://dx.doi.org/10.14336/AD.2017.0503] [PMID: 28966807]

[76] Jarrett P, Scragg R. A short history of phototherapy, vitamin D and skin disease. Photochem Photobiol Sci 2017; 16(3): 283-90.
[http://dx.doi.org/10.1039/c6pp00406g] [PMID: 27892584]

[77] Chen HY, Lin YH, Huang JW, Chen YC, Chen Y. Chinese herbal medicine network and core treatments for allergic skin diseases: Implications from a nationwide database. J Ethnopharmacol 2015; 168: 260-7.
[http://dx.doi.org/10.1016/j.jep.2015.04.002] [PMID: 25865681]

[78] Tan HY, Zhang AL, Chen DC, Xue CC, Lenon GB. Chinese herbal medicine for atopic dermatitis: A systematic review. J Am Acad Dermatol 2013; 69(2): 295-304.
[http://dx.doi.org/10.1016/j.jaad.2013.01.019]

[79] Findley K, Grice EA. The skin microbiome: a focus on pathogens and their association with skin disease. PLoS Pathog 2014; 10(11): e1004436.
[http://dx.doi.org/10.1371/journal.ppat.1004436] [PMID: 25393405]

[80] Lallas A, Argenziano G, Zendri E, *et al.* Update on non-melanoma skin cancer and the value of dermoscopy in its diagnosis and treatment monitoring 2013; 13(5): 541-58.
[http://dx.doi.org/10.1586/era.13.38]

[81] Napolitano M, Patruno C. Aryl hydrocarbon receptor (AhR) a possible target for the treatment of skin disease. Med Hypotheses 2018; 116: 96-100.
[http://dx.doi.org/10.1016/j.mehy.2018.05.001] [PMID: 29857917]

[82] Frech TM, Shanmugam VK, Shah AA, *et al.* Treatment of early diffuse systemic sclerosis skin disease. Clin Exp Rheumatol 2013; 31(2) (Suppl. 76): 166-71.
[PMID: 23910619]

[83] Yokogawa N, Tanikawa A, Amagai M, *et al.* Response to hydroxychloroquine in Japanese patients with lupus-related skin disease using the cutaneous lupus erythematosus disease area and severity index (CLASI). Mod Rheumatol 2013; 23(2): 318-22.
[http://dx.doi.org/10.3109/s10165-012-0656-3] [PMID: 22581095]

[84] Laldingliani TBC, Thangjam NM, Zomuanawma R, Bawitlung L, Pal A, Kumar A. Ethnomedicinal study of medicinal plants used by Mizo tribes in Champhai district of Mizoram, India. J Ethnobiol

Ethnomed 2022; 18(1): 22.
[http://dx.doi.org/10.1186/s13002-022-00520-0] [PMID: 35331291]

[85]　Bhowmik D, Yadav J, Tripathi KK, *et al.* Herbal Remedies of Azadirachta indica and its Medicinal Application. J Chem Pharm Res 2010; 2(1): 62-72.

[86]　Sachan AK, Gupta A. A review on nanotized herbal drugs. Int J Pharm Sci Res 2015; 6(63): 961-70.

[87]　Balick MJ, Cox PA. Plants That Heal Plants, People, Cult Garland Science; 2020.

[88]　Che CT, George V, Ijinu TP, Pushpangadan P, Marobela AK. Traditional Medicine. Pharmacogn Fundam Appl Strateg 2017; pp. 15-30.

[89]　Gurib-Fakim A, Sewraj M, Gueho J, Dulloo E. Medicalethnobotany of some weeds of Mauritius and Rodrigues. J Ethnopharmacol 1993; 39(3): 175-85.
[http://dx.doi.org/10.1016/0378-8741(93)90034-3] [PMID: 8258975]

[90]　Buchness MR. Alternative medicine and dermatology. Semin Cutan Med Surg 1998; 17(4): 284-90.
[http://dx.doi.org/10.1016/S1085-5629(98)80025-4] [PMID: 9859916]

[91]　Kuhnert N, Karar MGE. Herbal drugs from Sudan: Traditional uses and phytoconstituents. Pharmacogn Rev 2017; 11(22): 83-103.
[http://dx.doi.org/10.4103/phrev.phrev_15_15] [PMID: 28989244]

[92]　Mativandlela SPN, Lall N, Meyer JJM. Antibacterial, antifungal and antitubercular activity of (the roots of) Pelargonium reniforme (CURT) and Pelargonium sidoides (DC) (Geraniaceae) root extracts. S Afr J Bot 2006; 72(2): 232-7.
[http://dx.doi.org/10.1016/j.sajb.2005.08.002]

[93]　Duke JA. Zulu medicinal plants: an inventory. Choice Rev Online 1997; 40: 62.

[94]　Eldeen IMS, Van Staden J. *In vitro* pharmacological investigation of extracts from some trees used in Sudanese traditional medicine. S Afr J Bot 2007; 73(3): 435-40.
[http://dx.doi.org/10.1016/j.sajb.2007.03.009]

[95]　Chen W, Van Wyk BE, Vermaak I, Viljoen AM. Cape aloes—a review of the phytochemistry, pharmacology and commercialisation of Aloe ferox. Phytochem Lett 2012; 5(1): 1-12.
[http://dx.doi.org/10.1016/j.phytol.2011.09.001]

[96]　Kambizi L, Sultana N, Afolayan AJ. Bioactive compounds isolated from Aloe ferox: A plant traditionally used for the treatment of sexually transmitted infections in the Eastern Cape, South Africa. Pharm Biol 2005; 42(8): 636-9
[http://dx.doi.org/10.1080/13880200490902581]

[97]　Jia Y, Zhao G, Jia J. Preliminary evaluation: The effects of Aloe ferox Miller and Aloe arborescens Miller on wound healing. J Ethnopharmacol 2008; 120(2): 181-9.
[http://dx.doi.org/10.1016/j.jep.2008.08.008] [PMID: 18773950]

[98]　Sparg SG, van Staden J, Jäger AK. Efficiency of traditionally used South African plants against schistosomiasis. J Ethnopharmacol 2000; 73(1-2): 209-14.
[http://dx.doi.org/10.1016/S0378-8741(00)00310-X] [PMID: 11025158]

[99]　Patnam R, Kadali SS, Koumaglo KH, Roy R. A chlorinated coumarinolignan from the African medicinal plant, Mondia whitei. Phytochemistry 2005; 66(6): 683-6.
[http://dx.doi.org/10.1016/j.phytochem.2004.11.012] [PMID: 15771890]

[100]　Doughari JH, J H, Pukuma , M S, De , N . Antibacterial effects of Balanites aegyptiaca L. Drel. and Moringa oleifera Lam. on Salmonella typhi. Afr J Biotechnol 2007; 6(19): 2212-5.
[http://dx.doi.org/10.5897/AJB2007.000-2346]

[101]　Musa MS, Abdelrasool FE, Elsheikh EA, *et al.* Ethnobotanical study of medicinal plants in the Blue Nile State, South-eastern Sudan. J Med Plants Res 2011; 5(17): 4287-97.

[102]　Ragasa CY, Nacpil ZD, Natividad GM, Tada M, Coll JC, Rideout JA. Tetranortriterpenoids from

Azadirachta indica. Phytochemistry 1997; 46(3): 555-8.
[http://dx.doi.org/10.1016/S0031-9422(97)87092-6]

[103] Elegami AA, Almagboul AZ, Omer MEA, El Tohami MS. Sudanese plants used in folkloric medicine: screening for antibacterial activity. Part X. Fitoterapia 2001; 72(7): 810-7.
[http://dx.doi.org/10.1016/S0367-326X(01)00310-0] [PMID: 11677021]

[104] El Hadi A, Bashir A, El Kheir Y. Investigations of molluscicidal activity of certain Sudanese plants used in folk-medicine. Part IV. Planta Med 1984; 50(1): 74-7.
[http://dx.doi.org/10.1055/s-2007-969625]

[105] Elhassan GOM, Yagi SM. Nutritional composition of Grewia species (Grewia tenax (Forsk.) Fiori, G. flavescens Juss and G. Villosa willd) fruits. Adv J Food Sci Technol 2010; 2(3): 159-62.

[106] van Vuuren SF, Naidoo D. An antimicrobial investigation of plants used traditionally in southern Africa to treat sexually transmitted infections. J Ethnopharmacol 2010; 130(3): 552-8.
[http://dx.doi.org/10.1016/j.jep.2010.05.045] [PMID: 20561928]

[107] Kouam SF, Yapna DB, Krohn K, *et al.* Antimicrobial prenylated anthracene derivatives from the leaves of Harungana madagascariensis. J Nat Prod 2007; 70(4): 600-3.
[http://dx.doi.org/10.1021/np060556l] [PMID: 17352491]

[108] Moulari B, Pellequer Y, Lboutounne H, *et al.* Isolation and *in vitro* antibacterial activity of astilbin, the bioactive flavanone from the leaves of Harungana madagascariensis Lam. ex Poir. (Hypericaceae). J Ethnopharmacol 2006; 106(2): 272-8.
[http://dx.doi.org/10.1016/j.jep.2006.01.008] [PMID: 16483735]

[109] Rangasamy O, Raoelison G, Rakotoniriana FE, *et al.* Screening for anti-infective properties of several medicinal plants of the Mauritians flora. J Ethnopharmacol 2007; 109(2): 331-7.
[http://dx.doi.org/10.1016/j.jep.2006.08.002] [PMID: 17011733]

[110] Walter A, Samuel W, Peter A, Joseph O. Antibacterial activity of Moringa oleifera and Moringa stenopetala methanol and *n*-hexane seed extracts on bacteria implicated in water borne diseases. Afr J Microbiol Res 2011; 5: 153-7.

[111] Konning GH, Agyare C, Ennison B. Antimicrobial activity of some medicinal plants from Ghana. Fitoterapia 2004; 75(1): 65-7.
[http://dx.doi.org/10.1016/j.fitote.2003.07.001] [PMID: 14693222]

[112] Adetutu A, Morgan WA, Corcoran O. Ethnopharmacological survey and *in vitro* evaluation of wound-healing plants used in South-western Nigeria. J Ethnopharmacol 2011; 137(1): 50-6.
[http://dx.doi.org/10.1016/j.jep.2011.03.073] [PMID: 21501678]

[113] Pittler MG, Ed. Herbal Drugs and Phytopharmaceuticals Focus Altern Complement Ther. 3rd ed. Medpharm 2000; pp. 1-565.

[114] Lu Y, Lou YR, Xie JG, Yen P, Huang MT, Conney AH. Inhibitory effect of black tea on the growth of established skin tumors in mice: effects on tumor size, apoptosis, mitosis and bromodeoxyuridine incorporation into DNA. Carcinogenesis 1997; 18(11): 2163-9.
[http://dx.doi.org/10.1093/carcin/18.11.2163] [PMID: 9395217]

[115] Katiyar SK, Ahmad N, Mukhtar H. Green tea and skin. Arch Dermatol 2000; 136(8): 989-94.
[http://dx.doi.org/10.1001/archderm.136.8.989] [PMID: 10926734]

[116] Somboonwong J, Thanamittramanee S, Jariyapongskul A, Patumraj S. Therapeutic effects of *Aloe vera* on cutaneous microcirculation and wound healing in second degree burn model in rats. J Med Assoc Thai 2000; 83(4): 417-25.
[PMID: 10808702]

[117] Oreagba IA, Oshikoya KA, Amachree M. Herbal medicine use among urban residents in Lagos, Nigeria. BMC Complement Altern Med 2011; 11(1): 117.
[http://dx.doi.org/10.1186/1472-6882-11-117] [PMID: 22117933]

[118] Oyelami OA, Onayemi A, Oyedeji OA, Adeyemi LA. Preliminary study of effectiveness of *Aloe vera* in scabies treatment. Phytother Res 2009; 23(10): 1482-4.
[http://dx.doi.org/10.1002/ptr.2614] [PMID: 19274696]

[119] El Hajj M, Sitali DC, Vwalika B, Holst L. Herbal medicine use among pregnant women attending antenatal clinics in Lusaka Province, Zambia: A cross-sectional, multicentre study. Complement Ther Clin Pract 2020; 40: 101218.
[http://dx.doi.org/10.1016/j.ctcp.2020.101218] [PMID: 32891293]

[120] Rakotondrafara A, Rakotondrajaona R, Rakotoarisoa M, Ratsimbason M, Rasamison VE, Rakotonandrasana SR. Ethnobotany of medicinal plants used by the Zafimaniry clan in Madagascar. J Phytopharmacol 2018; 7(6): 483-94.
[http://dx.doi.org/10.31254/phyto.2018.7606]

[121] Picot-Allain MCN. *Aphloia theiformis* (Vahl.) Benn.: a plant with various therapeutic properties. J Soil Plant Biol 2018; 1: 16-20.

[122] Hamdy AA, Kassem HA, Awad GEA, *et al. In-vitro* evaluation of certain Egyptian traditional medicinal plants against Propionibacterium acnes. S Afr J Bot 2017; 109: 90-5.
[http://dx.doi.org/10.1016/j.sajb.2016.12.026]

[123] Aboelsoud NH. Herbal medicine in ancient Egypt. J Med Plants Res 2010; 4: 82-6.

[124] Hwang LC, Juliani HR, Govindasamy R, Simon JE. Traditional botanical uses of non-timber forest products (NTFP) in seven counties in Liberia. ACS Symp Ser 2020; 1361: 3-43.
[http://dx.doi.org/10.1021/bk-2020-1361.ch001]

[125] Chakraborty R, Sen S, Chanu NR, *et al.* An ethnobotanical survey of medicinal plants used by ethnic people of thoubal and kakching district, Manipur, India. In: Sen S, Chakraborty R, Eds. Herbal Medicine in India. Singapore: Springer 2020; pp. 41-9.
[http://dx.doi.org/10.1007/978-981-13-7248-3_4]

[126] Kaushik PK, Saha P. Home herbal garden for promotion of herbal health care system in Tripura. H. In: Sen S, Chakraborty R, Eds. Herbal Medicine in India. Singapore: Springer 2020; pp. 89-100.
[http://dx.doi.org/10.1007/978-981-13-7248-3_7]

[127] Minwuyelet T, Sewalem M, Gashe M. Review on therapeutic uses of *Aloe vera*. Glob J Pharmacol 2017; 11(2): 14-20.

[128] Maroyi A, Cheikhyoussef A. A comparative study of medicinal plants used in rural areas of Namibia and Zimbabwe. Indian J Tradit 2015; 14(3): 401-6.

[129] Alves de Medeiros AK, Speeckaert R, Desmet E, Van Gele M, De Schepper S, Lambert J. JAK3 as an emerging target for topical treatment of inflammatory skin diseases. PLoS One 2016; 11(10): e0164080.
[http://dx.doi.org/10.1371/journal.pone.0164080] [PMID: 27711196]

[130] Desmet E, Bracke S, Forier K, *et al.* An elastic liposomal formulation for RNAi-based topical treatment of skin disorders: Proof-of-concept in the treatment of psoriasis. Int J Pharm 2016; 500(1-2): 268-74.
[http://dx.doi.org/10.1016/j.ijpharm.2016.01.042] [PMID: 26806466]

[131] Jarnagin K, Chanda S, Coronado D, *et al.* Crisaborole topical ointment, 2%: a nonsteroidal, topical, anti-inflammatory phosphodiesterase 4 inhibitor in clinical development for the treatment of atopic dermatitis. J Drugs Dermatol 2016; 15(4): 390-6.
[PMID: 27050693]

[132] Limón D, Talló Domínguez K, Garduño-Ramírez ML, Andrade B, Calpena AC, Pérez-García L. Nanostructured supramolecular hydrogels: Towards the topical treatment of Psoriasis and other skin diseases. Colloids Surf B Biointerfaces 2019; 181: 657-70.
[http://dx.doi.org/10.1016/j.colsurfb.2019.06.018] [PMID: 31212138]

[133] Kim JE, Kim HJ, Lew BL, *et al.* Consensus guidelines for the treatment of atopic dermatitis in Korea (part I): general management and topical treatment. Ann Dermatol 2015; 27(5): 563-77.
[http://dx.doi.org/10.5021/ad.2015.27.5.563] [PMID: 26512171]

[134] Legendre L, Barnetche T, Mazereeuw-Hautier J, Meyer N, Murrell D, Paul C. Risk of lymphoma in patients with atopic dermatitis and the role of topical treatment: A systematic review and meta-analysis. J Am Acad Dermatol 2015; 72(6): 992-1002.
[http://dx.doi.org/10.1016/j.jaad.2015.02.1116] [PMID: 25840730]

[135] Dixon LJ, Witcraft SM, McCowan NK, Brodell RT. Stress and skin disease quality of life: the moderating role of anxiety sensitivity social concerns. Br J Dermatol 2018; 178(4): 951-7.
[http://dx.doi.org/10.1111/bjd.16082] [PMID: 29078254]

[136] Alikhan A, Felsten LM, Daly M, Petronic-Rosic V. Vitiligo: A comprehensive overview. J Am Acad Dermatol 2011; 65(3): 473-91.
[http://dx.doi.org/10.1016/j.jaad.2010.11.061] [PMID: 21839315]

[137] Boehncke WH, Menter A. Burden of disease: psoriasis and psoriatic arthritis. Am J Clin Dermatol 2013; 14(5): 377-88.
[http://dx.doi.org/10.1007/s40257-013-0032-x] [PMID: 23771648]

[138] Gieler U, Gieler T, Kupfer JP. Acne and quality of life - impact and management. J Eur Acad Dermatol Venereol 2015; 29 (Suppl. 4): 12-4.
[http://dx.doi.org/10.1111/jdv.13191] [PMID: 26059729]

[139] Akintunde TY, Akintunde OD, Musa TH, *et al.* Expanding telemedicine to reduce the burden on the healthcare systems and poverty in Africa for a post-coronavirus disease 2019 (COVID-19) pandemic reformation. Glob Heal J 2021; 5(3)

[140] Kamsu-Foguem B, Foguem C. Telemedicine and mobile health with integrative medicine in developing countries. Health Policy Technol 2014; 3(4): 264-71.
[http://dx.doi.org/10.1016/j.hlpt.2014.08.008]

[141] Littman-Quinn R, Chandra A, Schwartz A, *et al.*

[142] Hashmani MA, Jameel SM, Rizvi SSH, Shukla S. An adaptive federated machine learning-based intelligent system for skin disease detection: a step toward an intelligent dermoscopy device. Appl Sci (Basel) 2021; 11(5): 2145.
[http://dx.doi.org/10.3390/app11052145]

[143] Feldmeier H, Heukelbach J. Epidermal parasitic skin diseases: a neglected category of poverty-associated plagues. Bull World Health Organ 2009; 87(2): 152-9.
[http://dx.doi.org/10.2471/BLT.07.047308] [PMID: 19274368]

[144] Guy GP, Machlin SR, Ekwueme DU, Yabroff KR. Prevalence and costs of skin cancer treatment in the U.S., 2002–2006 and 2007–2011. Am J Prev Med 2015; 48(2): 183-7.

CHAPTER 7

Skin Cancer as an Emerging Global Threat and Potential Natural Therapeutic

Nadia Mushtaq[1], Aqsa Arooj[2], Areeba Akhtar[3] and Abdul Jabbar[4,*]

[1] *Department of Life Sciences, Syed Babar Ali School of Science and Engineering, Lahore University of Management Sciences, 54792, Lahore, Pakistan*

[2] *College of Earth and Environmental Sciences, Faculty of Environmental Sciences, University of the Punjab, 54590, Lahore, Punjab, Pakistan*

[3] *Department of Biotechnology, Kinnaird College Lahore, Punjab, Pakistan*

[4] *Department of Veterinary Medicine, Faculty of Veterinary Science, University of Veterinary and Animal Sciences, 54000, Lahore, Punjab, Pakistan*

Abstract: Background and Aim: Global advancement is facing a huge threat due to the increased number of skin cancer cases and potential health-system costs. Perception of skin cancer prevalence is important for the treatment, prevention strategies, and administration of medical allowances. In addition to fair and tanned skin, the risk factor for the development of disease is sedentary lifestyle habits, and the reduction in physical activities has risen the mortalities worldwide. This effort signifies information on incidence, risk factors, and mortality rates across six continents.

Methodology: The scientific literature was illustrated to find the correlation between the risk factors and resulting data to map, the approaches practiced concerning certain prevention strategies, in particular to alteration in behaviors such as reduction to UV-light exposure, screening and prevention in the progression of the disease.

Results: The incidence of the disease is highest in Australia and New Zealand and lowest in Asian countries. A global survey was done on disease burden in 2018, in which signposts Incidence and mortality are 33.3 ASR and 4.8 ASR, respectively, in New Zealand and 33.6 ASR and 3.2 ASR, respectively, in Australia for melanoma skin cancer. The resistance of skin cancer to topical chemotherapy has turned the attention to natural therapeutics, including herbs, plant extracts and nutraceuticals.

Conclusion: In difficult circumstances, a change in adaptive behavior and cognitive development can reduce the disease burden worldwide. Natural therapeutics can be used to exert anti-inflammatory, anti-proliferative and anti-tumorigenic by modulating the signaling pathways and other physiological effects.

* **Corresponding author Abdul Jabbar:** Department of Veterinary Medicine, Faculty of Veterinary Science, University of Veterinary and Animal Sciences, Lahore Punjab, Pakistan; Tel: +923454501318; E-mail: vet.drabduljabbar@gmail.com

Keywords: Apoptosis, Anti-inflammatory, Incidence, Melanoma skin cancer, Mortality, Melanocytes, Non- melanoma skin cancer, Natural therapeutics, preventive approaches, Signaling pathways, Risk factors, UV- radiation exposure.

INTRODUCTION

The biggest organ in the human body is skin, which plays an essential role in human health and survival by providing a physical obstruction between humans and the outer environment. This physical barrier formulates a critical first-line defense counter by attacking pathogens and must also protect against a variety of physiochemical factors [1]. Skin cancer is considered the most important type of cancer in Canada which is considered a noteworthy and emergent issue for public health. The Canadian Cancer Society has paid exceptional attention to the statistics report on cancer for 2014. For non-melanoma cancer, 76,100 cases and 440 deaths were calculated, and for melanoma skin cancer, there were about 6,500 new cases and 1,050 deaths [2].

Principal factors of risk for the advancement of numerous kinds of skin cancer include genetic constituents, nature of skin (associated with the capability to tan or burn), and ethnicity or race (strictly connected with melanoma). Compounding the elementary aspects is the extreme exposure to ultraviolet rays, which is among the big physical threats to the advancement of skin cancer in certain racial assemblages. Being the chief professional risk aspect, outdoor employees are more susceptible to emerging skin cancer [3].

Skin cancer has advanced as the most communal malignant disease accounting for 4.5% of all novel cancer cases with an average addition of about a million new cases annually. This prevalence is more supplementary than any other cancer category. It is a life frightening lethal disease whose risk and prevalence has been growing over the last three decades, triggering substantial cost to human well-being and the economy throughout the globe [4].

The highest prevalence of cases of skin cancer in Asia is documented in Kazakhstan, with a population of 23.3 per 100,000 [5]. The approximation for the United States is that one out of five Americans will diagnose with skin cancer throughout their lifespan. In the year 2012, approximately 5.4 million basal cell carcinomas (BCC) and spinocellular carcinomas (SCC) were diagnosed [2]. Every year the appearance of additional cases of skin cancer occurs than all the collective incidences of cancers of the lungs, breast, colon, and prostate. The latest study in the US predicted that in 2012, 5.4 million new cases were spotted among more than 3.3 million individuals [6].

The incidence of skin cancer is very high in many countries, out of which most cases are avoidable. Regardless, the struggles of addressing skin cancer risk factors like intentional tanning activities, insufficient sun protection, rates of skin cancer, and rates of melanoma skin cancer have continued to escalate worldwide. It is important to work with a unified approach, adequate support, and comprehensive and communitywide struggles to eliminate this cancer. Through this kind of commitment and coordination, there can be an achievement in the significant reduction of illness, death rates, and healthcare costs.

Variants of Skin Cancer

Skin cancer is typically assembled into non-melanoma (NMSC) and melanoma (MM). NMSC is further divided into squamous cell carcinoma (SCC) and basal cell carcinoma (BCC). Both types of carcinomas advance from the epidermis and contribute 25% and 70%, correspondingly [5].

The (NMSCs) non-melanoma skin cancers include basal cell carcinoma (BCC), which is the most common human cancer in white people. Non-melanoma skin cancer is most commonly diagnosed in men instead of women, and its chances increase with growing age [7]. In the year 2017, there were almost 24.5 million occurrences of cancer cases globally (16.8 million cases without non-melanoma skin cancer (NMSC) and 9.6 million cases of cancer expiries [8].

Melanoma is a destructive malignancy that emerges from the unrestrained division of melanocytes. It contributes to the greater part of skin cancer deaths [9]. A study illustrated that 1% deaths (3000/ annum) were caused by skin cancer in Germany in both men and women, out of which 80% deaths were caused by melanoma cancer [10].

Melanocytes are neural apex-derived pigment cells that are inherent at the dermal–epidermal interface and make straight contact with just about 20–30 keratinocytes *via* the nerve, for instance, dendritic projections. Melanocytes protect the keratinocytes from UV radiation *via* the amalgamation of the melanin polymer in particular organelles which are labelled as melanosomes and are shifted to related keratinocytes *via* the dendritic processes. Malignant alteration of melanocytes gives intensification to the most violent form of skin cancer, melanoma [1]. Fig. (**1**) demonstrates the types of skin cancer.

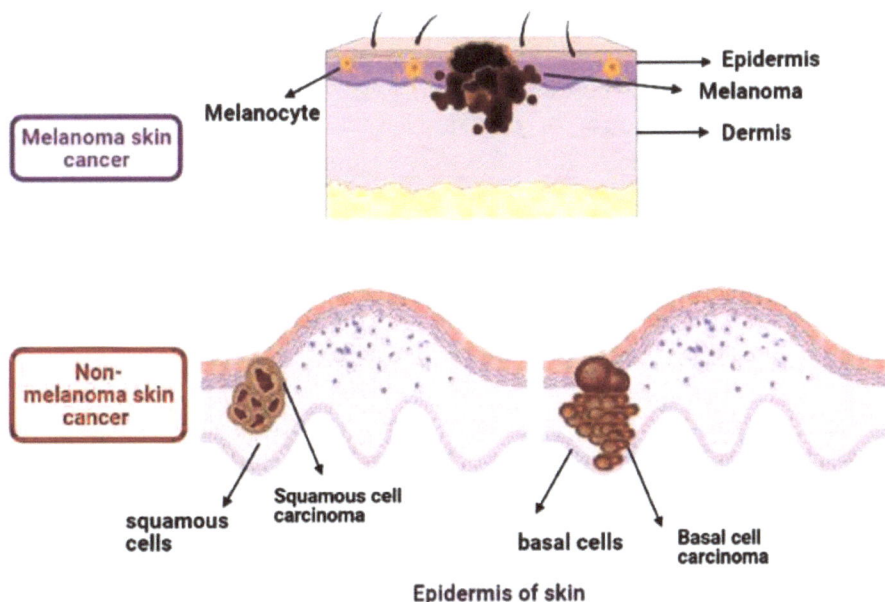

Fig. (1). Variants of skin cancer.

Non-melanoma type of skin cancer has the maximum occurrence in the global population, but its mortality rate is very less, and the patient can recover in a short time if diagnosed at an early stage. On the other hand, in relation to nationwide data on epidemiology, melanoma (MM) skin cancer is expected to symbolize just 3% of the malignant neoplasm while brutally disturbing the quality of life, which leads to metastases and eventually death [2].

Risk Factors

A Lighter Natural Skin Color

The most important environmental risk factor is the vulnerable coverage of fair skin people from the sun: irregular extreme exposure, cumulative lifetime exposure for SCC, predominantly during infancy and puberty, for basal cell carcinoma (BCC). The prevalence of both BCC and SCC has been gradually increasing universally through the past sixty years, especially in countries where fair-skinned inhabitants are predominant. Great risk backgrounds where people with lighter skin tones are comparatively at great risk of skin cancer comprising entertaining localities like gardens, parks, sports grounds, swimming pools and beaches [11].

People with fair to olive skin need some minutes of mid-morning or afternoon sun exposure to the arms, hands, and face (or correspondent part of the skin) to accomplish satisfactory levels of vitamin D from the month of September to April. In months of winter, such as from May to August, people having fair to olive skin need just 2–3 hours of mid-day sun contact throughout the week. People with a naturally darker skin tone may require up to 3–6 times more sun exposure than people with fair skin to level vitamin D [12]. Skin cancer has the most vulnerable phenotype (fair-colored eyes, hair, or skin) as a risk factor for skin cancer (for example, people with comparatively fair skin tone are more exposed to skin cancer) [2].

Skin that Burns, Freckles, Reddens Easily, or Becomes Painful in the Sun

Sunburn was more prevalent among individuals with an education of 10 to 12 years and among persons taking part in deliberated tanning activities like sunbed use, sunny vacations and sunbathing [13]. Although sunlight is advantageous to human health, solar exposure can be a source of harmful radiation. UVB is the most detrimental wavelength for keratinocyte DNA and it is considered a total hazard. This type of radiation is accountable for the sunburn reaction and photocarcinogenesis and this radiation constitutes the growth of skin cancers stimulated by UVR. Most of these damages are produced by indirect or direct photosensitive responses, which encourage DNA breaking and base destruction, becoming fatal and mutagenic [14]. Activities for sun protection have been considerably greater than before because of the introduction of skin cancer campaigns all over the world. Sunburn incidences, the percentage of intentional tanning and unprotected skin have also dropped over time [15]. For a number of years, New Zealand has depended on introducing sun defensing activities from Australia and using Australian skin cancer investigation to lead the health policy and promotion course on the statement that its developments of melanoma would reflect those in Australia. The first skin cancer prevention campaign in New Zealand began during the mid of 1980s, and in 1987 this transformed to a bigger stress on melanoma specific inhibition. In New Zealand, the leading skin cancer prevention campaign, called, 'Slip! Slop! Slap!' took place during the mid-1980s but this reformed in 1987 to a greater intensive message on prevention of melanoma [16].

Older Age

Universally, the chances of emerging cancer through a lifespan (ages 0-79 years) were 1 out of 4 for women and 1 out of 3 for men. In New Zealand, mortality due to melanoma considerably decreased in women of 15–34 ($p = 0.009$) and 35–44 years of age ($p = 0.04$), with insignificant change in women aged 45–64 years, and increased in women with 65 or more years of age ($p < 0.001$) from 1968–72 to 2003–07. In Australia, on the other hand, over the same time, the female mortality rate of melanoma has declined significantly in 3 youngest age groups (15–34 years, $p < 0.001$; 35–44 years, $p < 0.001$; and 45–64 years, $p = 0.008$), but increased expressively for women with age of 65 or more years ($p < 0.001$) [8].

A report of the annual melanoma death rate from Australia, established from 1931 to 2002, showed that mortality rates were highest in 1985 but considerably declined after 1985 in individuals aged less than 55 years and became stable at the age of 55–79 years [16]. Although skin cancer can occur at any age, it is most prevalent after 40 [4], and unnecessary exposure to UV rays before 18 years of age is a risk factor, similar to regular visits to tanning salons or sunbathing [2].

In Germany, the prevalence of melanoma in people with the age of more than 30 is just over 10 per 100,000, but it rises to about 70 in every 100,000 populations in people over 70 years of age. Till the age of 55 years, women have particularly higher rates of melanoma illness. However, this relationship is contrary in men above 55 years. Therefore, melanoma is cultivated in women with an average age of 60 years, prior to men with an average age of 66 years [10].

Ultraviolet Radiation Exposure

Skin malignant growth is the most well-known sort of disease. Since the skin is the biggest organ in the body, it also serves as the first line of defense against infections. Indeed, most skin-related harms are an immediate after-effect of contact with the UV radiation in the daylight. Overexposure to the UV- radiations can cause DNA harm in skin cells, bringing about uncontrolled development, cell expansion, and eventually malignancy [17]. The main reasons for developing skin cancer include needless exposure to the UV- radiation and harmful chemicals such as artificial foundations like sun beds. Although regular exposure to the sun maintains a healthy level of vitamin D in the body, sun protection is a major need for skin cancer prevention [12].

Undoubtedly, exposure to ultraviolet radiation is the most substantial cause of developing melanoma and non-melanoma skin carcinomas. Foundations of UV radiation include the sun (most commonly) and internal tanning equipment. WHO has recognized the exposure to UV- radiation both from the sun as well as the cancer-causing tanning beds [2].

The prevalence rate of skin disease exceptionally relies upon skin appearance and geographic dissimilarities, which characterizes the measure of UV radiation. A few components, including ethnic and geographic variety, should be viewed as important factors while concluding data related to skin diseases [18].

The harming impacts of UV- radiation on the skin have been broadly recorded. The harmful effects include scars on skin, allergy to light, hyperpigmentation, photoaging, damage to the skin and skin cancer. The most important preventive approaches used widely comprise clothing that can provide protection against UV-rays, change in adaptive behavior and sunscreens usage. Although numerous genetic and phenotypic risk factors have been acknowledged throughout the literature, the main casual factor remains sun exposure, specifically ultraviolet (UV) radiation; UV radiation has been publicized to exert a direct magnetic effect, emphasizing its part in melanoma pathogenesis [6].

The Incidence of Skin Cancer and Mortality Across the Globe

Incidence

The methods that measure the factors such as age and gender for particular cancer in a specific country can be grouped into the following broad categories:

- The 2018 (national) national event estimates were reviewed.
- Recent event estimates (national or regional) were applied to the 2018 population (50 countries), which signposted that prices were based on the national mortality model, using the number of event deaths at cancer registration centers in 14 countries.
- Cases were estimated from national mortality rates by modeling through using the death rates by stages of cancer registration in neighboring countries (37 countries).
- The rate of national incidences of national and gender-related cases of all combined cancers was determined on the basis of results from neighboring countries. These standards were categorized to determine the national incidence of specific sites using the most commonly cancer-related data (7 countries).
- Estimated evaluations of those from selected neighboring countries (32 countries) [19]. The incidence of skin cancer among different continents is shown in Fig. (**2**).

Mortality

The methods that are used to measure the mortality rates in people of different ages with sexually transmitted cancer in a particular country fall into the following broad categories priority-wise:

- It was anticipated that national mortality rates would be considered in 2018 (81 countries).
- The latest national mortality rate applied to the people of 2018 (20 countries.

- Estimated estimates from corresponding national models used death rates based on cancer records in neighboring countries (81 countries). Estimated ratings of those were from selected neighboring countries (3 countries) [20, 21]. The incidence and mortality rates among different continents are demonstrated in Table **1**.

HDI (Human Development Index)

The factor HDI is the cumulative result of indices of three dimensions: longevity, level of study, and dominance in the necessary sources of balanced health. All groups and regions, with significant progress in all aspects of HDI, have developed much faster as compared to lower or middle HDI countries. As this guide points out, the world is unequal because the national scale hides a lot of differences in human life.

There is an outpouring of inequality in the northern and southern provinces. Economic inequality has risen within all countries and also among many other countries as well [19, 22].

Table 1. **Predictable incidence and mortality rates for skin cancer around the world in 2018 [19].**

Countries	Melanoma of Skin Cancer						Non-Melanoma Skin Cancer						HDI
	Incidence (ASR)			Mortality (ASR)			Incidence (ASR)			Mortality (ASR)			
	M	F	Total	M	F	Total	M	F	Total	M	F	Total	
ASIA	-	-	-	-	-	-	-	-	-	-	-	-	-
Afghanistan	0.3	0.3	0.3	0.2	0.2	0.2	1.4	1.3	1.4	0.7	0.5	0.6	0.479
China	0.4	0.3	0.4	0.2	0.1	0.2	1.1	0.9	1.0	0.5	0.4	0.5	0.738
India	0.2	0.3	0.2	0.2	0.1	0.2	0.9	0.7	0.8	0.5	0.3	0.4	0.624
Pakistan	0.3	0.2	0.3	0.2	0.2	0.2	2.1	1.7	1.9	1.1	0.6	0.8	0.55
Japan	0.6	0.6	0.6	0.2	0.2	0.2	2.1	1.2	1.6	0.2	0.2	0.2	0.903
Korea Republic of	0.7	0.7	0.7	0.1	0.3	0.3	2.4	2.4	2.4	0.2	0.2	0.2	0.901
AFRICA	-	-	-	-	-	-	-	-	-	-	-	-	-
Nigeria	0.5	0.7	0.6	0.4	0.5	0.4	3.1	1.8	2.5	2.3	0.9	1.6	0.527
South Africa	2.9	1.9	2.2	1.5	0.8	1.1	17.4	7.5	11.3	1.5	0.8	1.0	0.666
Kenya	0.6	1.9	1.3	0.4	1.2	0.8	2.5	3.6	3.1	2.1	1.8	1.9	0.555
Ethiopia	0.4	0.1	0.2	0.3	0.1	0.2	1.6	3.4	2.6	1.2	1.7	1.5	0.448
Sudan	0.5	0.5	0.5	0.3	0.3	0.3	1.8	1.7	1.7	1.2	1.1	1.1	0.49
OCEANIA	-	-	-	-	-	-	-	-	-	-	-	-	-

(Table 1) cont.....

Countries	Melanoma of Skin Cancer						Non-Melanoma Skin Cancer						HDI
	Incidence (ASR)			Mortality (ASR)			Incidence (ASR)			Mortality (ASR)			
	M	F	Total	M	F	Total	M	F	Total	M	F	Total	
Fiji	0.3	1.3	0.9	0	0	0	1.3	1.0	1.1	0	0.4	0.2	0.736
New Zealand	**35.8**	**31.1**	**33.3**	**7.2**	**2.8**	**4.8**	**205.1**	**77.0**	**138.4**	**1.8**	**0.7**	**1.2**	**0.915**
Papua New Guinea	3.3	3.8	3.6	1.0	0.7	0.8	15.0	12.0	13.3	9.5	5.5	7.2	0.516
Samoa	0.0	0	0	2.4	0	1.2	0	0	0	0	0	0	0.704
NORTH AMERICA	-	-	-	-	-	-	-	-	-	-	-	-	-
United States of America	14.9	11.0	12.7	2.0	0.9	1.7	78.9	36.8	55.8	1.0	0.3	0.6	0.92
Canada	13.4	11.7	12.4	2.3	1.0	1.6	62.3	36.8	48.5	0.9	0.3	0.5	0.92
Jamaica	0.2	0.2	0.2	0.1	0.1	0.1	2.5	1.5	2.0	0.1	0.1	0.1	0.73
Mexico	2.1	2.3	2.2	0.6	0.4	0.5	6.7	5.0	5.8	0.9	0.6	0.7	0.762
SOUTH AMERICA	-	-	-	-	-	-	-	-	-	-	-	-	-
Argentina	3.8	2.2	2.9	1.4	0.6	0.9	7.9	4.2	5.7	0.9	0.3	0.5	0.827
Bolivia	2.0	3.3	2.7	0.7	0.9	0.8	4.0	3.0	3.5	0.8	0.6	0.7	0.674
Chile	2.7	2.4	2.5	1.0	0.6	0.8	9.8	5.3	7.3	1.2	0.4	0.7	0.847
Colombia	3.4	3.2	3.3	1.1	0.7	0.9	9.6	6.2	7.7	1.2	0.5	0.8	0.727
Brazil	2.9	2.8	2.8	1.0	0.6	0.8	14.5	9.1	11.4	1.2	0.6	0.8	0.754
AUSTRALIA	**40.4**	**27.5**	**33.6**	**4.3**	**2.2**	**3.2**	**233.8**	**64.7**	**147.5**	**2.0**	**0.5**	**1.2**	**0.939**
EUROPE	-	-	-	-	-	-	-	-	-	-	-	-	-
Germany	19.6	24.0	21.6	2.1	1.3	1.6	36.9	20.4	27.5	0.4	0.2	0.3	0.926
France	14.4	12.9	13.6	2.1	1.2	1.6	29.8	14.1	21.1	0.5	0.3	0.2	0.897
Italy	14.0	11.0	12.4	2.1	1.1	1.6	19.2	9.1	13.6	0.6	0.2	0.4	0.887
UK	15.0	15.3	15.0	2.3	1.3	1.8	33.2	14.1	22.8	0.6	0.2	0.4	0.909
Switzerland	23.4	19.5	21.3	2.7	1.2	1.9	55.1	35.6	44.4	0.6	0.2	0.4	0.939
ANTARCTICA	This is an ice land with no population.												

Table 2. Estimated new skin cancer cases and deaths by sex, United States, 2019 [23].

	Estimated New Cases			Estimated New Deaths		
-	Both Sexes	Male	Female	Both Sexes	Male	Female
Skin (excluding basal and squamous)	104,350	62,320	42,030	11,650	8,030	3,620
Melanoma of skin	96,480	57,220	39,260	7,230	4,740	2,490
Other non-epithelial skin	7,870	5,100	2,770	4,420	3,290	1,130

The non-melanoma type skin cancer incidence rate was reported highest in Australia, North America, and Eastern and Western Europe. Melanoma skin cancer incidence rate continued to increase in US and worldwide. The estimated new deaths and cases in the US are illustrated in Table **2**. The mortality rates came out to be higher in males as compared to females, as they were found more stable. Besides this, many other outcomes for skin cancer death were reported, such as health status prior to disease development and lifestyle habits [24].

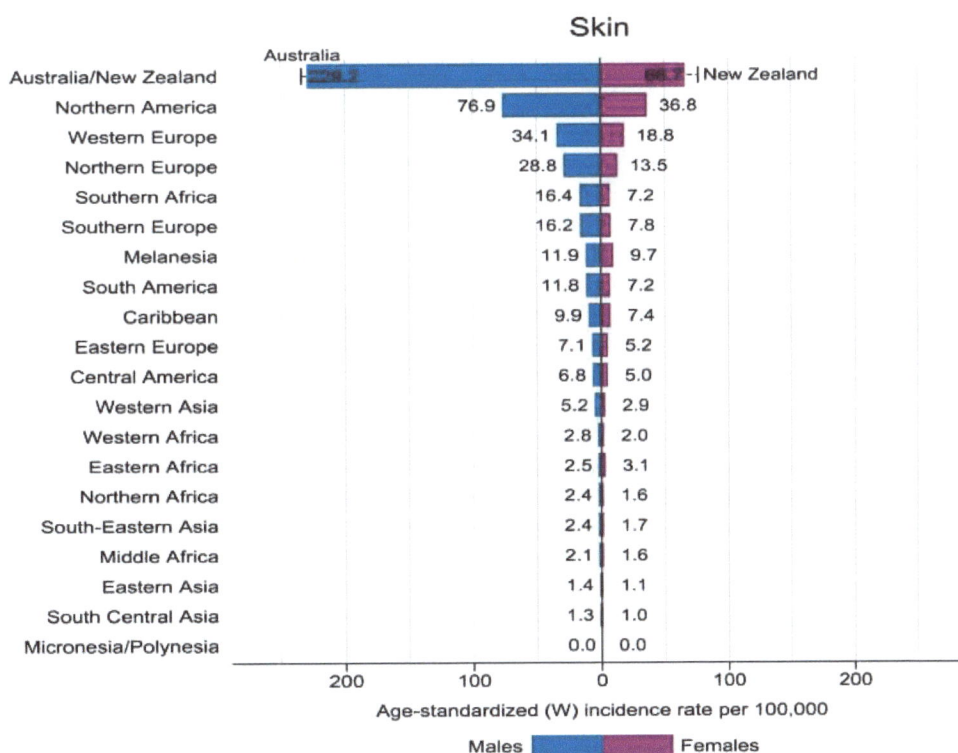

Fig. (2). Bar chart showing the incidence of skin cancer among different continents in descending order [20].

Health System Costs

Economic assessments were conducted in 2015 by using a number of methods, including cost-effectiveness, cost analysis, a variety of methods ('public', 'health sector', 'third party sponsor') and counter-analysis of cancer findings between 1982 and 2011. Outcomes include 'preventable cases', 'preventable deaths', and 'planned years of life'. On the global economy, the cost-benefit analysis, like the effects of productivity, was performed [15] with an additional $ AUD 0.16 ($ USD 0.12) per person on future skin cancer prevention throughout Australia, 140,000 skin cancer cases will be prevented over a 20-year period (2011 to 2030). Depending on the perspective and learning method, an improved system can be more powerful (both health benefits and costs) or more expensive (lower health benefits). The return on investment (ROI) was $ AUD 3.20 per dollar invested, with a total public benefit of $ AUD 1.43 billion [15].

The effort provided strong economic evidence for practicing prevention approaches for skin cancer. A good case analysis gives a significant standard for other countries to develop their skin cancer prevention programs, funding, and design [15].

The estimated annual cost of treating skin cancer in South Africa was ZAR 92.4 million (2015) (or US $ 15.7 million). Sensitivity analysis showed that the total amount may vary between ZAR 89.7 to 94.6 million (US $ 15.2 to $ 16.1 million) when melanoma-related variables were reversed and between ZAR 78.4 to 113.5 million ($ 13.3 to $ 19.3 million) when no melanoma-related changes were reversed [25].

Skin Cancer Prevention and Control Strategies

The circumvention of diseases is coined as prevention. To maintain a good health at older ages, measures have been taken to prevent ailments that play a critical role in health promotion and early diagnosis of diseases. Taking into account the approaches for disease prevention, not only the quality of life and life span prospect of the individual is upgraded, but also the community expense systems are also replaced [26]. The prevention encompasses three main strategies:

Primary Prevention of Skin Cancer (Avoiding the Development of Diseases)

The primary prevention approach makes use of the perception to avoid the behavior that can prove risky for skin cancer development, such as the insight into the dangers associated with UV rays exposure and knowledge about proper handling of UV radiation for both natural as well as artificial UV rays [26]. Some of the preventive measures that were taken to reduce the risk of getting skin cancer are as follows:

- The regular use of creams that provide UV protection.
- Reduction in outdoor activities from 11-16 O'clock so as to avoid UV rays exposure.
- The regular use of UV- protective clothing while going outside, staying under the shade and minimal or no visits to tanning parlors.

People under 30 years of age are advised not to use tanning beds, as 43- 76% of the risk for acquiring melanoma is evident with the usage of these beds [27].

Secondary Prevention of Skin Cancer (Early Detection and Treatment of Diseases)

The secondary prevention strategy focuses on self-examination and medical advice consultation. This strategy is encouraged to be followed in the areas where it is less commonly found. The awareness and proper guidance on the preliminary identification of signs of skin cancer are important for reducing the prognosis of the disease as the disease prognosis goes in parallel with the stage of cancer. Secondary prevention is highly related to screening [6].

Tertiary Prevention of Skin Cancer (Prevention of Progression and Complications)

Tertiary prevention emphasizes follow-up visits to the doctor if the patient has skin cancer prior with the objective of a preliminary diagnosis for the reoccurrence of the disease. The recommended follow-up examinations are clinical checkups and laboratory diagnostics regularly. The first three years after the incidence of the disease is a crucial time period for the reoccurrence of skin cancer, as 80% of cases confirmed the scenario [26]. Fig. (**3**) illustrates the various approaches for skin cancer prevention.

Control Strategies

The adaptation of behavioral changes and utilization of extracts that are light protective can control the increased number of skin cancer cases all around the globe. The UV radiation that evokes the body to show inflammatory responses is highly reduced using *Polypodium leucotomos* extracts. Moreover, the extract quickens the elimination of the photo products that were produced as a result of UV ray- exposure, and a decrease in the risk for DNA mutations takes place, which exerts protective effects that are beneficial for the prevention of skin cancer. Topical sunscreens are most commonly used for creating a shield for the skin to avoid UV- induced skin damage [28].

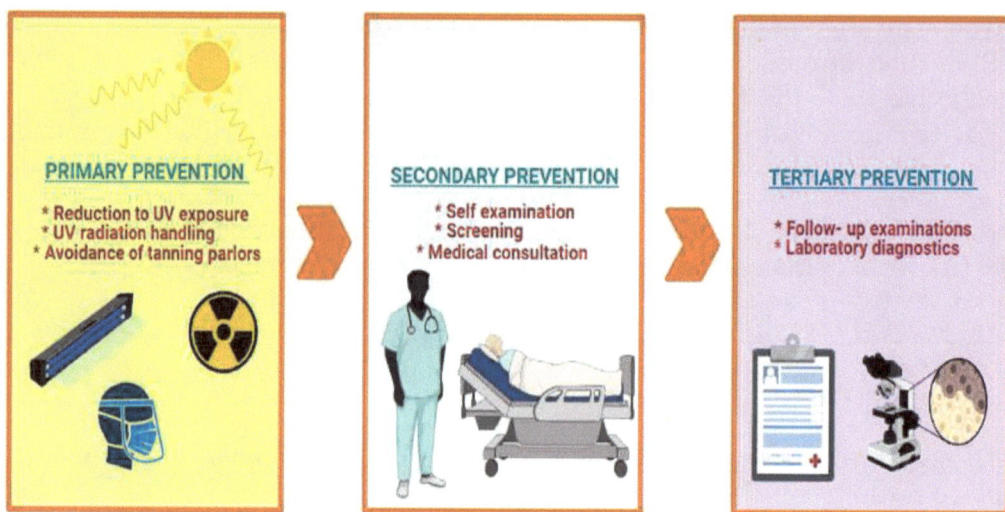

Fig. (3). Approaches for prevention of skin cancer.

For the previous several decades, public health movements have gained a lot of attention as they raise wakefulness in the general public about the consequences of excessive sun exposure and skin cancer protection strategies. Australia conducted a huge skin cancer prevention programme named Australia's Sun Smart programme which was a long-standing and multi-focused community-wide awareness campaign [29].

Treatment Through Natural Therapeutics-Nutraceuticals

Chemotherapy, radiotherapy and surgery are the few treatment options that are practiced for cancer patients. Unfortunately, these treatment strategies pose some serious risks to the well-being of the person and badly affect the quality of life. Subsequently, the natural herbal and plant extracts utilization proved to be a safer treatment for patients with skin, prostrate, lungs and other types of cancers. These medicines are termed natural therapeutics or nutraceuticals, which are natural active products that exert therapeutic effects for the promotion of better health and avoidance of wide-scale diseases [17]. Alkaloids, flavonoids, polyphenolics, sesquiterpenes and terpenoids altogether, known by the name phytochemicals, are therapeutic constituents of various medicinal plants, vegetables and fruits that exert effects by their anti-cancer properties [30].

Kaempferol-with Anti-Cancer Potential

Kaempferol, an aglycone flavonoid also known as tetrahydroxyflavone, is a chemical compound with a yellow hue. The four hydroxyl groups are placed at positions 3, 5, 7 and 40 [31]. The most common sources of Kaempferol are the parts of plants such as leaves, seeds, fruits, flowers and vegetables [32]. Kaempferol and its glycosylated derivatives are well-known for showing anti-inflammatory, antitumor, anticancer, apoptotic and antimicrobial activities in the human body.

Kaempferol and the byproducts released by the reaction of glycosyl donor and hydroxyl group are important for initiating various physiological activities in the human body, such as reduction in inflammation, inhibition of tumor growth, initiation of programmed cell death, and halting bacterial growth [33]. Various signaling pathways are targeted by the chemical for the inhibition of tumor growth. The development of skin cancer due to solar UV- radiations targets the Ribosomal S6 Kinase 1 RSK1 and Mitogen as well as Stress Activated protein Kinase 1 MSK1. RSK2 and MSK1 targeted skin cancer in a mouse model, and both significantly inhibited skin cancer development due to UV- exposure [34].

Magnolol-Prevention and Treatment of Cancer

Chinese and Japanese herbal plants such as *Magnolia officinalis*, *Magnolia obovata* and *Magnolia grandiflora* are essential plants because of holding massive medicinal properties. Magnolol (MAG) which is the bioactive chemical obtained from the roots, stem and bark of the Magnolia tree, is hydroxylated biphenyl. MAG reveals various biological activities as it initiates a reduction in inflammation, prevents fat development in arteries and inhibits oxidation. MAG controls cell survival, cell endurance, cell growth, spread of cancer to other parts of the body and new blood vessel development. MAG prevents the resistance against chemotherapy for various types of cancers by directly regulating the signaling pathways [35]. The long non-coding RNA for factor growth arrest-specific 5 (GAS5) is overexpressed by MAG, which upregulates it to induce the programmed cell death [36]. Further, MAG treatment can prevent chemically and UVB-induced skin cancer by inducing apoptosis.

The UVB- induced skin carcinogenesis is prevented by MAG treatment by initiating apoptosis- the programmed cell death [37]. MAG works by enhancing caspases-3,-8,-9 activities, changing the expression of factor, named as mitochondrial protein Bcl-2, which is anti-apoptotic through reducing the expression of pro-apoptotic factor Bax when the human malignant skin cancer A375-S2 cell line was exposed to MAG treatment which consequently repressed the cell growth [38]. The studies conducted on *in vivo* treatment of MAG on various animal models demonstrated that it repressed the cancer development, initiated apoptosis and stopped the cell cycle at G2/M phase [35].

Honokiol-Potent at Oncogenic Targets

Magnolia officinalis, *Magnolia obovate*, and *Magnolia grandiflora* are recognized as potential medicinal plants that release Honokiol (HNKL) from their bark and leaves. Honokiol is a biphenolic chemical compound that acts against a variety of tumors such as lung, skin, prostate, breast, gall bladder and colon. The *in vitro* and *in vivo* studies confirmed the anti-tumorigenic property of HNKL [39]. Like other therapeutic agents, HNKL treatment induces apoptosis in the skin cancer cells through a variety of ways, such as the activation of caspases and mitochondrial release of Cyt-c. HNKL down-regulates the cyclin-D1, mTOR and Akt phosphorylation levels in the cell which leads to cell cycle arrest. γ-secretase complex protein expression is also inhibited by HNKL [40, 41].

Noth-2 signaling pathway induces cellular proliferation and multiplication and inhibits apoptosis or programmed cell death. HNKL treatment suppressed the Notch-2 signalling pathway and initiated apoptosis in melanoma stem cells [42]. In a study that was conducted to see the synergistic effects of HNKL, magnolol and α-santalol were given in combination to the human epidermoid carcinoma A431 cells. HNKL altered cell viability and cell duplication and significantly enhanced the rate of apoptosis [37].

Black Salve-An Escharotic

Black salve is prepared by adding innocuous elements to zinc chloride or bloodroot (*Sanguinaria canadensis*). The ingredients make it a corrosive agent that extensively damages healthy and unhealthy or diseased tissue. This, when applied topically, forms a scar called eschar (dead tissue) as a result. Sanguinarine is more potent as it possesses a differential response for the non-melanoma skin cancer and the epidermal keratinocytes. Black salve is now widely marketed as an eschortic for the skin cancer treatment [43]. As black salve destroys both the normal and pathological tissues, patients may remain confuse clinical clearance of skin cancer with histological clearance. Black salve treatment leaves a person in confusion about the clearance of skin cancer and histological clearance as it indiscriminately damages the healthy and pathological tissues alike. As salve has many damaging effects to skin hence it's never considered a choice for primary treatment of skin cancer [44].

Pomegranate-A Potent Natural Therapeutic

Pomegranate fruit extract (PFE), pomegranate juice (PJ), and pomegranate seed oil (PSO) have been tested in cell culture, reconstituted human skin models, animal models of skin cancer and exhibit immense potential for preventing UVB-induced skin cancer.

The pomegranate fruit and its derivatives, such as juice, extracts and pomegranate seed oil, are believed to be a chemotherapeutic agent that targets various signaling pathways, evokes inhibition of inflammation, decreases cell growth, and controls the inhibition for tumor development. Pomegranate and its derivatives (PFE, PJ, and PSO) are widely tested in cell culture labs and showed vast potential for the prevention of skin cancer growth and development, especially the UVB- induced skin cancer [45].

Furthermore, the fruit extract of pomegranate also inhibits the addition of phosphate groups in the MAPK pathway in the human epidermal cells [46]. Fruit extract of pomegranate was also found to be inhibitory for the NFκB (nuclear factor kappa B), whose activation is mediated by UVB. Consequently, the phosphorylation of IκBα is reduced, the IκBα protein gets stabilized, and the stimulation of the IKKα factor is reduced [45].

Euphorbiaceae

Euphorbiaceae is the third main genus of flower-producing plants with nearly 2000 species and highly diversified in its habitat and growth forms. In Australia, people practice to apply the sap of *Euphorbia peplus L.* as a home treatment for curing skin cancer [47].

Curcumin

Curcumin, a bright yellow chemical compound, is a bioactive compound that targets various pathways. Curcumin selectively prevents the activation of COX-2 and prostaglandin production. These factors up-regulate the AMPK (activated protein kinases), which consequently suppresses COX-2 production. Moreover, it activates the p53 gene, which is a renowned anti-oncogenic element that subsequently initiates apoptotic activity in the cells. Furthermore, curcumin accumulates ceramide, a lipid molecule that implicates various biological activities such as programmed cell death, cell transformation and aging. Curcumin also overexpresses the gene that encodes TRAIL, which is a receptor for apoptosis. The chemical also inhibits the NF-κB, which in turn also up-regulates TRAIL [48].

Hypericum Perforatum L. – A Photomedicine

Hypericin- a Photosensitizer obtained from *Hypericum perforatum L* is significant in clinical settings for Photodynamic therapy. It is an extract that initiates the inhibition of new blood vessel development and the spread of cancer to other parts of the body by altering the intracellular pathways. In an *in vitro* experimental setting for detecting the response mechanism for melanoma and non-melanoma cells for human culture, the dose-specific treatment of hypericin-PDT indicated the killing of the cells by initiating programmed cell death. The melanoma cells were more responsive to initiating cell death mechanisms in a dose-dependent manner of hypericin [49].

CONCLUSION

Skin cancer is the biggest threat to global advancement. The rising cases and mortality across the globe pose to be a risk for economic stability as health system costs put a huge burden on the nations. The disease is highly prevalent in New Zealand and Australia and significantly lower in Asian countries. The predicted new cases can be controlled by adopting some prevention approaches and control strategies, including wearing sunscreens, medical consultation, screening and reducing UV exposure. Due to potential aftereffects of surgery, chemotherapy and radiography, natural therapeutics such as plant extracts, herbs and nutraceuticals are generally used worldwide. They evoke physiological responses by altering the signaling pathways, initiating apoptosis, decreasing cell growth and proliferation, and reducing the inflammation in the body.

REFERENCES

[1]   Yin K, Smith AG. Nuclear receptor function in skin health and disease: therapeutic opportunities in the orphan and adopted receptor classes. Cell Mol Life Sci 2016; 73(20): 3789-800.
        [http://dx.doi.org/10.1007/s00018-016-2329-4] [PMID: 27544210]

[2]   McWhirter JE, Hoffman-Goetz L. Skin deep: Coverage of skin cancer and recreational tanning in Canadian women's magazines (2000–2012). Can J Public Health 2015; 106(4): e236-43.
        [http://dx.doi.org/10.17269/cjph.106.4795] [PMID: 26285196]

[3]   Miolo N, Rodrigues RF, Silva ERD, Piati PK, Campagnolo OA, Marques LF. Skin cancer incidence in rural workers at a reference hospital in western Paraná. An Bras Dermatol 2019; 94(2): 157-63.
        [http://dx.doi.org/10.1590/abd1806-4841.20197335] [PMID: 31090820]

[4]   Ijaz S, Akhtar N, Khan MS, *et al.* Plant derived anticancer agents: A green approach towards skin cancers. Biomed Pharmacother 2018; 103: 1643-51.
        [http://dx.doi.org/10.1016/j.biopha.2018.04.113] [PMID: 29864953]

[5]   Iqbal J, Abbasi BA, Ahmad R, *et al.* Potential phytochemicals in the fight against skin cancer: Current landscape and future perspectives. Biomed Pharmacother 2019; 109: 1381-93.
        [http://dx.doi.org/10.1016/j.biopha.2018.10.107] [PMID: 30551389]

[6]   Seité S, del Marmol V, Moyal D, Friedman AJ. Public primary and secondary skin cancer prevention, perceptions and knowledge: an international cross☐sectional survey. J Eur Acad Dermatol Venereol 2017; 31(5): 815-20.

[http://dx.doi.org/10.1111/jdv.14104] [PMID: 28045207]

[7]   Newlands C, Currie R, Memon A, Whitaker S, Woolford T. Non-melanoma skin cancer: United
        Kingdom National Multidisciplinary Guidelines. J Laryngol Otol 2016; 130(S2): S125-32.
        [http://dx.doi.org/10.1017/S0022215116000554] [PMID: 27841126]

[8]   Fitzmaurice C, Allen C, Baber RM, *et al.* Global burden of disease cancer collaboration. global,
        regional, and national cancer incidence, mortality, years of life lost, years lived with disability, and
        disability-adjusted life-years for 32 cancer groups, 1990 to 2015: a systematic analysis for the global
        burden of disease study. JAMA Oncol 2017; 3(4): 524-48.
        [http://dx.doi.org/10.1001/jamaoncol.2016.5688] [PMID: 27918777]

[9]   Parashar K, Sood S, Mehaidli A, *et al.* Evaluating the anti-cancer efficacy of a synthetic curcumin
        analog on human melanoma cells and its interaction with standard chemotherapeutics. Molecules
        2019; 24(13): 2483.
        [http://dx.doi.org/10.3390/molecules24132483] [PMID: 31284561]

[10]   Kornek T, Augustin M. Skin cancer prevention. J Dtsch Dermatol Ges 2013; 11(4): 283-98.
        [http://dx.doi.org/10.1111/ddg.12066] [PMID: 23574893]

[11]   Wright CY, du Preez DJ, Millar DA, Norval M. The epidemiology of skin cancer and public health
        strategies for its prevention in southern africa. Int J Environ Res Public Health 2020; 17(3): 1017.
        [http://dx.doi.org/10.3390/ijerph17031017] [PMID: 32041101]

[12]   Scully M, Makin J, Maloney S, Wakefield M. Changes in coverage of sun protection in the news:
        threats and opportunities from emerging issues. Health Educ Res 2014; 29(3): 378-87.
        [http://dx.doi.org/10.1093/her/cyu013] [PMID: 24650946]

[13]   Køster B, Meyer M, Andersson T, Engholm G, Dalum P. Development in sunburn 2007–2015 and
        skin cancer projections 2007–2040 of campaign results in the Danish population. Medicine
        (Baltimore) 2018; 97(41): e12738.
        [http://dx.doi.org/10.1097/MD.0000000000012738] [PMID: 30313078]

[14]   Coutinho RCS, Santos AFD, Costa JGD, Vanderlei AD. Sun exposure, skin lesions and vitamin D
        production: evaluation in a population of fishermen. An Bras Dermatol 2019; 94(3): 279-286.
        [http://dx.doi.org/10.1590/abd1806-4841.20197201] [PMID: 31365655]

[15]   Shih STF, Carter R, Sinclair C, Mihalopoulos C, Vos T. Economic evaluation of skin cancer
        prevention in Australia. Prev Med 2009; 49(5): 449-53.
        [http://dx.doi.org/10.1016/j.ypmed.2009.09.008] [PMID: 19747936]

[16]   Sneyd MJ, Cox B. A comparison of trends in melanoma mortality in New Zealand and Australia: the
        two countries with the highest melanoma incidence and mortality in the world. BMC Cancer 2013;
        13(1): 372.
        [http://dx.doi.org/10.1186/1471-2407-13-372] [PMID: 23915380]

[17]   Sreedhar A, Li J, Zhao Y. Next-gen therapeutics for skin cancer: nutraceuticals. nutr cancer 2018;
        70(5): 697-709.
        [http://dx.doi.org/10.1080/01635581.2018.1470651] [PMID: 29764209]

[18]   Park E, Lee Y, Jue MS. Hydrochlorothiazide use and the risk of skin cancer in patients with
        hypertensive disorder: a nationwide retrospective cohort study from Korea. Korean J Intern Med
        (Korean Assoc Intern Med) 2020; 35(4): 917-28.
        [http://dx.doi.org/10.3904/kjim.2019.218] [PMID: 31842528]

[19]   Khazaei Z, Ghorat F, Jarrahi AM, Adineh HA, Sohrabivafa M, Goodarzi E. Global incidence and
        mortality of skin cancer by histological subtype and its relationship with the human development index
        (HDI); an ecology study in 2018. World Can Res J 2019; 6: e1265.
        [http://dx.doi.org/10.32113/wcrj_20194_1265]

[20]   Bray F, Ferlay J, Soerjomataram I, Siegel RL, Torre LA, Jemal A. Global cancer statistics 2018:
        GLOBOCAN estimates of incidence and mortality worldwide for 36 cancers in 185 countries. CA

Cancer J Clin 2018; 68(6): 394-424.
[http://dx.doi.org/10.3322/caac.21492] [PMID: 30207593]

[21] McGuire S. World Cancer Report 2014. Geneva, Switzerland: World Health Organization, International Agency for Research on Cancer, WHO Press, 2015. Adv Nutr 2016; 7(2): 418-9.
[http://dx.doi.org/10.3945/an.116.012211] [PMID: 26980827]

[22] Bray F, Jemal A, Grey N, Ferlay J, Forman D. Global cancer transitions according to the Human Development Index (2008–2030): a population-based study. Lancet Oncol 2012; 13(8): 790-801.
[http://dx.doi.org/10.1016/S1470-2045(12)70211-5] [PMID: 22658655]

[23] Siegel RL, Miller KD, Jemal A. Cancer statistics, 2019. CA Cancer J Clin 2019; 69(1): 7-34.
[http://dx.doi.org/10.3322/caac.21551] [PMID: 30620402]

[24] Rundle CW, Militello M, Barber C, Presley CL, Rietcheck HR, Dellavalle RP. Epidemiologic burden of skin cancer in the US and worldwide. Curr Dermatol Rep 2020; 9(4): 309-22.
[http://dx.doi.org/10.1007/s13671-020-00311-4]

[25] Gordon LG, Elliott TM, Wright CY, Deghaye N, Visser W. Modelling the healthcare costs of skin cancer in South Africa. BMC Health Serv Res 2016; 16(1): 113.
[http://dx.doi.org/10.1186/s12913-016-1364-z] [PMID: 27039098]

[26] Kornek T, Augustin M. Skin cancer prevention. J Dtsch Dermatol Ges 2013; 11(4): 283-96.
[PMID: 23574893]

[27] Doré JF, Chignol MC. Tanning salons and skin cancer. Photochem Photobiol Sci 2012; 11(1): 30-7.
[http://dx.doi.org/10.1039/c1pp05186e] [PMID: 21845253]

[28] Zattra E, Coleman C, Arad S, *et al.* Polypodium leucotomos extract decreases UV-induced Cox-2 expression and inflammation, enhances DNA repair, and decreases mutagenesis in hairless mice. Am J Pathol 2009; 175(5): 1952-61.
[http://dx.doi.org/10.2353/ajpath.2009.090351] [PMID: 19808641]

[29] Tabbakh T, Volkov A, Wakefield M, Dobbinson S. Implementation of the SunSmart program and population sun protection behaviour in Melbourne, Australia: results from cross-sectional summer surveys from 1987 to 2017. PLoS Med 2019; 16(10): e1002932.
[http://dx.doi.org/10.1371/journal.pmed.1002932]

[30] Yang SF, Weng CJ, Sethi G, Hu DN. Natural bioactives and phytochemicals serve in cancer treatment and prevention. Evid Based Complement Alternat Med 2013; 2013: 1.
[http://dx.doi.org/10.1155/2013/698190] [PMID: 24454507]

[31] Li H, Ji HS, Kang JH, *et al.* Soy leaf extract containing kaempferol glycosides and pheophorbides improves glucose homeostasis by enhancing pancreatic β-cell function and suppressing hepatic lipid accumulation in db/db mice. J Agric Food Chem 2015; 63(32): 7198-210.
[http://dx.doi.org/10.1021/acs.jafc.5b01639] [PMID: 26211813]

[32] Imran M, Salehi B, Sharifi-Rad J, *et al.* Kaempferol: a key emphasis to its anticancer potential. Molecules 2019; 24(12): 2277.
[http://dx.doi.org/10.3390/molecules24122277] [PMID: 31248102]

[33] Calderón-Montaño JM, Burgos-Morón E, Pérez-Guerrero C, López-Lázaro M. A review on the dietary flavonoid kaempferol. Mini Rev Med Chem 2011; 11(4): 298-344.
[http://dx.doi.org/10.2174/138955711795305335] [PMID: 21428901]

[34] Yao K, Chen H, Liu K, *et al.* Kaempferol targets RSK2 and MSK1 to suppress UV radiation-induced skin cancer. Cancer Prev Res (Phila) 2014; 7(9): 958-67.
[http://dx.doi.org/10.1158/1940-6207.CAPR-14-0126] [PMID: 24994661]

[35] Ranaware A, Banik K, Deshpande V, *et al.* Magnolol: a Neolignan from the Magnolia family for the prevention and treatment of cancer. Int J Mol Sci 2018; 19(8): 2362.
[http://dx.doi.org/10.3390/ijms19082362] [PMID: 30103472]

[36] Wang TH, Chan CW, Fang JY, *et al.* 2-O-Methylmagnolol upregulates the long non-coding RNA, GAS5, and enhances apoptosis in skin cancer cells. Cell Death Dis 2017; 8(3): e2638.
[http://dx.doi.org/10.1038/cddis.2017.66] [PMID: 28252643]

[37] Chilampalli C, Zhang X, Kaushik RS, *et al.* Chemopreventive effects of combination of honokiol and magnolol with α-santalol on skin cancer developments. Drug Discov Ther 2013; 7(3): 109-15.
[PMID: 23917859]

[38] You Q, Li M, Jiao G. Magnolol induces apoptosis *via* activation of both mitochondrial and death receptor pathways in A375-S2 cells. Arch Pharm Res 2009; 32(12): 1789-94.
[http://dx.doi.org/10.1007/s12272-009-2218-6] [PMID: 20162409]

[39] Chen SZ. [Research progress in anticancer effects and molecular targets of honokiol in experimental therapy]. Yao Xue Xue Bao 2016; 51(2): 202-7.
[PMID: 29856535]

[40] Mannal PW, Schneider J, Tangada A, McDonald D, McFadden DW. Honokiol produces anti-neoplastic effects on melanoma cells *in vitro.* J Surg Oncol 2011; 104(3): 260-4.
[http://dx.doi.org/10.1002/jso.21936] [PMID: 21472732]

[41] Kaushik G, Ramalingam S, Subramaniam D, *et al.* Honokiol induces cytotoxic and cytostatic effects in malignant melanoma cancer cells. Am J Surg 2012; 204(6): 868-73.
[http://dx.doi.org/10.1016/j.amjsurg.2012.09.001] [PMID: 23231930]

[42] Banik K, Ranaware AM, Deshpande V, *et al.* Honokiol for cancer therapeutics: A traditional medicine that can modulate multiple oncogenic targets. Pharmacol Res 2019; 144: 192-209.
[http://dx.doi.org/10.1016/j.phrs.2019.04.004] [PMID: 31002949]

[43] Eastman KL, McFarland LV, Raugi GJ. A review of topical corrosive black salve. J Altern Complement Med 2014; 20(4): 284-9.
[http://dx.doi.org/10.1089/acm.2012.0377] [PMID: 24175872]

[44] Lim A. Black salve treatment of skin cancer: a review. J Dermatolog Treat 2018; 29(4): 388-92.
[http://dx.doi.org/10.1080/09546634.2017.1395795] [PMID: 29098921]

[45] Sharma P, McClees S, Afaq F. Pomegranate for Prevention and Treatment of Cancer: An Update. Molecules 2017; 22(1): 177.
[http://dx.doi.org/10.3390/molecules22010177] [PMID: 28125044]

[46] Afaq F, Malik A, Syed D, Maes D, Matsui MS, Mukhtar H. Pomegranate fruit extract modulates UV-B-mediated phosphorylation of mitogen-activated protein kinases and activation of nuclear factor kappa B in normal human epidermal keratinocytes paragraph sign. Photochem Photobiol 2005; 81(1): 38-45.
[http://dx.doi.org/10.1562/2004-08-06-RA-264.1] [PMID: 15493960]

[47] Ernst M, Grace OM, Saslis-Lagoudakis CH, Nilsson N, Simonsen HT, Rønsted N. Global medicinal uses of Euphorbia L. (Euphorbiaceae). J Ethnopharmacol 2015; 176: 90-101.
[http://dx.doi.org/10.1016/j.jep.2015.10.025] [PMID: 26485050]

[48] Laura V, Mattia F, Roberta G, *et al.* Potential of Curcumin in Skin Disorders. Nutrients 2019; 11(9): 2169.
[http://dx.doi.org/10.3390/nu11092169] [PMID: 31509968]

[49] Kleemann B, Loos B, Scriba TJ, Lang D, Davids LM. St John's Wort (Hypericum perforatum L.) photomedicine: hypericin-photodynamic therapy induces metastatic melanoma cell death. PLoS One 2014; 9(7): e103762.
[http://dx.doi.org/10.1371/journal.pone.0103762] [PMID: 25076130]

CHAPTER 8

Skin Ulcers as a Painful Disorder with Limited Therapeutic Protocols

Thongtham Suksawat[1] and Pharkphoom Panichayupakaranant[1,*]

[1] *Department of Pharmacognosy and Pharmaceutical Botany, Faculty of Pharmaceutical Sciences, Prince of Songkla University, Hat-Yai 90112, Thailand*

Abstract: A skin ulcer is a type of open wound on the skin caused by injury, poor circulation, pressure, or infection. Specific forms of wounds are described using distinct terms, such as surgical incision, burn, and laceration. Skin ulcers can be extremely painful and take a long time to heal. They can become infected and cause other medical complications if left untreated. Treatment for skin ulcers is determined on the basis of the ulcer condition as well as the underlying cause. However, there is still a shortage of effective and safe medications for skin ulcer since current treatment guidelines for wound management consists only of wound dressing, antibiotics, and pain control. Wound healing and anti-inflammatory agents used for treating skin ulcers are quite limited. Recent revelations about natural compounds and their multifunctional pharmacological attributes, especially those with anti-inflammatory, antibacterial, antioxidant and wound-healing activities, have been very encouraging for therapeutic skin ulcer development. Various phytochemicals, such as curcuminoids, flavonoids, xanthones, polyphenolic compounds, saponins, and terpenoids, were reportedly used as alternative agents for the treatment of skin ulcers. This chapter describes skin ulcers, their pathophysiology, as well as current therapeutic protocols. In addition, some selected phytochemicals and herbal extracts with strong prospects as well as their commercially available products for the treatment of skin ulcers, are highlighted.

Keywords: Anti-inflammation, Antimicrobial, Antioxidant, Skin ulcer, Wound healing.

INTRODUCTION

Skin is the largest organ that covers the entire external surface of the human body and serves a significant biological function. The skin helps to maintain fluid homeostasis, regulates temperature and chemical metabolism, provides sensory

---

[*] **Corresponding author Pharkphoom Panichayupakaranant:** Department of Pharmacognosy and Pharmaceutical Botany, Faculty of Pharmaceutical Sciences, Prince of Songkla University, Hat-Yai 90112, Thailand; Tel: +66-74-288980; E-mail: pharkphoom.p@psu.ac.th

Heba Abd El-Sattar El-Nashar, Mohamed El-Shazly & Nouran Mohammed Fahmy (Eds.)

messages to the brain, and acts as the first line of the body's defense mechanism against pathogens, stress from the environment, and mechanical injury. Wounds are physical injuries that cause an opening or breaking of the skin or a break in the epithelial integrity of the skin, which may be accompanied by disruption of the structure and function of the underlying normal tissue. Wound infection is one of the most frequent illnesses in the world as a result of inadequate sanitary settings [1]. As a result, adequate healing procedures are required for the restoration of the skin and normal physiological conditions. Depending on the level of injury, the self-wound healing process begins with four stages, including hemostasis, inflammation, proliferation, and remodeling, and ultimately decides the look and strength of the tissue recovered [2].

Herbal medications have been traditionally used in wound therapy for disinfection, dressing, and debridement. All of which aid in the formation of an adequate physical healing process. A variety of plants are used in folklore cultures to cure incisions, wounds, and burns [3]. Recently, the mechanism of herbal extracts and phytochemicals in the wound healing process has attracted more attention since they can work *via* many mechanisms and demonstrate therapeutic characteristics at various phases of the wound healing process [4]. Various plant extracts have shown the ability to treat and cure skin ulcers through their biological effects, *i.e.*, wound healing, antimicrobial, and anti-inflammation, antioxidants and occasionally anti-allergy. Antimicrobial agents help in reducing tissue injury and inflammation caused by wound infection, while anti-inflammatory and antioxidant agents are capable of enhancing wound healing and protect tissues from oxidative damage. Therefore, phytochemicals that possess all these biological properties have a high potential to accelerate wound healing [5, 6].

This chapter aims to elucidate alternative skin ulcer therapy by describing targets for innovative pharmacological approaches against skin ulcers, herbal extracts or phytochemicals with high prospects, and their patented products that might be utilized as therapeutic alternatives. The typical features of skin ulcers, their pathogenesis, as well as current therapies are also described.

SKIN ULCERS AND PATHOPHYSIOLOGY

A skin ulcer is defined as any damage to the skin and, in most cases, to the epidermis of the skin that disturbs its regular function. Skin ulcers are classified as open or closed ulcers according to the etiology of ulcer formation, which is categorized by acute and chronic ulcers [7]. Acute ulcers, which consist of surgical and accidental ulcers, involve regular processes of inflammation, tissue proliferation, and remodeling. All of these processes take place on time [8].

Chronic ulcers are usually prolonged to heal because the healing process does not progress normally, and there is local infection. The most serious causes of chronic ulcers are diabetes mellitus, hypoxia, trauma, and inadequate treatment in the early stages of wounding [9]. Since chronic ulcers are frequently exposed to bacteria as a result of delayed wound healing, they progress to the infection stage. The pathogenic bacteria found in ulcers are *Staphylococcus aureus, S. epidermidis, Streptococcus pyogenes, Pseudomonas aeruginosa, Bacillus subtilis, Escherichia coli,* and *Enterococcus faecalis,* as well as pathogenic fungi such as *Candida albicans,* have been implicated as primarily responsible for chronic ulcer infections [10].

Skin, the largest organ in the human body, is vital to life's nourishment by regulating water and electrolyte balance, body temperature, and functioning as a frontier to external pathogens such as microorganisms. These functions are no longer efficiently performed when this shield is damaged due to ulcers or burns. As a result, restoring its integrity as quickly as feasible is critical [11]. A skin ulcer is an interruption in the skin's epithelial integrity. The disruption can also affect the dermis and subcutaneous tissue. Normal skin ulcer healing necessitates a complicated series of processes that culminate in the repair of wounded tissues. A healed wound can be defined as restoring to its normal anatomical structure and function within a regular period of time, usually following a small insult. Skin ulcer pathophysiology is thus a bodily wound-healing process that keeps skin functioning normally [12].

Based on the conventional classification, wound healing is classified into four processes, namely hemostasis, inflammation, proliferation, and remodeling. These stages usually happen in this order, with occasional overlap. Normally, an ulcer will heal within 4 to 6 weeks [13]. When part of the skin is damaged, the hemostasis phase is established. At this stage, a number of significant events occur. Vasoconstriction is initially used to keep the body from bleeding out rapidly. Platelets are infused into the wound to halt bleeding and create a clot. As a result, during the coagulation cascade, a fibrin mesh forms around the platelet plugs, assisting in clot formation. Subsequently, platelets start to release cytokines and growth factors that aid in the wound-healing process. Platelets also have dense compartments that store amines that improve microvascular permeability, such as serotonin. The inflammatory response is triggered, and inflammatory cells are activated. Angiogenesis and epithelization are promoted by neutrophils and cytokines. The ulcer starts to seal during the inflammatory phase. Bacteria and debris are eliminated, and the migration of cells is boosted. After granulocytes or polymorphonuclear leukocytes (PMNLs) infiltrate the wound, they phagocytose bacteria and other foreign particles in the wound environment and eliminate them by secretion of degrading enzymes and oxygen-derived free radical species.

Hemostasis and vascular permeability promotion are involved in this condition. The proliferative phase begins when granulation tissue is promoted. The fibrin matrix is replaced with newly generated granulation tissue in this condition. There is also fibroblast migration, collagen synthesis, granulation tissue creation, vascularization, and re-epithelialization. Macrophages are among the cells participating in this process of wound healing. Depending on the wound condition, concomitant medical disorders, and other risk factors, the remodeling phase begins around week 3 and lasts 12 to 24 months. The remodeling begins when excess collagen dissolves and wound contraction peaks. Matrix synthesis and remodeling begin simultaneously with the development of granulation tissue and last for a long time. Fibrin and hyaluronan are broken down as the matrix matures, and collagen bundles grow in diameter, resulting in increased wound tensile strength [14].

CURRENT TREATMENTS FOR SKIN ULCERS

Wounds are categorized into two types, namely acute and chronic wounds. Post-operative wounds, abrasions, mild burns, and some trauma wounds are examples of acute wounds that heal at an orderly rapid pace [15]. In contrast, chronic wounds may not heal in an orderly manner and are frequently characterized by delayed healing and recurring infections. The guideline treatment procedures for acute skin wound ulcers involve wound cleansing, debridement, dressing, and infection control.

Wound Cleansing

The main objective of wound cleansing is to remove wound debris and reduce the bacteria load in order to treat or prevent wound infection. In most conditions, a clean wound treatment technique, such as irrigation with tap water or wound bathing, should be used. Wounds should not be cleaned using items that may leave fibers in the wound, such as cotton wool or products containing cotton wool [16].

Wound Debridement

If debridement is indicated in any wound, first-line dressings such as a hydrogel sheet, an alginate, a gelling fiber, or a hydrocolloid dressing should be used to aid the process. Antimicrobial dressings should not be utilized unless the wound has been determined to be infected [17].

Wound Dressing

Traditional wound dressings, such as gauze, plasters, bandages, and cotton wool, are used as primary dressings to protect the wound from environmental contamination. Novel wound dressings have been devised to aid wound healing. These new techniques are designed to protect the wound from drying out and to encourage healing. Interactive dressings are semi-occlusive or occlusive and come in films, foam, hydrogel, and hydrocolloid forms. These dressings function as a barrier to bacterial infiltration into the wound environment [18].

Infection Control

Infectious skin ulcers have a specific treatment plan. Antibiotics, both topical and systemic, can be beneficial. To treat serious colonization or compartment infection, topical antibiotics should be explored. The choice of topical treatment is determined by the bacteria found by culture or clinical examination, as well as the risk of topical sensitization. Agents such as neomycin, bacitracin, lanolin-containing products and fucidin ointment might amplify the inflammatory response and act as sensitizers. Topical aminoglycosides, such as gentamicin, have been linked to an increase in the likelihood of microbial resistance [19]. Systemic antibiotics show level I evidence of efficacy for the treatment of sepsis or bacteremia from wound infections, cellulitis, and osteomyelitis. Infections in the deep compartment may not respond to topical therapies, while infections in the superficial compartment may require oral or parenteral antibiotics if they do not react to topical medications. Systemic antibiotics are used when evidence of infection expands beyond the ulcer edges, or when the ulcer is growing or generating satellite ulcers. Antibiotic medicines can be selected based on both culture and clinical data [20].

Treatments for chronic ulcers are determined based on their cause. The most prevalent causes of chronic ulcers are venous leg ulcers (VLUs), pressure ulcers (PRUs), diabetic neuropathic foot ulcers (DFUs), and arterial insufficiency leg ulcers. The conventional treatment modalities for this chronic condition include compression, basic wound dressing, debridement, moisture-retentive dressings, patient nutrition management, infection control, and dressings to keep the wound bed wet [21].

ALTERNATIVE THERAPEUTIC PROTOCOLS FOR ALLEVIATION OF SKIN ULCERS

Nutrition and medicinal herbs are examples of complementary and alternative therapeutic interventions that have received medical attention. Certain herbal medicines may provide symptom alleviation and aid in the healing of wounds.

Herbs are commonly offered in the form of pills, capsules, tablets, teas, and tinctures [22]. In recent years, there has been a lot of interest in the underlying mechanisms of herbal medicines and phytochemicals in skin wound healing. Some herbal extracts appear to act through multiple mechanisms and exhibit healing properties at various stages of the wound-healing process. Flavonoids, polyphenols, anthraquinones, and naphthoquinones promote fibroblast cell proliferation, antimicrobial activity, and anti-inflammatory effects, all of which hasten wound healing [5]. Considering the current limitations of conventional skin ulcer treatment guidelines with regards to the wound healing process, seeking herbal extracts and phytochemicals with desirable, beneficial biological activities against skin ulcers is, therefore worthwhile in the context of delivering better, safe, and efficacious skin ulcer treatment [23].

Table 1. Plant extracts and phytochemicals with potential for the treatment of skin ulcers.

Plant Name	Family	Tested Compounds	Expected Active Compounds	Activity/Mechanism of Action
Aloe vera	Liliaceae	Leaf extract	Aloin, aloe-emodin, and acemannan	Increase wound closure and collagen production, decrease Multidrug-resistant *P. aeruginosa*
Azadirachta indica	Meliaceae	Leaf extract, seed oil	Nimbidin	Possess wound healing through edema suppressing, and reduction of NO and PGE-2
Centella asiatica	Apiaceae	Leaf extract	Asiaticoside, madecassoside, and asiatic acid	Promote secretion of hyaluronan, decrease pro-inflammatory cytokines and antibacterial against *E. coli*, *P. aeruginosa*, and *S. aureus*
Curcuma longa	Zingiberaceae	Rhizome extract	Curcumin	Promote collagenization and angiogenesis, suppress COX-2, LOX and iNOS, and antibacterial against MRSA
Embelia ribes	Myrsinaceae	Fruit extract	Embelin	Exhibit epithelialization and collagen formation, decrease inflammatory mediator, TNF-alpha, and antibacterial against *B. subtilis* and *S. aureus*, *E. coli* and *P. aeruginosa*
Garcinia mangastana	Clusiaceae	Peel extract	Alpha-mangostin	Promote epithelialization and dermal-epidermal junction, down-regulate pro-inflammatory cytokines, and antibacterial against MRSA and VRE

(Table 1) cont.....

Plant Name	Family	Tested Compounds	Expected Active Compounds	Activity/Mechanism of Action
Lawsonia inermis	Lythraceae	Leaf extract	Lawsone	Improve wound contraction and decrease epithelialization time, Suppressed TGF-1, VEGF-A, Inhibited *B. subtilis, E. coli, S. aureus, S. paratyphi, C. albicans*
Phoenix dactylifera	Arecaceae	Fruit extract	Tannins, carotenoids, hydroxy cinnamic acids, hydroxy benzoic acids, polyphenols	Decreased COX-1 and COX-2, Inhibited *S. aureus, S. epidermidis, E. coli*
Picrorhiza kurroa	Scrophulariaceae	Rhizome extract	Picroside I-V, kutkoside, minecoside, veronicoside, pikuroside, cucurbitacin glycosides	Promoted re-epithelialization, neovascularization, and cell migration, Decreased cytokines and COX-2 and iNOS, Inhibited *S. aureus, S. pyogenes, P. aeruginosa, E. coli*
Piper betle	Piperaceae	Leaf and stem extract	Betel-phenol, chavicol	Promoted wound closure and epithelialization, Inhibited *S. aureus, S. pyogenes, T. mentagrophytes, C. albicans*
Punica granatum	Punicaceae	Peel extract	Ellagic acid	Increased collagen production and wound healing time, Reduced pro-inflammatory mediators, Inhibited *S. aureus* and *P. aeruginosa*
Terminalia spp.	Combretaceae	Fruit extract	Tannic acid, chebulagic acid	Promoted collagen cross-linking and stabilized collagen scaffolds, Inhibited pro-inflammatory mediators, Inhibited *E. coli*
Zingiber officinale	Zingiberaceae	Rhizome extract	6-Gingerol	Stimulated collagen deposition, wound contraction and re-epithelialization, Decreased pro-inflammatory cytokines, Inhibited *P. aeruginosa*

HERBAL EXTRACTS AND PHYTOCHEMICALS AS MULTITARGET THERAPEUTIC AGENTS

The usage of herbal treatments has grown at an exponential rate in recent years. Due to their inexpensive cost, natural nature, and lack of negative side effects, these agents are gaining acceptance in both developed and developing countries.

Plants have been used extensively in traditional wound care [23]. Various phytochemicals have been identified as active compounds that possess anti-inflammatory, antioxidant, and antimicrobial activity, as well as the ability to positively impact inflammation, epithelialization, collagenization, and wound contraction. The biological activities and mechanisms of action of some plant extracts and phytochemicals that have been considered for the treatment of skin ulcers are highlighted in Table **1**.

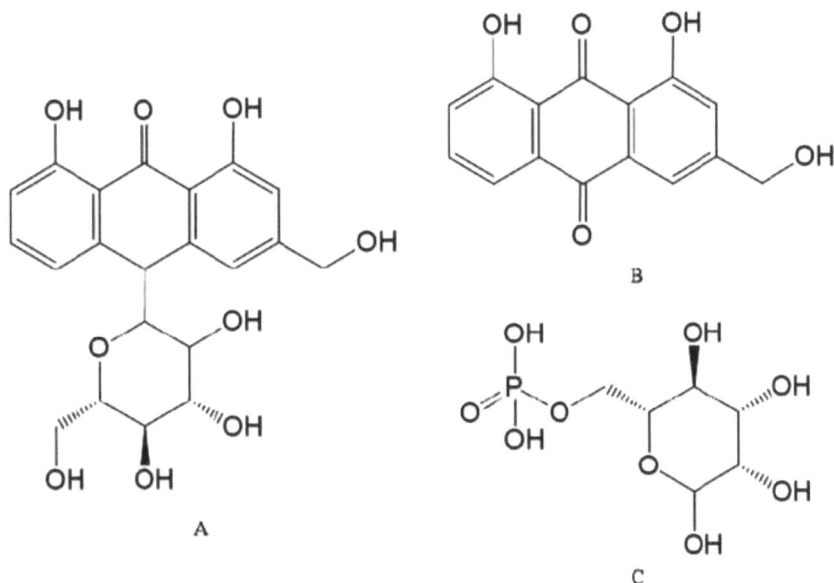

Fig. (1). Chemical structures of aloin (**A**) and aloe-emodin (**B**) and mannose-6-phosphate (**C**).

Aloe Vera

Aloe vera is a member of the Liliaceae family and has long been used to treat burns, ulcers, and surgical wounds as a first-line therapy. It is a medicinal plant with complex constituents and various biological activities. *A. vera* has been shown to exhibit pharmacological activities relevant to the treatment of skin ulcers, including skin protection and healing, anti-inflammatory, antibacterial, antioxidant, and regenerative effects. *A. vera* leaf extracts promoted cell proliferation in fibroblast cells *via* up-regulation of TGFβ1 and bFGF genes [24]. Treatment with *A. vera* gel has been demonstrated to enhance the healing process of wound lesions, increase wound contraction *via* increased collagen production and fibroblast proliferation as well as modify the extracellular matrix during wound healing [25]. Gram-positive bacteria tend to be more susceptible to *A. vera* leaf extracts than Gram-negative bacteria. *A. vera* leaf extracts and gel exhibited antibacterial activity against *S. aureus*, *S epidermidis*, *S. pyogenes*, and *P.*

aeruginosa isolated from human skin ulcers, with the MIC values of 100-500 µg/ml [26]. Some bioactive compounds have been identified in *A. vera*, including aloin, aloe-emodin, mannose-6-phosphate (Fig. **1**), acemannan (Fig. **2**), glucomannan, saponins, anthraquinones, and oleic acid [27].

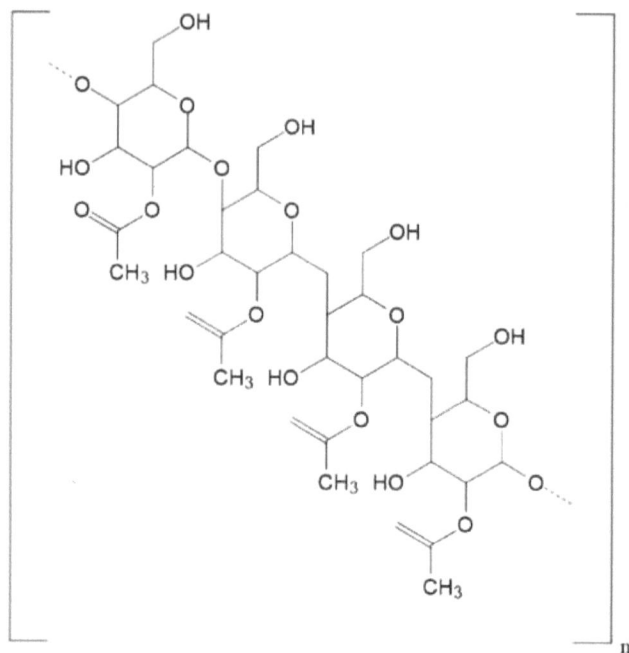

Fig. (2). Chemical structure of acemannan.

Acemannan or mesoglycan or acetylated glucomannan, a primary mucopolysaccharide derived from *A. vera*, possessed anti-inflammatory effects *via* inhibition of macrophage and T-cell activity and suppression in the production of proinflammatory mediators and cytokines, including interleukin-1 (IL-1), interleukin-6 (IL-6), tumor necrosis factor-alpha (TNF-alpha), prostaglandin E2 (PGE2), and nitrous oxide [28]. Acemannan also enhanced the proliferation of skin fibroblasts and increased wound healing rate by shifting the cell cycle process and boosting vascular endothelial growth factor (VEGF), a potent proangiogenic growth factor in the skin, which significantly impact wound repair *via* neovascularization and encouraging endothelial cell proliferation and migration and type I collagen production [29]. In addition, acemannan interacted and entrapped endogenous mitogen inhibitors as well as reactive oxygen species, resulting in increased phagocytosis. Furthermore, *A. vera* glycans have also been shown to dramatically promote *de novo* granulation tissue development [30]. *A. vera* extract containing deacetylation of acemannan exhibited antibiofilm formation against *Escherichia coli* and *Enterococcus faecalis* with the biofilm inhibitory concentrations, BIC_{50} and BIC_{90} of $\leq 7.6\%$ and $\leq 68.2\%$, respectively [31]. In addition, *A. vera* gel exhibited antibacterial activity against multidrug-resistant *P. aeruginosa* isolated from skin infection ulcers, with an MIC of 400 µg/ml [31].

Mannose-6-phosphate is the major sugar derivative in Aloe gel. This compound plays an important function in the epithelialization process. Mannose-6-phosphate reportedly binds to fibroblast receptors and effectuates fibroblast proliferation resulting in collagen production and skin proliferation. This sugar also suppressed transforming growth factor (TGF-1 and TGF-2) activation, resulting in increased epithelialization [32].

It has been reported that glucomannan increased fibroblast proliferation by stimulating the production of epidermal growth factor, resulting in wound healing, while aloin and aloe-emodin exhibited anti-inflammatory activity [33]. Aloin reduced inflammatory mediator production, TNF-alpha, IL-6, nitric oxide synthase (iNOS), and cyclooxygenase-2 (COX-2) [34]. Aloin also maintained the skin's collagen fibers within normal range and protected the skin through its antioxidant activity *via* inhibition of lipid peroxidation and reactive oxygen species, as well as enhancing glutathione peroxidase concentration and superoxide dismutase activity [35].

Therapeutic benefits of *A. vera* were also explored in patients with acute and chronic ulcers, and it found that *A. vera* helps to prevent skin ulcers. Its active compound was identified as mucopolysaccharides, which were responsible for improving skin integrity, reducing erythema, retaining moisture, and wound healing [36].

Recently, various nanofibrous preparations have been developed for tissue engineering, including a nanofibrous scaffold loaded with 8% w/w *A. vera* extract. The nanofiber containing *A. vera* extract showed better cell adhesion and proliferation of fibroblast cells compared to the nanofibrous scaffold alone. Moreover, the antimicrobial activities of nanofiber-containing *A. vera* extract against *S. aureus* and *E. coli* were better than the nanofibrous scaffold alone. Therefore, the *A. vera* nanofibrous scaffold was suggested to be suitable for wound healing applications [37].

Azadirachta Indica

Azadirachta indica or neem is an evergreen plant in the Meliaceae family and native to Southeast Asia and India. This plant has long been used to treat skin ulcers. Various phytochemicals have been reported in neem, such as alkaloids, flavonoids, triterpenoids, and triterpenoid glycosides. Nimbidin (Fig. **3**), a triterpenoid compound, has been identified as a major active compound of neem that exhibited antioxidant, anti-inflammatory, and antibacterial activities, which were beneficial in the healing process [38]. Based on the topical method of excision wound, the ethanol extract of *A. indica* leaves exhibited a significant reduction in wound diameter and increased wound healing rate [39], while neem seed oil (2 ml/kg body weight) possessed anti-inflammatory activity by suppressing edema in edema-induced mice. The beneficial effects of neem oil on chronic ulcer therapy have been evaluated clinically and indicated that after 8 weeks of neem oil treatment, 44% of patients displayed more than 50% wound healing [40].

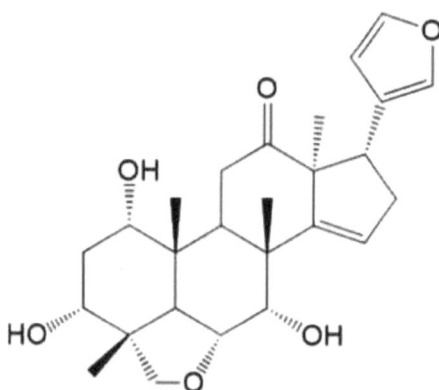

Fig. (3). Chemical structure of nimbidin.

The anti-inflammatory effect of nimbidin has been determined in a mouse model using an oral administration and found that nimbidin suppressed phagocytosis through inhibiting migration of macrophages to their peritoneal cavities in response to inflammatory induction as well as decreases in nitric oxide and PGE2 productions and releases from macrophages [40]. An emollient cream containing neem extract (2.5% w/v) has been formulated and exhibited an anti-inflammatory effect on paw edema by 39-60% after 3 h treatment, and also showed skin ulcer re-epithelization within 10-14 days [41]. Neem seed extract also exhibited antifungal activity against dermatophytes (*Trichophyton rubrum, T. mentagrophytes*, and *Microsporum nanum)*, with an MIC of 31 µg/ml for all tested dermatophytes [41].

Centella Asiatica

Centella asiatica is a popular medicinal plant in the family of Apiaceae. It has been traditionally used for a variety of medical purposes, including memory enhancement, antidepressants, antimicrobial infection, and treatment of psoriasis as well as skin wound healing [42]. *C. asiatica* extracts possess wound-healing properties *via* various mechanisms in different phases of the wound-healing process. Oral and topical applications of 1% *C. asiatica* alcoholic extract in rats revealed an increase of collagen synthesis in granulation tissues at wound sites, resulting in a faster wound-healing process [43]. *C. asiatica* extracts also inhibited the growth of *E. coli, P. aeruginosa,* and *S. aureus*, with the MIC values of 0.04-1.25 mg/ml [44].

Various phytochemicals have been isolated from *C. asiatica*, including triterpenoid saponins, essential oils, flavonoids, and phytosterols. Triterpenoids, namely asiaticoside, madecassoside, asiatic acid (Fig. **4**), and centelloside, have been identified as active compounds with wound-healing effects [45].

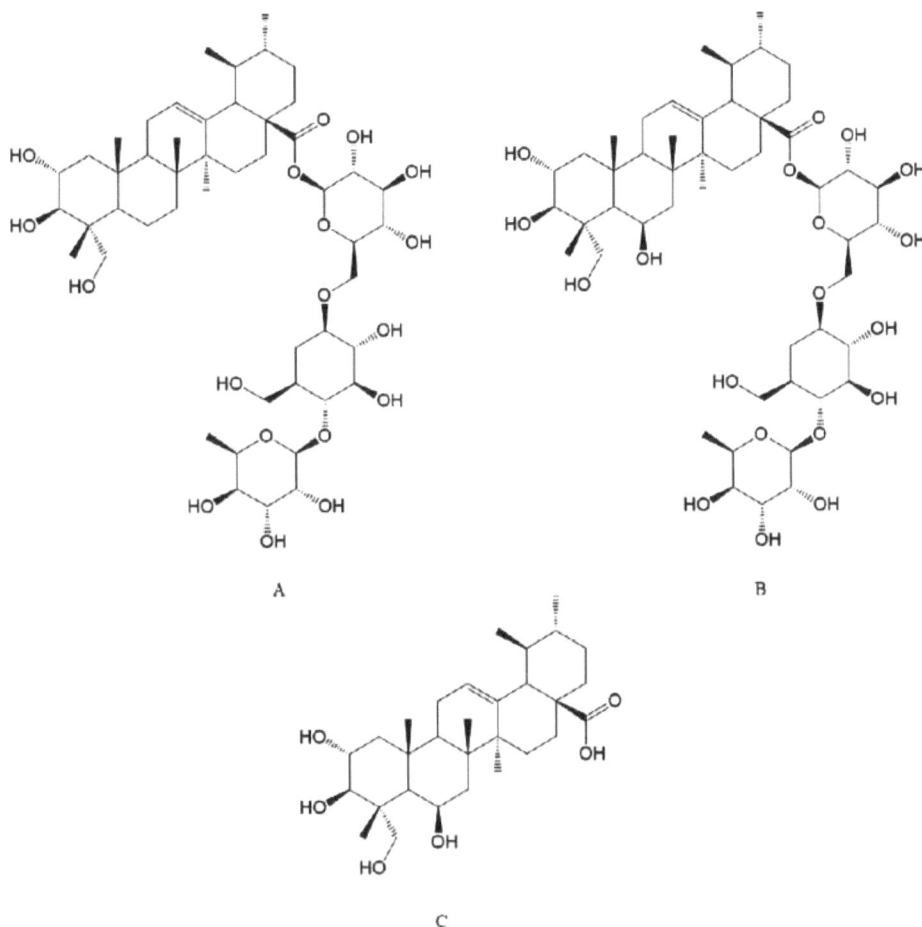

Fig. (4). Chemical structures of asiaticoside (**A**), madecassoside (**B**) and asiatic acid (**C**).

Asiaticoside is a pentacyclic triterpenoid glycoside comprising two glucose and one rhamnose sugar molecule. Asiaticoside works to strengthen skin cells and promote healing, stimulate blood cells and the immune system, and acts as a natural antibacterial agent [46]. Asiaticoside enhanced wound healing by increasing skin cell migration rate and the number of normal human dermal fibroblasts, and improving initial skin cell adhesion. Furthermore, asiaticoside has been recommended for the treatment of scars and keloids because it increases the production of skin aging inhibitor type I collagen in human dermal fibroblast cells [47].

Madecassoside has been reported to aid in the wound healing of cell injury by making collagen and also inhibiting keloid development in primary fibroblasts derived from human keloids [48]. In the treatment of dermatitis, madecassoside also reduced pro-inflammatory cytokines and significantly improved skin hydration by increasing the secretion of keratinocytes and hyaluronan in human skin fibroblasts [49].

Asiatic acid has been shown to induce the generation of neuroglia and cuticle cornification, and stimulate granulation, all of which are involved in wound healing. Moreover, it exhibits antinociceptive action and anti-inflammatory activity, which can elevate wound healing treatment [50]. Additionally, Asiatic acid plays an important role in antimicrobial activity in the wound healing treatment. For instance, the triterpenoid has been reported to inhibit *E. faecalis* with an MIC value of 64 µg/ml as well as inhibits biofilm formation [33].

A method for the preparation of pentacyclic triterpene enriched extract has been developed in order to produce a high-quality extract of *C. asaitica* using a green microwave extraction [51]. The extract was standardized to contain 65% w/w total pentacyclic triterpenes (asiaticoside, madecassoside, asiatic acid, and madecassic acid). This extract has been reported to exhibit anti-inflammatory activity through inhibition of nitric oxide inhibitory action, with an IC_{50} of 64.6 µg/ml, and tyrosinase inhibitory effects, with an IC_{50} of 104.8 µg/ml. On the other hand, the extract possessed relatively little antioxidant effect [52].

Recently, a 3-month, split-face, double-blind, randomized, placebo-controlled trial indicated a topical administration of 0.05% w/w *C. asiatica* gel formulation containing 51% w/w madecassoside and 38% w/w asiaticoside improved skin erythema and wound appearance after laser resurfacing for acne scars. This treatment regimen may be used as an alternative treatment for post-laser resurfacing [53]. In addition, transdermal patches made from 0.34% standardized *C. asiatica* extract containing 57% pentacyclic triterpenes exhibited good wound healing properties [54].

Curcuma Longa

Curcuma longa or turmeric, has long been topically used in the Indian subcontinent for the treatment of skin lesions, particularly ulcers. Turmeric contains curcuminoids, namely curcumin, desmethoxycurcumin, and bisdemethoxycurcumin (Fig. **5**), as the major active compounds, which exhibit various biological activities that are beneficial to skin diseases [55]. Curcumin possesses anti-inflammatory, antioxidant, and antiproliferative activities by interacting with important cellular pathways during transcription, translation, and post-translational processes [56]. Curcumin promotes the wound-healing process by increasing collagenization and angiogenesis in gastric tissues. It has been shown that curcumin administration in mice at a dosage of 40 mg/kg for 11 days exhibited a good wound-healing effect as well as reduced healing time [57]. Curcumin exhibited anti-inflammatory activity by suppressing key enzymes in skin ulcers mediating inflammatory reactions, namely COX-2, lipoxygenase, and iNOS. A topical gel containing 1% curcumin showed improvement of psoriasis in psoriasis patients after 2-6 weeks of therapy, and promoted plaque improvement by 25-70% after 3-4 weeks of treatment [58]. Curcumin also exhibited potent antibacterial activity against MRSA with an MIC value of 18.4 µg/ml *via* interfering with bacterial cell membranes, DNA, proteins, and cell walls [58].

Several clinical investigations have shown the safety of curcumin in humans at 12 g/day. Curcuminoids have low GI absorption, therefore, curcumin blood and tissue levels appear to be of inadequate bioavailability [60]. Several studies have attempted to increase curcumin bioavailability. Solid dispersion of curcuminoids-polyvinylpyrrolidone K30 and a ternary inclusion complex of curcuminoids-hydroxypropyl-β-cyclodextrin-polyvinylpyrrolidone K30 have been successfully prepared to enhance water-solubility and dissolution rate of curcuminoids [60, 61].

Embelia Ribes

Embelia ribes is a plant of the Myrsinaceae family, which has a number of medicinal uses, including the treatment of gastrointestinal problems and inflammatory illnesses [59]. Interestingly, treatment with *E. ribes* ethanol extract in rat wound ulcers exhibited epithelialization, and collagen formation. Furthermore, embelin (Fig. **6**), a benzoquinone isolated from *E. ribes* fruits, showed full wound healing, with higher fibroblasts and a considerable increase in collagen levels [60]. Embelin also exhibited a wide range of biological actions, including anti-inflammatory, analgesic, antibacterial, and antioxidant properties. The anti-inflammatory effect of embelin in the wound healing process is associated with a decrease in TNF-alpha, an inflammatory mediator.

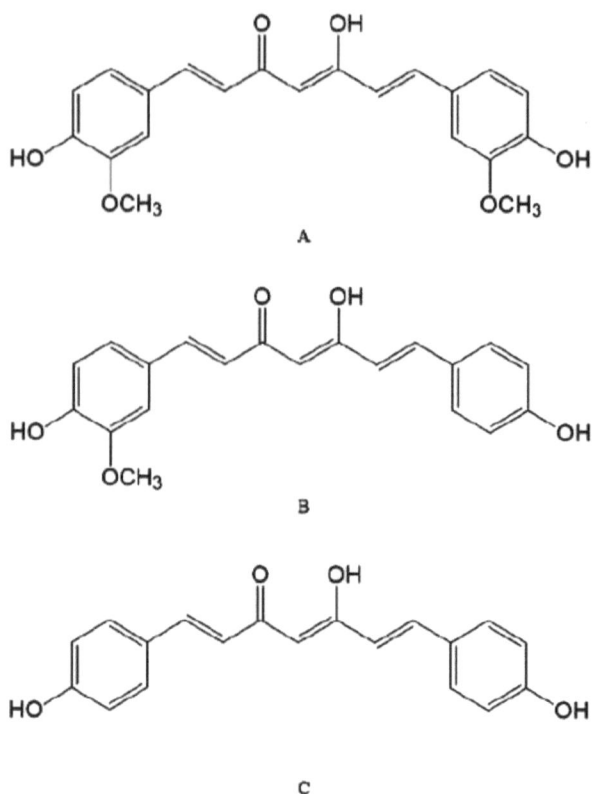

Fig. (5). Chemical structures of curcumin (**A**), desmethoxycurcumin (**B**), and bisdemethoxycurcumin (**C**).

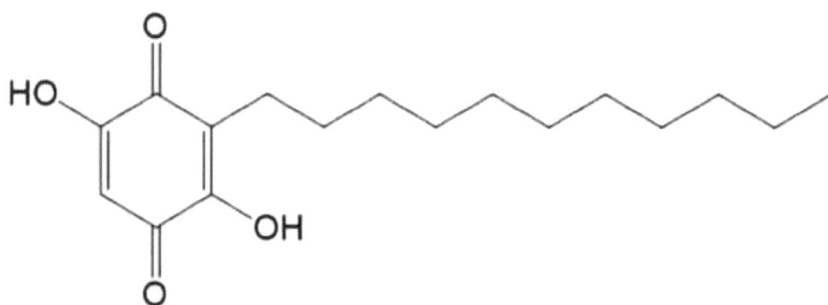

Fig. (6). Chemical structure of embelin.

A hydrogel made from embelin (0.2%) was developed as a pharmaceutical product for wound healing. *In vitro* study on the drug release profile of the hydrogel revealed that more than 80% of embelin was released after 12 h. In addition, the wound healing efficiency of the hydrogel was investigated *in vivo*, and showed a reduced healing time [60]. Also, in excision, incision, and dead space wound models, rats treated with embelin (4 mg/ml) were found to require less time to complete epithelialization of the ulcers than those treated with ethanol extract of *E. ribes* (30 mg/ml) [59]. Furthermore, 5% embelin topical ointment and 25 and 50 mg/kg embelin oral formulation increased the proportion of epithelialization and collagenization in diabetic rats, highlighting its beneficial wound-healing effect [61].

Embelin also exhibited antibacterial activity against *B. subtilis* and *S. aureus*, *E. coli* and *P. aeruginosa*, with the MIC and MBC values of 50 µg/ml and 400 µg/ml, respectively [62].

Garcinia Mangostana

Garcinia mangostana is a tropical plant that has been traditionally used to treat skin ulcers. It has been reported that topical application of *G. mangostana* extract (0.2-0.4 g/dose) on burn ulcers promoted epidermal re-epithelialization in the wound healing process [63]. A variety of compounds in *G. mangostana* have been isolated and identified, such as xanthones, flavonoids, saponins, and tannins. However, the major active compounds that play an important role in skin ulcer treatment are xanthones, especially α-mangostin (Fig. **7**), which has been reported to exert various biological effects, including anti-inflammatory, antibacterial, antioxidant, and analgesic effects [64].

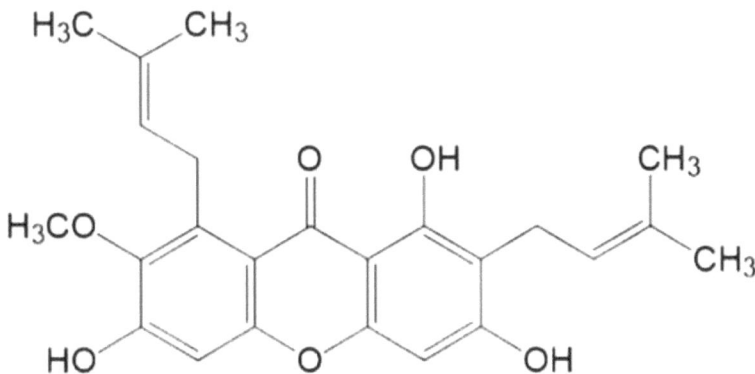

Fig. (7). Chemical structure of α-mangostin.

α-Mangostin exhibited anti-inflammation in the wound healing process through mast cell formation and by downregulating the expression of pro-inflammatory cytokines. During the proliferation phase of wound healing, α-mangostin decreased PGE2 production and exhibited antioxidant activity [65]. The molecular mechanism of α-mangostin in the wound healing process involves the reduction of total leukocyte migration, particularly neutrophil migration [66]. α-

Mangostin also possesses potent antibacterial activity, which is essential for an infectious wound. It exhibited inhibitory effects against methicillin-resistant *S. aureus* (MRSA) and vancomycin-resistant *Enterococci* (VRE) with the MIC values of 6.2-12.5 µg/ml. α-Mangostin exhibited antibacterial activity through cytoplasmic membrane alteration, resulting in intracellular content leakage and water diffusion across the membrane [67, 68] as well as the binding of isoprenyl moiety to phospholipids of the bacterial membrane, resulting in disturbance of metabolism *via* proton motive force dispersion [69].

Recently, a method for the preparation of α-mangostin-rich extracts containing 95% w/w α-mangostin has been developed using a green microwave extraction. The standardized extract exhibited antibacterial activity against MRSA with the MIC values of 7.8-31.2 µg/ml [70].

Lawsonia Inermis

Lawsonia inermis or Henna, is a plant belonging to the Lythraceae family. This plant has been used to treat burn ulcers and skin infections due to its antibacterial and anti-inflammatory effects. This plant contains various phytochemicals, including carbohydrates, phenolic compounds, flavonoids, saponins, proteins, alkaloids, terpenoids, quinones, xanthones, lipids, resin, and tannins [71]. *L. inermis* leaf extract promotes the wound healing process through stimulation of keratinocyte re-epithelialization [72] and shortens the length of the inflammatory process through the production of growth factors, TGF-1 and VEGF-A in fibroblast cells [73]. *L. inermis* leaf extract also exhibited antibacterial action against a wide range of pathogenic microorganisms, including *B. subtilis, E. coli, S. aureus*, and *C. albicans* as well as bacteria that cause burn wound infections [74, 75]. Recently, a topical formulation of *L. inermis* leaf and stem decoction (1 g/ml) was reported to improve pressure ulcers by decreasing the average ulcer area in a grade-one pressure ulcer patient [76].

Lawsone or 2-hydroxy-1,4-naphthoquinone (Fig. **8**) is the major naphthoquinone found in dried powders of henna leaves (around 0.5 - 1.5% w/w). This active molecule has piqued the interest of researchers in pharmaceutical and biomedical fields due to its antibacterial, anti-inflammatory, and antioxidant properties, particularly for wound healing applications [77]. Lawsone promotes wound healing through its action on skin homeostasis by activating the aryl hydrocarbon receptor (AhR) pathway in keratinocytes. AhR is critical in protecting the skin's integrity against long-term environmental damage [78]. Moreover, lawsone exhibited antibacterial activity against *B. subtilis, E. coli, S. epidermidis,* and *S. aureus* with the MIC values of 187.5, 750, 187.5 and 375 µg/ml, respectively [79]. Recently, a topical lawsone gel (0.5-1.5%) was formulated and showed excellent wound healing characteristics, which improved wound contraction and decreased epithelialization time within 13 days in skin tissue [80].

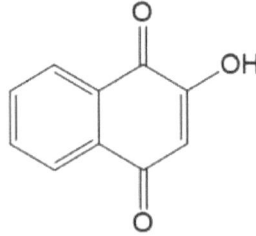

Fig. (8). Chemical structure of lawsone.

Phoenix Dactylifera

Phoenix dactylifera or date palm, is a tree native to Asia and commonly grown for its tasty, sweet fruit. Date palm has also been used in Ayurvedic medicine to treat lower respiratory tract infections, oedema, and microbial infections. Tannins, carotenoids, hydroxy cinnamic acids, hydroxybenzoic acids, and polyphenols are among the phytochemicals found in date palms. An ethanol extract from date palm seeds has been shown to decrease interferon-γ, COX-1 and COX-2 enzymes, the mediators involved in inflammatory signals [81, 82]. In addition, a polyphenol extract from date palm syrup exhibited antibacterial activity against *S. aureus* and *S. epidermidis*, with an MIC value of 500 μg/ml [83]. Furthermore, a flavonoid extract of date palm inhibited *E. coli* and *S. aureus*, with the MIC values of 30 and 20 μg/ml, respectively, through its hydrogen peroxide generating property, which resulted in increased oxidative stress to bacteria [84]. This may be an indication that the flavonoid group in date palms may play a critical role in wound healing properties.

Picrorhiza Kurroa

Picrorhiza kurroa is a member of the Scrophulariaceae family. This plant is a perennial herb found in Asian countries. The rhizomes of this plant have been traditionally used to treat infections and inflammatory disorders. *P. kurroa* leaf extract possessed an anti-inflammatory effect mediated by suppressing macrophage-derived cytokines and mediators (TNF-alpha, IL-1, IL-6) *via* NF-kB signaling as well as decreasing cyclooxygenase-2 and iNOS activities [85]. Moreover, an alcoholic extract of *P. kurroa* exhibited potent antibacterial activity against *S. aureus*, *S. pyogenes*, *P. aeruginosa*, and *E. coli* [86]. *P. kurroa* contains various phytochemicals, including iridoid glycosides (picroside I-V, kutkoside, minecoside, veronicoside, and pikuroside), cucurbitacin glycosides, and polyphenolic compounds [87].

A standardized extract of iridoid glycoside containing picroside I and kutkoside (Fig. **9**) at a ratio of 1:1.5 w/w exhibited wound healing activity through superoxide scavenger, hypoxia-protective action, and increased production of vascular endothelial growth factor [88]. Moreover, the standardized extract (12 mg/kg) promoted wound-healing effects in an animal model [89].

Piper Betle

Piper betle or Betel is a plant in the Piperaceae family and is wildly distributed in Southeast Asia. Betel leaves have shown potential for wound treatment. A methanol extract from betel leaves has been shown to boost wound healing through fibroblast cell proliferation and improve wound healing in mouse skin models with burn and excision wounds [90]. Moreover, an ointment formulation containing *P. betle* leaf and stem extract increased the rate of wound closure and reduced the healing phase in rats, which might be attributed to increased epithelialization [91]. Betel leaves contain phenolic compounds, including betel-phenol and chavicol, which may have substantial antifungal and antibacterial activities [92]. The betel oil, which mainly contains 5-(2-propenyl)-1, 3-benzodioxole, eugenol isomer, and caryophyllene, exhibited significant antimicrobial activity against *S. aureus*, *S. pyogenes*, and *C. albicans* with the MIC values of 125, 15.6, and 195 µg/ml, respectively [93].

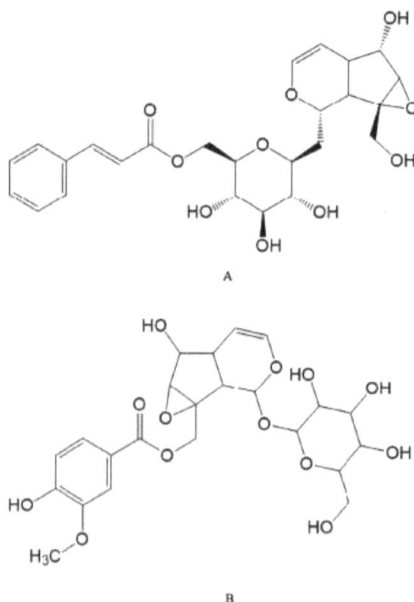

Fig. (9). Chemical structures of pricoside I (**A**) and kutkoside (**B**).

Punica Granatum

Punica granatum, or pomegranate, is a member of the Punicaceae family and has been exploited as a source of bioactive chemicals with various biological activities for treating skin ulcers. A topical gel containing 5% pomegranate peel extract increased collagen level in the excision wound, thereby shortening the wound healing time by 10 days in an animal model [94]. In addition, a topical gel containing 10% pomegranate peel extract exhibited good wound healing properties in minor aphthous stomatitis patients in a double-blind clinical trial [95].

P. granatum contains mainly phenolic compounds, such as polyphenols, tannins, flavonoids, ellagic acid, epicatechin, and epigallocatechin. Ellagic acid and punicalagin A (Fig. **10**) are the primary active compounds of pomegranate that have been reported for antioxidant, antibacterial, and anti-inflammatory effects [96].

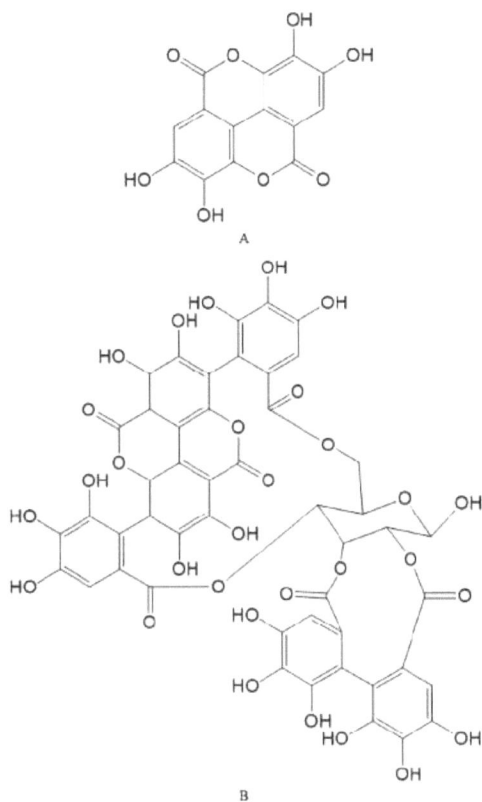

Fig. (10). Chemical structures of ellagic acid (**A**) and punicalagin A (**B**).

Ellagic acid exhibited anti-inflammatory effects *via* suppressing pro-inflammatory mediators, *i.e.*, IL-1, IL-6, NO, and NF-kB, myeloperoxidase (MPO) enzyme, apoptosis, DNA damage, and angiogenesis, and impact cell proliferation [97 - 100]. Furthermore, ellagic acid-loaded chitosan films have been shown to inhibit *S. aureus* and *P. aeruginosa* with an MIC value of 18 µg/ml [101]. A standardized pomegranate peel extract containing 13% ellagic acid exhibited wound healing activity through increased tensile strength, accelerated wound contraction, and facilitated collagen synthesis in both incision and burn wounds in rats [102]. The standardized extract also possessed an anti-inflammatory effect mediated by the inhibition of NO and exhibited potent antibacterial activity against *S. aureus* and *S. epidermidis* with the MIC values of 7.8-15.6 µg/ml [99]. Moreover, a topical formulation of the standardized extract presented an excellent effect against skin inflammatory disorder by reducing ear edema and MPO activity in mice [100].

Punicalagin is an ellagitannin found in *P. granatum*. Punicalagin exhibited anti-inflammatory activity through reduced production of pro-inflammatory cytokines, *i.e.*, IL-1, IL-6, IL-8 and IL-17, metalloproteinase, cytokine modulating enzyme, as well as antioxidant activity [103, 104]. Punicalagin also possessed antibacterial activity against *S. aureus* (MIC of 0.25 mg/ml) and inhibition of its biofilm formation [105].

Terminalia Spp.

The plants in the *Terminalia* genus have been historically used as traditional medicine in Southeast Asia for wound healing treatment, especially *T. arjuna* and *T. chebulu,* due to their wound-healing, antioxidant, and antibacterial effects. A polyherbal formulation containing 0.08% *T. chebula* extract has been shown to promote angiogenesis, epithelialization, and collagen production in fibroblast cells, which indicates its wound healing adjuvant [106].

Based on agar diffusion assay, ethanol extracts of *T. chebula* exhibited antibacterial activity against MRSA and multidrug-resistant *E. coli* [107]. In addition, tannic acid and chebulagic acid (Fig. **11**) isolated from *T. chebulu* possessed wound healing activities. Tannic acid promotes the wound-healing process by increasing collagen cross-linking and stabilizing collagen scaffolds in skin ulcers [108]. Furthermore, a hydrogels containing 5% w/w tannic acid exhibited anti-inflammatory effect *via* inhibiting NO generation in activated human macrophages. Additionally, based on the agar diffusion test, the tannic acid-loaded hydrogel exhibited antibacterial activity against *E. coli* [109].

Chebulagic acid also possesses antioxidant and anti-inflammatory activities. It exhibited potent anti-inflammatory effects by suppressing NF-kB, TNF-alpha and COX-2 during the wound healing process. Additionally, chebulagic acid plays an important role in the proliferation phase in the wound healing process through stimulation of angiogenesis by increasing vascular endothelial growth factor [110].

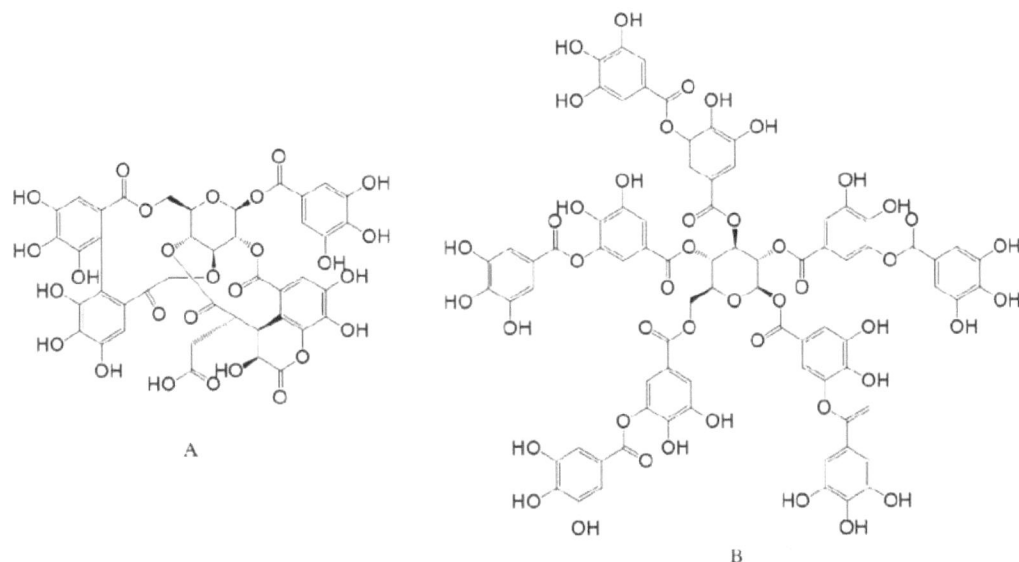

Fig. (11). Chemical structures of tannic acid (**A**) and chebulagic acid (**B**).

Zingiber Officinale

Ginger (*Zingiber officinale*) rhizome is widely used as a spice. The rhizome contains various biologically active compounds, including diterpenoids, flavonoids, gingerols, and shogaols. Ginger rhizome extract promotes the wound healing process *via* stimulating collagen deposition, wound contraction, re-epithelialization, and altering cell motility and heat tolerance [111]. An ethanol extract of ginger has been shown to increase wound healing characteristics in wound-infected albino rats, with percentages of 51% and 91% on days 4 and 8, respectively [112].

6-Gingerols (Fig. **12**) is the major active compound of ginger and responsible for its anti-inflammatory effect [113]. 6-Gingerol decreased pro-inflammatory cytokine production in LPS-stimulated macrophages [114]. Additionally, 6-gingerol (25 mg/kg) promoted higher amounts of hydroxyproline, fibronectin, and collagen expression in diabetic wound mice, resulting in a quicker rate of wound healing and complete epithelialization [115].

6-Gingerol (0.1-100 μM) also inhibited the biofilm formation of *P. aeruginosa*, a virulence factor involved in wound infection. Based on *in silico* study, 6-gingerol interacted with *P. aeruginosa* sensing receptor *via* the hydrophobic moiety of a long alkyl chain in conjunction with the carbonyl group and hydrogen bonding [116].

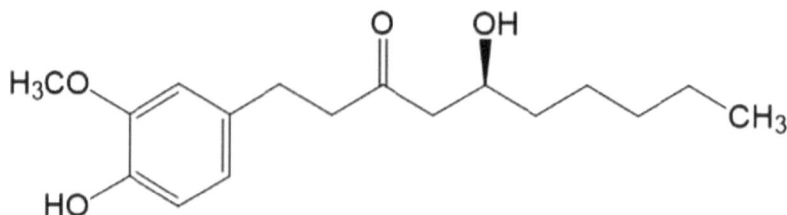

Fig. (12). Chemical structure of 6-gingerol.

In a prospective clinical trial, post-tonsillectomy patients treated with 500 mg ginger capsules for 10 days were found to expedite wound site epithelialization [117].

COMMERCIALLY AVAILABLE PRODUCTS AND PATENTS

Currently, many herbal-derived wound-healing preparations are readily available around the world. Table **2** highlights some innovative products for patients with skin ulcers. The patents were granted by the United States Patent and Trademark Office (USPTO) and Thailand's Department of Intellectual Property (DIP).

Table 2. Patents on herbal preparations for skin ulcer treatment.

Patent No.	Descriptions of Invention	References
8,709,509 (US patent)	A unique, synergistic, and effective herbal composition as a regenerative medicine, consisting of a combination of therapeutically effective levels of extracts produced from *C. longa* and other herbal extracts as a basis, beneficial for the treatment of wound healing.	[118]
11,154,533 (US patent)	Compositions and techniques for treating autoinflammatory skin illnesses such as psoriasis, dermatitis, pyoderma gangrenosum, palmoplantar pustulosis, prurigo nodularis, and/or hidradenitis suppurativa are presented. Curcumin is used as the agent in one embodiment.	[119]
11,071,786 (US patent)	A dermal skin protectant and carrier composed of two viscosity dimethicone components, containing *A. vera*.	[120]
11,154,583 (US patent)	An herbal cream formulation that may be used to treat skin illnesses and disorders, as well as for therapeutic and aesthetic purposes. The compound used in the present invention contains *G. mangostana* peels.	[121]
11,083,749 (US patent)	Methods and compositions are comprised of *P. granatum* treating a region of a patient's skin, *e.g.*, an itch, insect bite or sting, inflammation, discomfort, or irritation, by applying an effective quantity of a siliceous molecular sieve adsorbent to said area of the skin to address the ailment.	[122]

(Table 2) cont.....

Patent No.	Descriptions of Invention	References
78564 (Thai patent)	Microwave-assisted extraction techniques and formulations for preparing *P. betle* extract containing hydroxychavicol for topical formulation.	[123]
139379 (Thai patent)	Method and composition of *Z. officinale* gel for anti-inflammation and analgesic	[124]

CONCLUSION

Wound healing has been a clinical challenge for successful skin ulcer therapy since ancient times. Recent studies, including *in vitro*, *in vivo*, and clinical trials, supported the high potential of plant extracts and phytochemicals for the development of wound healing remedies because of their acceptable safety, and efficacy derived from multiple mechanisms, *i.e.*, antioxidant, anti-inflammatory, antibacterial, and wound healing actions. The most active phytochemicals for wound healing effects belong to phenolic and triterpenoid compounds. The effectiveness is attributable to antioxidant, anti-inflammatory, antibacterial, and skin regeneration activities. Furthermore, several plant constituent-based patented methods for wound healing applications have been developed. However, most of these still require clinical trials to establish their effectiveness and safety profiles for use in the treatment of skin ulcers.

ACKNOWLEDGEMENTS

The authors wish to thank Dr. Fredrick Eze for assistance with English editing.

REFERENCES

[1] Sorg H, Tilkorn DJ, Hager S, Hauser J, Mirastschijski U. Skin wound healing: an update on the current knowledge and concepts. Eur Surg Res 2017; 58(1-2): 81-94.
[http://dx.doi.org/10.1159/000454919] [PMID: 27974711]

[2] Rodero MP, Khosrotehrani K. Skin wound healing modulation by macrophages. Int J Clin Exp Pathol 2010; 3(7): 643-53.
[PMID: 20830235]

[3] Shedoeva A, Leavesley D, Upton Z, Fan C. Wound healing and the use of medicinal plants. Evid Based Complement Alternat Med 2019; 2019: 1-30.
[http://dx.doi.org/10.1155/2019/2684108] [PMID: 31662773]

[4] Dan MM, Sarmah P, Vana DR, Dattatreya A. Wound healing: concepts and updates in herbal medicine. Int J Med Res Health Sci 2018; 7: 170-81.

[5] Yazarlu O, Iranshahi M, Kashani HRK, *et al.* Perspective on the application of medicinal plants and natural products in wound healing: A mechanistic review. Pharmacol Res 2021; 174: 105841.
[http://dx.doi.org/10.1016/j.phrs.2021.105841] [PMID: 34419563]

[6] Elgohary H, Al Jaouni S, Selim S. Wound healing: In response to natural remedies and phototherapy. Int J Pharm Pharm Sci 2017; 8: 568-75.

[7] Kirsner RS, Eaglstein WH. The wound healing process. Dermatol Clin 1993; 11(4): 629-40.
[http://dx.doi.org/10.1016/S0733-8635(18)30216-X] [PMID: 8222347]

[8]   Li J, Chen J, Kirsner R. Pathophysiology of acute wound healing. Clin Dermatol 2007; 25(1): 9-18.
[http://dx.doi.org/10.1016/j.clindermatol.2006.09.007] [PMID: 17276196]

[9]   Han G, Ceilley R. Chronic wound healing: a review of current management and treatments. Adv Ther 2017; 34(3): 599-610.
[http://dx.doi.org/10.1007/s12325-017-0478-y] [PMID: 28108895]

[10]   Robson MC, Stenberg BD, Heggers JP. Wound healing alterations caused by infection. Clin Plast Surg 1990; 17(3): 485-92.
[http://dx.doi.org/10.1016/S0094-1298(20)30623-4] [PMID: 2199139]

[11]   Kondo T, Ishida Y. Molecular pathology of wound healing. Forensic Sci Int 2010; 203(1-3): 93-8.
[http://dx.doi.org/10.1016/j.forsciint.2010.07.004] [PMID: 20739128]

[12]   Broughton G 2nd, Janis JE, Attinger CE. The basic science of wound healing. Plast Reconstr Surg 2006; 117(7) (Suppl.): 12S-34S.
[http://dx.doi.org/10.1097/01.prs.0000225430.42531.c2] [PMID: 16799372]

[13]   Broughton G 2nd, Janis JE, Attinger CE. Wound healing: an overview. Plast Reconstr Surg 2006; 117 1e-S-32e-S.

[14]   Mercandetti M, Cohen A. Wound healing and repair. Emedicine 2017; 14: 12-20.

[15]   Witte MB, Barbul A. General principles of wound healing. Surg Clin North Am 1997; 77(3): 509-28.
[http://dx.doi.org/10.1016/S0039-6109(05)70566-1] [PMID: 9194878]

[16]   Atiyeh BS, Dibo SA, Hayek SN. Wound cleansing, topical antiseptics and wound healing. Int Wound J 2009; 6(6): 420-30.
[http://dx.doi.org/10.1111/j.1742-481X.2009.00639.x] [PMID: 20051094]

[17]   Attinger CE, Bulan EJ. Débridement. Foot Ankle Clin 2001; 6(4): 627-60.
[http://dx.doi.org/10.1016/S1083-7515(02)00010-4] [PMID: 12134576]

[18]   Abdelrahman T, Newton H. Wound dressings: principles and practice. Surgery 2011; 29: 491-5. [oxford].

[19]   Fay MF. Drainage Systems. AORN J 1987; 46(3): 442-56.
[http://dx.doi.org/10.1016/S0001-2092(07)66456-4] [PMID: 3307625]

[20]   Healy B, Freedman A. Infections. BMJ 2006; 332(7545): 838-41.
[http://dx.doi.org/10.1136/bmj.332.7545.838] [PMID: 16601046]

[21]   Markova A, Mostow EN. US skin disease assessment: ulcer and wound care. Dermatol Clin 2012; 30(1): 107-111, ix.
[http://dx.doi.org/10.1016/j.det.2011.08.005] [PMID: 22117872]

[22]   Thangapazham RL, Sharad S, Maheshwari RK. Phytochemicals in wound healing. Adv Wound Care 2016; 5(5): 230-41.
[http://dx.doi.org/10.1089/wound.2013.0505] [PMID: 27134766]

[23]   Shah A, Amini-Nik S. The role of phytochemicals in the inflammatory phase of wound healing. Int J Mol Sci 2017; 18(5): 1068.
[http://dx.doi.org/10.3390/ijms18051068] [PMID: 28509885]

[24]   Hormozi M, Assaei R, Boroujeni MB. The effect of *Aloe vera* on the expression of wound healing factors (TGFβ1 and bFGF) in mouse embryonic fibroblast cell: *In vitro* study. Biomed Pharmacother 2017; 88: 610-6.
[http://dx.doi.org/10.1016/j.biopha.2017.01.095] [PMID: 28142117]

[25]   Liang J, Cui L, Li J, Guan S, Zhang K, Li J. *Aloe vera*: a medicinal plant used in skin wound healing. Tissue Eng Part B Rev 2021; 27(5): 455-74.
[http://dx.doi.org/10.1089/ten.teb.2020.0236] [PMID: 33066720]

[26]   Haque SD, Saha SK, Salma U, Nishi MK, Rahaman MS. Antibacterial Effect of *Aloe vera* (*Aloe*

barbadensis) leaf gel against *Staphylococcus aureus, Pseudomonas aeruginosa, Escherichia coli* and *Klebsiella pneumoniae.* Mymensingh Med J 2019; 28(3): 490-6.
[PMID: 31391416]

[27]   Bendjedid S, Lekmine S, Tadjine A, Djelloul R, Bensouici C. Analysis of phytochemical constituents, antibacterial, antioxidant, photoprotective activities and cytotoxic effect of leaves extracts and fractions of *Aloe vera.* Biocatal Agric Biotechnol 2021; 33: 101991.
[http://dx.doi.org/10.1016/j.bcab.2021.101991]

[28]   Sadgrove NJ, Simmonds MSJ. Pharmacodynamics of *Aloe vera* and acemannan in therapeutic applications for skin, digestion, and immunomodulation. Phytother Res 2021; 35(12): 6572-84.
[http://dx.doi.org/10.1002/ptr.7242] [PMID: 34427371]

[29]   Liu C, Cui Y, Pi F, Cheng Y, Guo Y, Qian H. Extraction, purification, structural characteristics, biological activities and pharmacological applications of acemannan, a polysaccharide from *Aloe vera*: A review. Molecules 2019; 24(8): 1554.
[http://dx.doi.org/10.3390/molecules24081554] [PMID: 31010204]

[30]   Caley MP, Martins VLC, O'Toole EA. Metalloproteinases and wound healing. Adv Wound Care 2015; 4(4): 225-34.
[http://dx.doi.org/10.1089/wound.2014.0581] [PMID: 25945285]

[31]   Salah F, Ghoul YE, Mahdhi A, Majdoub H, Jarroux N, Sakli F. Effect of the deacetylation degree on the antibacterial and antibiofilm activity of acemannan from *Aloe vera.* Ind Crops Prod 2017; 103: 13-8.
[http://dx.doi.org/10.1016/j.indcrop.2017.03.031]

[32]   Dahms NM, Rose PA, Molkentin JD, Zhang Y, Brzycki MA. The bovine mannose 6-phosphate/insulin-like growth factor II receptor. The role of arginine residues in mannose 6-phosphate binding. J Biol Chem 1993; 268(8): 5457-63.
[http://dx.doi.org/10.1016/S0021-9258(18)53343-3] [PMID: 8449908]

[33]   Liu FW, Liu FC, Wang YR, Tsai HI, Yu HP. Aloin protects skin fibroblasts from heat stress-induced oxidative stress damage by regulating the oxidative defense system. PLoS One 2015; 10(12): e0143528.
[http://dx.doi.org/10.1371/journal.pone.0143528] [PMID: 26637174]

[34]   Park MY, Kwon HJ, Sung MK. Evaluation of aloin and aloe-emodin as anti-inflammatory agents in aloe by using murine macrophages. Biosci Biotechnol Biochem 2009; 73(4): 828-32.
[http://dx.doi.org/10.1271/bbb.80714] [PMID: 19352036]

[35]   Kaparakou EH, Kanakis CD, Gerogianni M, *et al.* Quantitative determination of aloin, antioxidant activity, and toxicity of*ALOE VERA* leaf gel products from Greece. J Sci Food Agric 2021; 101(2): 414-23.
[http://dx.doi.org/10.1002/jsfa.10650] [PMID: 32643805]

[36]   Dat AD, Poon F, Pham KBT, Doust J. *Aloe vera* for treating acute and chronic wounds. Sao Paulo Med J 2014; 132(6): 382-82.
[http://dx.doi.org/10.1590/1516-3180.20141326T1] [PMID: 25351761]

[37]   Ghorbani M, Nezhad-Mokhtari P, Ramazani S. *Aloe vera*-loaded nanofibrous scaffold based on Zein/Polycaprolactone/Collagen for wound healing. Int J Biol Macromol 2020; 153: 921-30.
[http://dx.doi.org/10.1016/j.ijbiomac.2020.03.036] [PMID: 32151718]

[38]   Ugoeze KC, Aja PC, Nwachukwu N, Chinko BC, Egwurugwu JN. Assessment of the phytoconstituents and optimal applicable concentration of aqueous extract of *Azadirachta indica* leaves for wound healing in male Wistar rats. Thaiphesatchasan 2021; 45.

[39]   Barua C, Talukdar A, Barua A, *et al.* Evaluation of the wound healing activity of methanolic extract of *Azadirachta indica* (Neem) and *Tinospora cordifolia* (Guduchi) in rats. Pharmacologyonline 2010; 1: 70-7.

[40]   Singh A, Singh A, Narayan G, Singh T, Shukla V. Effect of Neem oil and Haridra on non-healing wounds. Ayu 2014; 35(4): 398-403.
        [http://dx.doi.org/10.4103/0974-8520.158998] [PMID: 26195902]

[41]   Banerjee K, Thiagarajan N, Thiagarajan P. Formulation optimization, rheological characterization and suitability studies of polyglucoside-based *Azadirachta indica* a. Juss emollient cream as a dermal base for sun protection application. Indian J Pharm Sci 2018; 79: 914-22.

[42]   Bylka W, Znajdek-Awiżeń P, Studzińska-Sroka E, Dańczak-Pazdrowska A, Brzezińska M. *Centella asiatica* in dermatology: an overview. Phytother Res 2014; 28(8): 1117-24.
        [http://dx.doi.org/10.1002/ptr.5110] [PMID: 24399761]

[43]   Suguna L, Sivakumar P, Chandrakasan G. Effects of *Centella asiatica* extract on dermal wound healing in rats. Indian J Exp Biol 1996; 34(12): 1208-11.
        [PMID: 9246912]

[44]   Oyedeji OA, Afolayan AJ. Chemical composition and antibacterial activity of the essential oil of *Centella asiatica*. Growing in South Africa. Pharm Biol 2005; 43(3): 249-52.
        [http://dx.doi.org/10.1080/13880200590928843]

[45]   Wu F, Bian D, Xia Y, *et al.* Identification of major active ingredients responsible for burn wound healing of *Centella asiatica* herbs. Evid Based Complement Alternat Med 2012; 2012: 1-13.
        [http://dx.doi.org/10.1155/2012/848093] [PMID: 23346217]

[46]   Hou Q, Li M, Lu YH, Liu DH, Li CC. Burn wound healing properties of asiaticoside and madecassoside. Exp Ther Med 2016; 12(3): 1269-74.
        [http://dx.doi.org/10.3892/etm.2016.3459] [PMID: 27588048]

[47]   Kaur G, Sarwar Alam M, Athar M. Nimbidin suppresses functions of macrophages and neutrophils: relevance to its antiinflammatory mechanisms. Phytother Res 2004; 18(5): 419-24.
        [http://dx.doi.org/10.1002/ptr.1474] [PMID: 15174005]

[48]   Song J, Dai Y, Bian D, *et al.* Madecassoside induces apoptosis of keloid fibroblasts *via* a mitochondrial-dependent pathway. Drug Dev Res 2011; 72(4): 315-22.
        [http://dx.doi.org/10.1002/ddr.20432]

[49]   Shen X, Guo M, Yu H, Liu D, Lu Z, Lu Y. *Propionibacterium acnes* related anti-inflammation and skin hydration activities of madecassoside, a pentacyclic triterpene saponin from *Centella asiatica*. Biosci Biotechnol Biochem 2019; 83(3): 561-8.
        [http://dx.doi.org/10.1080/09168451.2018.1547627] [PMID: 30452312]

[50]   Lv J, Sharma A, Zhang T, Wu Y, Ding X. Pharmacological review on asiatic acid and its derivatives: a potential compound. SLAS Technol 2018; 23(2): 111-27.
        [http://dx.doi.org/10.1177/2472630317751840] [PMID: 29361877]

[51]   Puttarak P, Panichayupakaranant P. A new method for preparing pentacyclic triterpene rich *Centella asiatica* extracts. Nat Prod Res 2013; 27(7): 684-6.
        [http://dx.doi.org/10.1080/14786419.2012.686912] [PMID: 22577972]

[52]   Puttarak P, Brantner A, Panichayupakaranant P. Biological activities and stability of a standardized pentacyclic triterpene enriched *Centella asiatica* extract. Nat Prod Sci 2016; 22(1): 20-4.
        [http://dx.doi.org/10.20307/nps.2016.22.1.20]

[53]   Damkerngsuntorn W, Rerknimitr P, Panchaprateep R, *et al.* The Effects of a standardized extract of *Centella asiatica* on postlaser resurfacing wound healing on the face: a split-face, double-blind, randomized, placebo-controlled trial. J Altern Complement Med 2020; 26(6): 529-36.
        [http://dx.doi.org/10.1089/acm.2019.0325] [PMID: 32310680]

[54]   Puttarak P, Pichayakorn W, Sripoka K, Chaimud K, Panichayupakaranant P. Preparation of Centella extracts loaded Aloe vera transdermal patches for wound healing purpose. Adv Mater Res 2015; 1060: pp. 54-7.

[55] Maheshwari RK, Singh AK, Gaddipati J, Srimal RC. Multiple biological activities of curcumin: A short review. Life Sci 2006; 78(18): 2081-7.
[http://dx.doi.org/10.1016/j.lfs.2005.12.007] [PMID: 16413584]

[56] Akbik D, Ghadiri M, Chrzanowski W, Rohanizadeh R. Curcumin as a wound healing agent. Life Sci 2014; 116(1): 1-7.
[http://dx.doi.org/10.1016/j.lfs.2014.08.016] [PMID: 25200875]

[57] Soleimani H, Amini A, Taheri S, *et al.* The effect of combined photobiomodulation and curcumin on skin wound healing in type I diabetes in rats. J Photochem Photobiol B 2018; 181: 23-30.
[http://dx.doi.org/10.1016/j.jphotobiol.2018.02.023] [PMID: 29486459]

[58] Teow SY, Liew K, Ali SA, Khoo ASB, Peh SC. Antibacterial action of curcumin against *Staphylococcus aureus*: a brief review. J Trop Med 2016; 2016: 1-10.
[http://dx.doi.org/10.1155/2016/2853045] [PMID: 27956904]

[59] Kumara Swamy HM, Krishna V, Shankarmurthy K, *et al.* Wound healing activity of embelin isolated from the ethanol extract of leaves of Embelia ribes Burm. J Ethnopharmacol 2007; 109(3): 529-34.
[http://dx.doi.org/10.1016/j.jep.2006.09.003] [PMID: 17034970]

[60] Shrimali H, Mandal UK, Nivsarkar M, Shrivastava N. Fabrication and evaluation of a medicated hydrogel film with embelin from *Embelia ribes* for wound healing activity. Future J Pharm Sci 2019; 5(1): 12.
[http://dx.doi.org/10.1186/s43094-019-0011-z]

[61] Deshmukh PT, Gupta VB. Embelin accelerates cutaneous wound healing in diabetic rats. J Asian Nat Prod Res 2013; 15(2): 158-65.
[http://dx.doi.org/10.1080/10286020.2012.758634] [PMID: 23327735]

[62] Radhakrishnan N, Gnanamani A, Mandal A. A potential antibacterial agent Embelin, a natural benzoquinone extracted from *Embelia ribes.* Biol Med (Aligarh) 2011; 3: 1-7.

[63] Swastini DA, Udayana INK, Arisanti CIS. Cold cream combination of *Garcinia mangostana* L. *Anredera cordifolia* (Ten.) and *Centella asiatica* extracts on Burn Healing Activity Test. Res J Pharm Technol 2021; 14: 2483-6.
[http://dx.doi.org/10.52711/0974-360X.2021.00437]

[64] Mahabusarakam W, Wiriyachitra P, Phongpaichit S. Antimicrobial activities of chemical constituents from *Garcinia mangostana* Linn. J Siam Soc 1986; 12: 239-42.

[65] Herrera-Aco DR, Medina-Campos ON, Pedraza-Chaverri J, Sciutto-Conde E, Rosas-Salgado G, Fragoso-González G. Alpha-mangostin: Anti-inflammatory and antioxidant effects on established collagen-induced arthritis in DBA/1J mice. Food Chem Toxicol 2019; 124: 300-15.
[http://dx.doi.org/10.1016/j.fct.2018.12.018] [PMID: 30557668]

[66] Mohan S, Syam S, Abdelwahab SI, Thangavel N. An anti-inflammatory molecular mechanism of action of α-mangostin, the major xanthone from the pericarp of *Garcinia mangostana* : an *in silico*, *in vitro* and *in vivo* approach. Food Funct 2018; 9(7): 3860-71.
[http://dx.doi.org/10.1039/C8FO00439K] [PMID: 29953154]

[67] Koh JJ, Qiu S, Zou H, *et al.* Rapid bactericidal action of alpha-mangostin against MRSA as an outcome of membrane targeting. Biochim Biophys Acta Biomembr 2013; 1828(2): 834-44.
[http://dx.doi.org/10.1016/j.bbamem.2012.09.004] [PMID: 22982495]

[68] Sakagami Y, Iinuma M, Piyasena KGNP, Dharmaratne HRW. Antibacterial activity of α-mangostin against vancomycin resistant *Enterococci* (VRE) and synergism with antibiotics. Phytomedicine 2005; 12(3): 203-8.
[http://dx.doi.org/10.1016/j.phymed.2003.09.012] [PMID: 15830842]

[69] Song M, Liu Y, Li T, *et al.* Plant natural flavonoids against multidrug resistant pathogens. Adv Sci (Weinh) 2021; 8(15): 2100749.
[http://dx.doi.org/10.1002/advs.202100749] [PMID: 34041861]

[70]   Meah MS, Lertcanawanichakul M, Pedpradab P, *et al.* Synergistic effect on anti-methicillin-resistant *Staphylococcus aureus* among combinations of α-mangostin-rich extract, lawsone methyl ether and ampicillin. Lett Appl Microbiol 2020; 71(5): 510-9.
        [http://dx.doi.org/10.1111/lam.13369] [PMID: 32770753]

[71]   Sakarkar D, Sakarkar U, Shrikhande V, *et al.* Wound healing properties of Henna leaves. Indian J Nat Prod Resour 2004; 3: 406-12.

[72]   Daemi A, Farahpour MR, Oryan A, Karimzadeh S, Tajer E. Topical administration of hydroethanolic extract of *Lawsonia inermis* (henna) accelerates excisional wound healing process by reducing tissue inflammation and amplifying glucose uptake. Kaohsiung J Med Sci 2019; 35(1): 24-32.
        [http://dx.doi.org/10.1002/kjm2.12005] [PMID: 30844141]

[73]   Sultana T, Hossain M, Rahaman S, Kim YS, Gwon JG, Lee BT. Multi-functional nanocellulose-chitosan dressing loaded with antibacterial lawsone for rapid hemostasis and cutaneous wound healing. Carbohydr Polym 2021; 272: 118482.
        [http://dx.doi.org/10.1016/j.carbpol.2021.118482] [PMID: 34420741]

[74]   Babu PD, Subhasree R. Antimicrobial activities of *Lawsonia inermis*-a review. Am J Plant Sci 2009; 2: 231-2.

[75]   Muhammad H, Muhammad S. The use of *Lawsonia inermis* Linn.(henna) in the management of burn wound infections. Afr J Biotechnol 2005; 4: 1-9.

[76]   Eghbali-Babadi M, Rafiei Z, Mazaheri M, Yazdannik A. The effect of henna (*Lawsonia Inermis*) on preventing the development of pressure ulcer grade one in intensive care unit patients. Int J Prev Med 2019; 10(1): 26.
        [http://dx.doi.org/10.4103/ijpvm.IJPVM_286_17] [PMID: 30967912]

[77]   Kamal M. Pharmacological activities of *Lawsonia inermis* Linn.: a review. Molecules 2010; 15: 2139-51.

[78]   Lozza L, Moura-Alves P, Domaszewska T, *et al.* The Henna pigment Lawsone activates the Aryl Hydrocarbon Receptor and impacts skin homeostasis. Sci Rep 2019; 9(1): 10878.
        [http://dx.doi.org/10.1038/s41598-019-47350-x] [PMID: 31350436]

[79]   Sakunphueak A, Panichayupakaranant P. Comparison of antimicrobial activities of naphthoquinones from *Impatiens balsamina*. Nat Prod Res 2012; 26(12): 1119-24.
        [http://dx.doi.org/10.1080/14786419.2010.551297] [PMID: 21895457]

[80]   Adeli-Sardou M, Yaghoobi MM, Torkzadeh-Mahani M, Dodel M. Controlled release of lawsone from polycaprolactone/gelatin electrospun nano fibers for skin tissue regeneration. Int J Biol Macromol 2019; 124: 478-91.
        [http://dx.doi.org/10.1016/j.ijbiomac.2018.11.237] [PMID: 30500508]

[81]   Abdul-Hamid NA, Abas F, Ismail IS, *et al.* ^{1}H-NMR-based metabolomics to investigate the effects of Phoenix dactylifera seed extracts in LPS-IFN-γ-induced RAW 264.7 cells. Food Res Int 2019; 125: 108565.
        [http://dx.doi.org/10.1016/j.foodres.2019.108565] [PMID: 31554083]

[82]   Saryono S, Warsinah W, Isworo A, Efendi F. Anti-inflammatory effect of date seeds (*Phoenix dactylifera* L) on carrageenan-induced edema in rats. Trop J Pharm Res 2019; 17(12): 2455-61.
        [http://dx.doi.org/10.4314/tjpr.v17i12.22]

[83]   Taleb H, Maddocks SE, Morris RK, Kanekanian AD. Chemical characterisation and the anti-inflammatory, anti-angiogenic and antibacterial properties of date fruit (*Phoenix dactylifera* L.). J Ethnopharmacol 2016; 194: 457-68.
        [http://dx.doi.org/10.1016/j.jep.2016.10.032] [PMID: 27729284]

[84]   Abdennabi R, Bardaa S, Mehdi M, *et al. Phoenix dactylifera* L. sap enhances wound healing in Wistar rats: Phytochemical and histological assessment. Int J Biol Macromol 2016; 88: 443-50.
        [http://dx.doi.org/10.1016/j.ijbiomac.2016.04.015] [PMID: 27064088]

[85]   Kumar R, Gupta Y, Singh S, Raj A. Anti-inflammatory effect of *Picrorhiza kurroa* in experimental models of inflammation. Planta Med 2016; 82(16): 1403-9.
[http://dx.doi.org/10.1055/s-0042-106304] [PMID: 27163229]

[86]   Usman MRM, Surekha Y, Chhaya G, Devendra S. Preliminary screening and antimicrobial activity of *Picrorhiza kurroa* royle ethanolic extracts. Int J Pharm Sci Rev Res 2012; 14: 73-6.

[87]   Masood M, Arshad M, Rahmatullh Q, *et al.* Picrorhiza kurroa: An ethnopharmacologically important plant species of Himalayan region. Pure Appl Biol 2015; 4(3): 407-17.
[http://dx.doi.org/10.19045/bspab.2015.43017]

[88]   Singh AK, Warren J, Sharma A, Steele K, Maheshwari RK. Picroliv, a phytochemical enhances wound healing in rats. J Ilmu Kesehat Farm Wound Repair Regen 2005; 13(2): A4-A27.
[http://dx.doi.org/10.1111/j.1067-1927.2005.130215c.x]

[89]   Singh A, Sharma A, Warren J, *et al.* Picroliv accelerates epithelialization and angiogenesis in rat wounds. Planta Med 2007; 73(3): 251-6.
[http://dx.doi.org/10.1055/s-2007-967119] [PMID: 17318779]

[90]   Lien LT, Tho NT, Ha DM, Hang PL, Nghia PT, Thang ND. Influence of phytochemicals in *Piper betle* Linn leaf extract on wound healing. Burns Trauma 2015; 3: s41038-015-0023-7.
[http://dx.doi.org/10.1186/s41038-015-0023-7] [PMID: 27574669]

[91]   Darmawan A, Yusuf S, Tahir T, Syahriyani S. Betel leaf extract efficacy on wound healing: a systematic review. J Ilmu Kesehat Farm 2021; 10: 526-36.

[92]   Santhanam G, Nagarajan S. Wound healing activity of *Curcuma aromatica* and *Piper betle*. Fitoterapia 1990; 61: 458-9.

[93]   Thuy BTP, Hieu LT, My TTA, *et al.* Screening for *Streptococcus pyogenes* antibacterial and *Candida albicans* antifungal bioactivities of organic compounds in natural essential oils of *Piper betle* L., *Cleistocalyx operculatus* L. and *Ageratum conyzoides* L. Chem 2021; 75: 1507-19.

[94]   Karim S, AlKreathy H, Ahmad A, Khan MI. Effects of methanolic extract based-gel from Saudi–pomegranate (*Punica granatum* L.) peels with enhanced *in vivo* healing potential on excision wounds in diabetic rats. Front Pharmacol 2021; 12: 1337.
[http://dx.doi.org/10.3389/fphar.2021.704503]

[95]   Tavangar A, Soleymani B, Ghalayani P, Zolfaghary B, Farhad AR. The efficacy of *Punica granatum* extract in the management of recurrent aphthous stomatitis. J Res Pharm Pract 2013; 2(2): 88-92.
[http://dx.doi.org/10.4103/2279-042X.117389] [PMID: 24991610]

[96]   Chidambara Murthy KN, Reddy VK, Veigas JM, Murthy UD. Study on wound healing activity of *Punica granatum* peel. J Med Food 2004; 7(2): 256-9.
[http://dx.doi.org/10.1089/1096620041224111] [PMID: 15298776]

[97]   Ghorbanzadeh B, Mansouri MT, Hemmati AA, Naghizadeh B, Mard SA, Rezaie A. A study of the mechanisms underlying the anti-inflammatory effect of ellagic acid in carrageenan-induced paw edema in rats. Indian J Pharmacol 2015; 47(3): 292-8.
[http://dx.doi.org/10.4103/0253-7613.157127] [PMID: 26069367]

[98]   Ríos JL, Giner R, Marín M, Recio M. A pharmacological update of ellagic acid. Planta Med 2018; 84(15): 1068-93.
[http://dx.doi.org/10.1055/a-0633-9492] [PMID: 29847844]

[99]   Panichayupakaranant P, Tewtrakul S, Yuenyongsawad S. Antibacterial, anti-inflammatory and anti-allergic activities of standardised pomegranate rind extract. Food Chem 2010; 123(2): 400-3.
[http://dx.doi.org/10.1016/j.foodchem.2010.04.054]

[100]   Mo J, Panichayupakaranant P, Kaewnopparat N, Songkro S, Reanmongkol W. Topical anti-inflammatory potential of standardized pomegranate rind extract and ellagic acid in contact dermatitis. Phytother Res 2014; 28(4): 629-32.

[http://dx.doi.org/10.1002/ptr.5039] [PMID: 23873506]

[101] Tavares WS, Tavares-Júnior AG, Otero-Espinar FJ, Martín-Pastor M, Sousa FFO. Design of ellagic acid-loaded chitosan/zein films for wound bandaging. J Drug Deliv Sci Technol 2020; 59: 101903.
[http://dx.doi.org/10.1016/j.jddst.2020.101903]

[102] Mo J, Panichayupakaranant P, Kaewnopparat N, Nitiruangjaras A, Reanmongkol W. Wound healing activities of standardized pomegranate rind extract and its major antioxidant ellagic acid in rat dermal wounds. J Nat Med 2014; 68(2): 377-86.
[http://dx.doi.org/10.1007/s11418-013-0813-9] [PMID: 24407977]

[103] Huang M, Wu K, Zeng S, *et al.* Punicalagin inhibited inflammation and migration of fibroblast-Like synoviocytes through NF-κB pathway in the experimental study of rheumatoid arthritis. J Inflamm Res 2021; 14: 1901-13.
[http://dx.doi.org/10.2147/JIR.S302929] [PMID: 34012288]

[104] Kulkarni AP, Mahal HS, Kapoor S, Aradhya SM. *In vitro* studies on the binding, antioxidant, and cytotoxic actions of punicalagin. J Agric Food Chem 2007; 55(4): 1491-500.
[http://dx.doi.org/10.1021/jf0626720] [PMID: 17243704]

[105] Xu Y, Shi C, Wu Q, *et al.* Antimicrobial activity of punicalagin against *Staphylococcus aureus* and its effect on biofilm formation. Foodborne Pathog Dis 2017; 14(5): 282-7.
[http://dx.doi.org/10.1089/fpd.2016.2226] [PMID: 28128637]

[106] Krishnamoorthy J, Sumitira S, Ranjith M, *et al.* An *in vitro* study of wound healing effect of a poly-herbal formulation as evidenced by enhanced cell proliferation and cell migration. Egypt Dermatol Online J 2012; 8: 1-7.

[107] Sato Y, Oketani H, Singyouchi K, *et al.* Extraction and purification of effective antimicrobial constituents of *Terminalia chebula* RETS against methicillin-resistant *Staphylococcus aureus.* Biol Pharm Bull 1997; 20(4): 401-4.
[http://dx.doi.org/10.1248/bpb.20.401] [PMID: 9145218]

[108] Natarajan V, Krithica N, Madhan B, Sehgal PK. Preparation and properties of tannic acid cross-linked collagen scaffold and its application in wound healing. J Biomed Mater Res B Appl Biomater 2013; 101B(4): 560-7.
[http://dx.doi.org/10.1002/jbm.b.32856] [PMID: 23255343]

[109] Ninan N, Forget A, Shastri VP, Voelcker NH, Blencowe A. Antibacterial and anti-inflammatory pH-responsive tannic acid-carboxylated agarose composite hydrogels for wound healing. ACS Appl Mater Interfaces 2016; 8(42): 28511-21.
[http://dx.doi.org/10.1021/acsami.6b10491] [PMID: 27704757]

[110] Reddy DB, Reddanna P. Chebulagic acid (CA) attenuates LPS-induced inflammation by suppressing NF-κB and MAPK activation in RAW 264.7 macrophages. Biochem Biophys Res Commun 2009; 381(1): 112-7.
[http://dx.doi.org/10.1016/j.bbrc.2009.02.022] [PMID: 19351605]

[111] Rahayu K, Suharto I, Etika A, Nurseskasatmata S. The effect of ginger extract (*Zingiber officinale Roscoe*) on the number of neutrophil cells, fibroblast and epithelialization on incision wound. J Phys Conf Ser 2020; 1569: 032063.
[http://dx.doi.org/10.1088/1742-6596/1569/3/032063]

[112] Mohamed AHB, Osman AAF. Antibacterial and wound healing potential of ethanolic extract of *Zingiber Officinale* in albino rats. J Med Plants Res 2017; 3: 1-6.

[113] Kazerouni A, Kazerouni O, Pazya N. Effects of Ginger (*Zingiber officinale*) on skin conditions: A non quantitative review article. J Turk Acad Dermatol 2013; 7: 137-222.

[114] Tripathi S, Maier KG, Bruch D, Kittur DS. Effect of 6-gingerol on pro-inflammatory cytokine production and costimulatory molecule expression in murine peritoneal macrophages. J Surg Res 2007; 138(2): 209-13.

[http://dx.doi.org/10.1016/j.jss.2006.07.051] [PMID: 17291534]

[115] Al-Rawaf HA, Gabr SA, Alghadir AH. Molecular changes in diabetic wound healing following administration of vitamin D and ginger supplements: biochemical and molecular experimental study. Evid Based Complement Alternat Med 2019; 2019: 1-13.
[http://dx.doi.org/10.1155/2019/4352470] [PMID: 31428171]

[116] Prateeksha , Singh BR, Shoeb M, *et al.* Scaffold of selenium nanovectors and honey phytochemicals for inhibition of *Pseudomonas aeruginosa* quorum sensing and biofilm formation. Front Cell Infect Microbiol 2017; 7: 93.
[http://dx.doi.org/10.3389/fcimb.2017.00093] [PMID: 28386534]

[117] Koçak İ, Yücepur C, Gökler O. Is ginger effective in reducing post-tonsillectomy morbidity? a prospective randomised clinical trial. Clin Exp Otorhinolaryngol 2018; 11(1): 65-70.
[http://dx.doi.org/10.21053/ceo.2017.00374] [PMID: 28877566]

[118] Patankar S. Herbal composition for the treatment of wound healing. A regenerative medicine. Patent No. US20148709509B2, 2014.

[119] Davidson M, Saiki J, Andreasson J. Topical compositions and methods for treating inflammatory skin diseases. Patent No. US20210186931A1, 2021.

[120] Latta M. Dermal skin protectant and carrier. Patent No. US20200138958A1, 2020.

[121] Laddha UD. Composition and method of skin relief cream useful for eczema, psoriasis, lipoma, burn wounds, scars, keloids, shingles, dry skin disorders, and skin allergies. Patent No. US20200061144A1, 2020.

[122] Gioffre AJ. Methods and compositions for treating skin. Patent No. US20200215104A1, 2020.

[123] Panichayupakaranant P. Methods and compositions of preparation of Piper betle extract containing hydroxychavicol for topical formulation. Patent No. 78564, 2020.

[124] Attatippaholkun M. Method and composition of *Zingiber officinale* gel for antiiinflammation and analgesic. Patent No. 139379, 2016.

SUBJECT INDEX

A

Acid(s) 15, 16, 18, 24, 34, 35, 52, 80, 87, 100, 116, 139, 151, 152, 153, 215, 221, 228, 229, 230
  arachidonic 34
  ascorbic 116
  azelaic 52, 87
  chebulagic 215, 229, 230
  dicarboxylic 52
  dihomo-gamma-linolenic 35
  ellagic 80, 215, 228, 229
  fatty 35, 100, 152
   free fatty (FFAs) 15, 139
  fusidic 18, 151
  gallic 80
  glutamic 16
  glycyrrhetinic 35
  glycyrrhizinic 34
  linoleic 35, 153
  madecassic 221
  mycophenolic 24
Acne 80, 81, 82, 83, 84, 85, 86, 87, 88, 102, 164, 168, 172
  and eczema treatment 84
  and leprosy management 84
  and nappy rash treatment 84
  pathogenesis of 83, 84
Action 16, 17, 85, 102
  anti-inflammatory 85
  immunosuppressive 16, 17, 102
Activation 2, 8, 9, 11, 13, 84, 99, 109, 113, 140, 146, 150, 203, 204
  enzymatic 13
  immune 2, 9
  inflammasome 84
  -regulated chemokine 146
Activity 11, 12, 34, 35, 52, 57, 59, 60, 69, 82, 101, 110, 113, 150, 152, 153, 193, 202, 209, 218, 222, 232
  antagonizing cytokine 150
  anti-oxidative 152

antiandrogen 82
antiproliferative 222
  deliberated tanning 193
  display anti-oxidant 34
  enzymatic 153
  immune 101
  oestrogenic 35
  skin regeneration 232
  superoxide dismutase 218
  wound-healing 209
Adaptive immune systems 27, 28, 141
Adiponectin 138
Adipose tissue 138
Agar diffusion assay 229
Agents 1, 9, 26, 149, 204
  chemotherapeutic 204
  immunomodulatory 1
  immunosuppressive 149
  infectious 9, 26
Allergen-specific immune therapy (ASIT) 28
Allergic 8, 13, 28, 109, 117, 144, 135, 137, 142
  reaction 109
  responses 117, 144
  rhinitis 8, 13, 28, 135, 142
  rhinoconjunctivitis 137
Allergies, peanut 8
Amino acids, hygroscopic 7
Anemia 174
Angelica sinensis 36
Angiogenesis 211, 214, 222, 229, 230
Anti-acne activity 84, 85
Anti-inflammatory 34, 35, 122, 143, 148, 149, 153, 174, 209, 214, 219, 221, 222, 225, 226, 228, 229, 230
  activity 34, 221, 229
  agents 34, 148, 174, 209
  effects 143, 153, 214, 219, 222, 225, 226, 228, 229, 230
  properties 35, 122, 149, 153
Anti-tumorigenic property 203
Antibacterial 84, 85, 86, 166, 219, 227